POCKET MEDICAL REFERENCE SERIES

Ear, Nose and Throat
J. A. S. CARRUTH

Rheumatology
A. K. CLARKE

Intensive Care
G. R. PARK and A. R. MANARA

Clinical Oncology
GARETH J. G. REES

Ophthalmology
NICHOLAS EVANS

Oxford University Press, Walton Street, Oxford OX2 6DP

Oxford   New York   Toronto
Delhi   Bombay   Calcutta   Madras   Karachi
Kuala Lumpur   Singapore   Hong Kong   Tokyo
Nairobi   Dar es Salaam   Cape Town
Melbourne   Auckland   Madrid
and associated companies in
Berlin   Ibadan

Oxford is a trade mark of Oxford University Press

Published in the United States
by Oxford University Press Inc., New York

Second edition published by Oxford University Press 1991
Reprinted 1993

British Library Cataloguing in Publication Data
A catalogue record for this book is
available from the British Library

Library of Congress Cataloging in Publication Data

ISBN 0-19-263000 8

Typeset by Footnote Graphics, Warminster, Wiltshire
Printed and bound by Biddles Ltd, Guildford and King's Lynn

Accidents and Emergencies

Second Edition

Major-general N. G. KIRBY OBE OStJ FRCS FRCS (Ed)

Consultant Accident and Emergency Surgeon
Guy's Hospital, London, UK

Oxford New York Tokyo
OXFORD UNIVERSITY PRESS

Preface

Newly appointed Casualty Officers have the formidable task of dealing, many for the first time, with a wide variety of traumatic and medical conditions which present in the Accident and Emergency Department of an acute general hospital.

This pocket book is an attempt to present a brief survey of the many conditions you will encounter with advice on how to deal with these patients. It is not possible to include everything in a pocket book but I took advice from succeeding cohorts of my Casualty Officers and Registrars on topics they wished to see covered. Diagrams and flow charts are given for quick and easy reference.

Read this quickly before you start your job—the introduction at least—and familiarize yourself with the contents: this will give you a good idea of what to expect in your new job and ease reference when you need advice. A call for a second edition has enabled me to carry out a tidying up and revision. I have had many comments from reviewers, fellow Accident and Emergency consultants as well as Casualty Officers who have had to use the book: with this advice I have clarified obscure sections.

London   N.G.K.
May 1991

Acknowledgements

The Resuscitation Council of Great Britain revised their recommendations for cardio-pulmonary resuscitation and have kindly given me permission to use this in this edition.

'*Guidelines for the management of acute severe asthma*' has been published by the British Thoracic Society, Research Unit of the Royal College of Physicians of London, the King's Fund Centre, and the National Asthma Campaign. Dr G. M. Cochrane, Consultant Respiratory Physician of Guy's Hospital, who has advised on this section kindly arranged permission to use these guidelines in this book.

As before I have had advice, criticism, and suggestions for updating from many consultant colleagues. Fellow consultants in Accident and Emergency Mrs Anne McGuiness of the Royal Free Hospital, Dr Tanya Malpass, High Wycombe General Hospital, and Mr Tony Martin of the Galway University Hospital, as with the first edition, have given me good support and advice on the whole book.

More specialist advice has come from Mr Robert Kirby, Consultant General Surgeon, North Staffordshire Royal Infirmary; Dr John Henry, Consultant Physician, Guy's Hospital Poisons Unit; Mr Tony Rowsell, Consultant Plastic Surgeon, Guy's Hospital; Dr Norman Simmonds, Consultant Microbiologist and Dr Leo Stimmler, Consultant Paediatrician of Guy's Hospital. Other specialist chapters have been read and revised by Dr Stephen Beer, Senior Registrar in Metabolic Medicine; Dr Jonathan Barker, Senior Registrar in Dermatology; Dr Paul Crone, Registrar in A & E; Dr Cam Bhui, Psychiatric Registrar; Miss Janice Rymer, Senior Gynaecological Registrar; Dr John Watkinson, Senior Registrar in ENT; Dr Leyre Zabala, Casualty Officer, and Dr William Dunsmuir, Casualty Officer, all of Guy's Hospital. Mr Nick Gillham, Senior Orthopaedic Research Fellow of Royal College of Surgeons of England has given much useful advice on orthopaedics and trauma.

Mrs Wendy Reinders of Castle House Publications encouraged me to undertake this revision and the staff at Oxford University Press took over the difficult task of guiding my book through publication in Oxford. As before I am grateful to my Senior Registrar Mr Alan Montague and Mr David Watson, Senior Lecturer in Accident & Emergency, Guy's and

Lewisham Hospitals, for reading the proofs. The overall responsibility for final facts and their accuracy must be mine.

I have not cited all the authorities consulted or quoted in the writing of this pocket book; I hope that where work is recognized the author will take satisfaction in my need to repeat it for the benefit of Casualty Officers.

Drug dosages have been included for many drugs. While great care has been taken to ensure the accuracy of the book's content when it went to press, neither the author nor the publisher can be responsible for the accuracy and completeness of the information. If there is any doubt, the British National Formulary, manufacturers' current product literature, or other suitable reference should be consulted.

Contents

Abbreviations

AF	auricular fibrillation
AIDS	acquired immunodeficiency syndrome
AP	antero-posterior
ARC	AIDS-related complex
ATT	adsorbed tetanus toxoid
A-V	atrio-ventricular
aVF	ECG trace
aVL	ECG trace
BAEM	British Association for Accident and Emergency Medicine
BAPS	British Association of Paediatric Surgeons
BBB	bundle branch block
BCC	basal cell carcinoma
βHCG	beta human chorionic gonadotrophin
BNF	British National Formulary
BP	blood pressure
BPA	British Paediatric Association
BSB	body surface burnt
CCU	coronary care unit
CHB	complete heart block
COAD	chronic obstructive airway disease
COB	chronic obstructive bronchitis
CPK	serum creatinine phosphokinase
CPR	cardiopulmonary resuscitation
C&S	culture and sensitivity
CSA	Casualty Surgeons Association
CSF	cerebro-spinal fluid
CSOM	chronic suppurative otitis media
CT scan	computerised axial tomography
CVA	cerebro-vascular accident
CVP	central venous pressure
CXR	chest x-ray
C7/T1	intervertebral joint between 7th cervical and first thoracic vertebrae

DKA	diabetic ketoacidosis
DTs	delirium tremens
DU	duodenal ulcer
DVT	deep vein thrombosis
ECG	electrocardiogram
EDTA	editic acid (BNF)
ENT	ear, nose and throat
ERPC	evacuation of retained products of conception
E + U	electrolytes and urea
FB	foreign body
FBC	full blood count
FDP	flexor digitorum profundus
FDS	flexor digitorum superficialis
F waves	ECG, fibrillation waves
GI	gastrointestinal
GIB	gastrointestinal bleeding
GTN	glyceryl trinitrate
GU	gastric ulcer
GUM	genito-urinary medicine
HAS	high arm sling
HIV	human immunodeficiency virus
HVS	high vaginal swab
I&D	incision and drainage
IM	intramuscular
IPPR	intermittent positive pressure respiration
IUCD	intrauterine contraceptive device
IVP	intravenous pyelogram
IVU	intravenous urogram
LIF	left iliac fossa
LFT	liver function test
LPC	lotio picis carbonis
LV	left ventricle
LVF	left ventricular failure
MH	medical history
MI	myocardial infarction
MTP	metatarso-phalangeal
MUA	manipulation under anaesthetic

NAD	nothing abnormal detected
NSAID	non-steroidal anti-inflammatory drugs
OA	osteoarthritis
OE	otitis externa
OM X-ray	occipito-mental view of facial bones
OM	otitis media
PA	postero-anterior
PCC	post-coital contraception
PCV	packed cell volume
PE	pulmonary embolus
PEEP	positive end expiratory pressure
PEFR	peak expiratory flow rate
PGL	persistent generalised lymphadenopathy
PID	pelvic inflammatory disease
POP	plaster of Paris
POP	progesterone only pill
PR	per rectum examination
PSL	partial skin loss
PUO	pyrexia of unknown origin
PUVA	psoralan used in combination with UVA
PV	per vaginal examination
P waves	ECG, see fig. 3.2
QRS	ECG, see fig. 3.2
Q waves	ECG, see fig. 3.2
RA	rheumatoid arthritis
RAMP	rapid absorbent matrix pad (hCG assay)
RBBB	right bundle branch block
RBC	red blood cell
RIF	right iliac fossa
RMO	resident medical officer
RSO	resident surgical officer
R or T	ECG, see fig. 3.2
RTA	road traffic accident
RUQ	right upper quadrant
RV	right ventricular
SBE	subacute bacterial endocarditis
SCC	squamous cell carcinoma
SGOT	serum glutamic oxaloacetic acid transaminase

SLE	systemic lupus erythematosis
ST	ECG, see fig. 3.2
STD	sexually transmitted disease
SVE	supra-ventricular extrasystoles
TB	tuberculosis
TFT	thyroid function tests
TIA	transient ischaemic attacks
TTC	tetracycline
T waves	ECG, see fig. 3.2
URTI	upper respiratory tract infection
USS	ultrasound scan
UTI	urinary tract infection
UVA	ultra-violet A
VE	ventricular extrasystoles
VF	ventricular fibrillation
VHF	viral haemorrhagic fever
VPb	ventricular paroxysmal bradycardia
VT	ventricular tachycardia
WCC	white cell count
WSL	whole skin loss
%BSB	percentage body surface burnt

Introduction

Starting work in an accident and emergency department can be the most stimulating but worrying stage in your medical career. For the first time you are going to face the possibility of meeting any trauma or illness, usually acute but not infrequently chronic, from the whole range of medicine. Most casualty departments now have senior doctors to train and support you, but this varies considerably over the country. It is usual to give new casualty officers the opportunity to attend a special course before starting their new appointment, with regular postgraduate training periods while in post. However, the time soon arrives when you are the spearhead doctor and have to make vital life- or limb-saving decisions on your own, and if necessary to ask for help. More often than not the conditions seen are those not covered in your medical course and often not severe. Nevertheless the patient is worried and is requesting treatment. This book is intended to give you advice on a comprehensive range of the A & E situations you might possibly meet. It is not feasible to cover the whole range of cases you could see, but I have tried to make this book useful as a pocket reference, and by asking my registrars and casualty officers to contribute, have included those topics on which they wanted practical advice. It is not possible to give a wide choice of treatments either, but I have included the range of techniques which are used in my department. I have also given advice on cases that are best referred — it is often a case of 'the sooner the better' until you have gained experience. All A & E departments should have a library available, day and night, of practical reference books for when this book has been exhausted or found wanting. At the end of the book there is a list of these volumes, which should be available on a shelf, battered, dog-eared and chained if need be, but there to be referred to quickly.

Before starting your job, read:

    (i) A first-aid book if you have not before. Few students have the opportunity to do so at medical school, and they are soon coming into contact with the most experienced first-aiders and para-medics in the country — those who man the emergency ambulances.

    (ii) If you do not have it already, get a copy of the British National Formulary (BNF) — it is reliable, practical, updated every 6 months, and free. You should refer to it when you are treating the elderly, young, pregnant, and using drugs with which you are not familiar.

(iii) Next you should quickly read through this pocket reference, to learn a few tips, but more importantly to know where to look late at night when you are alone and perplexed.

Communication

Most doctors learn to take histories, examine patients, make a diagnosis, prescribe treatment, but rarely how to communicate with the patient. Do revise your clinical examination notes, but please do also learn how to take time and communicate with the patient, his relatives and friends. So often people complain that the doctor was brusque, barked questions without apparently listening to the answers, did not realise why the patient was worried and asking for help. Dr Tony Martin of Sunderland Royal Infirmary gives the following advice:

- Look at patients and give them your full attention.
- Watch for signs of incongruity between what they say and what you see.
- Make them feel you are not in a hurry — even if you are.
- Let them do the talking.
- Explore their fears; it's the anxiety cycle that accentuates illness.
- Explain things clearly.
- Attune your language and approach to the patient.
- Remember, the first thing you say is what they remember.
- Take into account the patient's environment and way of life.
- Watch out for the patient's last remark — it could well be the most important information.

To that I would add: make sure they understand the diagnosis, treatment, prognosis, and the need for further visits to hospital or GP. If you want to make sure, write it down and explain to their relatives or friends. Most A & E departments have printed instruction cards to be given to patients in POP (plaster of paris) or with head injuries. The use of these cards is to be encouraged as most patients remember only about 40 per cent of what you tell them.

If there has been a mistake made in your handling or treatment of a patient, do not be too proud to say sorry; the patient will always appreciate your frankness. The Medical Defence Union's view is 'that the patient is entitled to a prompt, sympathetic and above all truthful account of what has occurred. . . . It is very important that a sincere and honest apology is made.'

The record card

After taking the history, including a list of what drugs the patient is already taking, make sure the key factors, both positive and negative, are clearly and legibly written onto the casualty card. If the card has a duplicate sheet make sure that the permanent copy is legible. In these sad days with increasing litigation this is often the only record available for medico-legal reports — or your defence — later. Do not be afraid to use anatomical terms — these are precise. Draw diagrams of bruises, stab wounds and lacerations in assaults and RTAs (road traffic accidents). Ensure that you record the digits by name and that the correct side of the body is clearly seen. In lacerations over vital areas such as digits, wrist, ankle, and heel, ensure that you have tested and recorded function, present or lost, of the important nerves, arteries and tendons. X-ray readings are noted as positive with a diagnosis or negative. Any investigations done are recorded with results.

Write down your provisional diagnosis — it may need reviewing after admission or further investigations but it is a starting-point for your decision to refer, treat or discharge.

Finally, sign your name clearly and with pride — not the usual illegible medical scrawl. If that is not possible, at least print your initials so that you can be traced several years later.

A & E departments have many different methods of communication but it is your responsibility to ensure:

   (i) that the patient knows what is happening to him and his treatment regime;
  (ii) that the A & E staff carry this out to the intended standard;
 (iii) that the GP is informed — preferably in writing;
 (iv) that district nurses and social services are notified — particularly with the elderly (see page 165).

Treatment delegated to nurses or medical students, such as suturing or application of POP splints, remains your responsibility so make sure that you supervise if necessary and check the final result.

X-rays: guidelines on the referral of patients

These guidelines, used in Guy's Hospital, are to help reduce cost and unnecessary patient irradiation. 1 CXR = 300 mega Becquerels. The doctor on duty in the A & E department should request an x-ray wherever his clinical judgement suggests it is indicated. The guidelines may help in the timing of such examinations. They are not meant to be a rigid set of rules.

Unnecessary x-ray examinations make no contribution to patient management; they are costly in time and films; they also may lead to delays in the A & E department. They educate the patient into bad habits; always expecting, even demanding, x-rays. Exposure to ionising radiation is harmful, so adhere to clinical indications and limit the examination to the area that has been injured.

Medico-legal aspects

Following a recent test case, the Courts, Defence Societies, and the Royal College of Radiology confirm that x-rays should be taken only when clinically indicated, and not as a protection against future litigation. Negligence does not occur when the decision is taken after a proper clinical examination and is recorded as not being necessary on clinical grounds.

Emergency services

Many patients seen outside normal working hours are not emergencies; they should be referred during the normal hours to the main x-ray department.

Clinical details on the request form

The request form should be legible, and give a summary of the clinical problem with the precise area to be x-rayed. If you are not sure which films are required, discuss it with the radiographer or look it up in 'Positioning In Radiography' (see list of further reading).

Criteria for skull x-ray after recent head injury

Skull x-ray can be helpful but clinical judgement is necessary. The presence of one or more of the following indicates a need for skull x-ray in patients with a history of head injury.

  (i) Loss of consciousness, confusion or amnesia at any time.
 (ii) Neurological symptoms or signs.
(iii) Cerebro-spinal fluid or blood from the nose or ear.
(iv) Suspected penetrating injury, scalp bruising or swelling.
 (v) Alcohol intoxication.
(vi) Difficulty in assessing the patient (e.g. the young, epileptics).

N.B. Simple scalp laceration by itself is not a criterion for skull x-ray.

Skull radiography

Specify which side the injury is. Three views are necessary, PA, Townes, and horizontal beam lateral; the latter will show fluid levels and the upper cervical spine. In all patients with severe head injuries, ask for a lateral view of the whole cervical spine to include C7/T1 intervertebral space.

Facial bones

Request occipito-mental views (10 and 30 degrees OM). More complex views are best left to the maxillo-facial surgeons.

Mandible

Orthopantomography is the procedure of choice but is usually available only in dental departments. Ask for PA and obliques.

Chest

Routine chest radiography (CXR) has no place in A & E. CXR is for patients with acute problems and abnormal signs in the chest.

Oblique views of ribs to demonstrate fractures are needed only in the *left* lower chest where the underlying spleen is at risk.

If a pneumothorax or an inhaled endobronchial foreign body (FB) is suspected, request films in expiration and inspiration.

Shoulder and clavicles

Indications: suspected fracture or dislocation.

Elbows

Indications: swelling, restricted movement, evidence of distal ischaemia. In children obtain a comparison view of the other side if in doubt.

Hands

Specify precise nature and site of injury. For fingers ask for that named digit only. Minor lacerations and injuries do not justify x-ray.

Knees

Indications: acute injury with pain, effusion and swelling. Meniscal and ligamentous injuries are not demonstrated.

Ankles

Indications: swelling and localised tenderness over the malleoli. Those over 40 and patients falling down steps merit x-rays.

The absence of swelling excludes underlying fracture. Specify site, lateral or medial; do not ask for blanket films of 'ankle and foot'.

Foot

Specify the exact bones that are injured to ensure you get the correct view.

Calcaneal spur

A calcaneal spur, like a lumbar osteophyte, is a common occurrence in the older age group. The only significant finding is erosion or fracture of the spur.

Abdomen

Plain abdominal films are not usually of much help in suspected appendicitis, cholelithiasis, chronic abdominal pain, constipation, irritable bowel syndrome, haematemesis or melaena.

An erect CXR will show gas under the diaphragm best. The most sensitive study for free gas is a lateral decubitus film.

Reserve erect abdominal films for patients with suspected obstruction.

Emergency IVU

This study is used in suspected renal colic during an episode of pain. A delayed film is required if the kidney is obstructed and contrast is seen in the collecting system at 15 minutes.

X-rays of the spine

Lumbar spine

The majority of patients presenting with low back pain have soft tissue disorders of the ligaments, apophyseal joints or disc: these do not show on x-rays. Only x-ray to exclude other disorders:

  (a) Ankylosing spondylitis and congenital defects in the younger age group.
  (b) Infection, osteoporosis and secondary deposits with collapse in the older age group.
  (c) Remember however that there has been an increase in bone tuberculosis (TB) in immigrants from the Far East.

Patients with low back pain and without nerve root signs are best referred to the orthopaedic clinic for review and x-ray later. This x-ray gives a very high dose of radiation to the gonads.

Prolapsed intervertebral disc

Plain x-ray of the lumbar spine will not diagnose an acute disc prolapse. Degenerative changes and spondylosis of apophyseal joints are extremely common, x-ray degenerative changes are as common in asymptomatic patients as in those with backache. Patients with nerve root compression and with sciatic pain, with muscular weakness or sensory changes should be x-rayed.

The sacro-iliac joints are visible on the antero-posterior (AP) lumbar spine.

Cervical spine

Acute whiplash injury or sports injuries will often show loss of the normal cervical curve due to musculo-ligamentous injury. Severe head injuries will require x-ray of the cervical spine.

Plain x-rays are of no value in acute torticollis.

Coccyx

X-rays of the coccyx after injury are not helpful but give the patient's gonads a high dose of radiation.

Spine, hips and knees

Once the diagnosis of degenerative disease/spondylosis has been established follow-up x-rays are not required in A & E.

All x-rays should be reviewed promptly and any positive findings checked with the casualty card. A system for calling cases back for review should be easily and quickly available. Taking an x-ray is only part of the clinical examination and not the final step. The result should be discussed with the radiographer or a senior doctor if you are not sure of the diagnosis. You must learn to recognise the normal and abnormal radiological anatomy and, if not sure, ask. Even towards the end of appointments some do get over-confident and miss a fracture! Sometimes the fracture does not correspond with the site of maximum tenderness or there is a non-traumatic abnormality present, so do examine the whole film carefully. If you are taking over other people's patients on change of shift, pay especial attention and look at the patient and his injury.

Difficult patients

The violent patient

Violence towards the staff in A & E Departments is a problem. The vast majority of abuse is only verbal, but increasingly, violence is physical. The violent patients, relatives, or friends are usually under the influence of alcohol but may be psychologically unbalanced. Occasionally some cases are provoked by staff attitudes, usually unwittingly, and delays in being seen; but fear, disorientation, pain and underlying illness all make a patient more prone to violent outbursts. Tactful reassuring attitudes from nursing, reception and medical staff, accompanied by skilful management, will often avert incidents. It is unfortunate that security measures need to be introduced to protect members of the staff and other patients, but their presence needs to be discreet and not provocative. It often means furniture may be cut, but this is better than hurting the staff. An efficient alarm system needs to be installed in all areas of the department where staff may be alone with patients. When dealing with psychiatric patients particularly two doors are important.

At all times it must be appreciated that until these patients have been examined and a firm diagnosis been made the patient cannot safely be evicted or discharged from the department.

The drunk patient

It is dangerous to assume that changes either in the level of consciousness or abnormal behaviour in a drunk patient is due to alcohol alone, no matter what the blood/breath alcohol level is. A breathalyser measurement is useful only to *exclude* alcohol as a cause of coma/confusion.

Differential diagnosis of confusion/coma and abnormal behaviour in the patient who has been drinking:

    (a) head injury
    (b) hypoglycaemia

(c) overdosage with other drugs
(d) epilepsy — post-ictal state
(e) cerebral haemorrhage
(f) sub-arachnoid haemorrhage
(g) other toxic confusional states

Management of the drunk patient

1 Observation.
(a) All head injuries that are also drunk should be admitted.
(b) Regular frequent observations of the level of consciousness must be recorded.
(c) Repeated estimations of the levels of breath alcohol enable a trend to be established.
(d) Never discharge a patient until a definite upward trend is confirmed. Single readings are meaningless.

2 History.
(a) The drunk patient may not admit to an alcohol problem but information from relatives and friends can be useful.
(b) Is the patient likely to deteriorate further, bearing in mind the amount of alcohol still in the stomach?
(c) If he is to be admitted following trauma is there a risk of withdrawal fits, delirium tremens (DTs) etc.?

3 Examination and investigation — look for underlying pathology.
(a) Skull x-ray is indicated where head injury is suspected. However it is useless to attempt on an unco-operative patient, poor films neither prove nor disprove fractures. Admit and observe patient until decent films can be obtained.
(b) Screening:
   (i) Blood glucose, hypoglycaemia often masquerades as alcohol intoxication. Serial blood levels should be taken. Hypoglycaemia may also occur in alcoholic liver diseases.
   (ii) Toxicology — other drugs may have been ingested.
(c) Haematology and biochemistry — acute confusion/hepatic coma may be precipitated in those with liver damage by minor stress, drugs, intercurrent infection, gastro-intestinal (GI) bleeds, myocardial infarction, alcohol excess. FBC, LFT, electrocardiogram (ECG), etc. may also be needed to exclude other causes of coma/confusion.

The drug addict

Frequently drug addicts attend an A & E Department with carefully rehearsed and convincing stories of acute back or chest pain, gallstone or renal colic. These patients often show evidence of injections in the arms, subcutaneous abscesses or loss of fat and thrombosed superficial veins. Most hospitals keep a record of these cases who regularly receive 'pain relief' from an unwitting Casualty officer.

The Misuse of Drugs (Notification of and Supply to Addicts) Regulations 1973

With an increased spread of human immunodeficiency virus between drug misusers who share injecting equipment, the Chief Medical Officer (CMO) has reminded doctors of the regulation to notify him in writing at the Home Office, within seven days of attendance, any person he considers, or has reasonable grounds to suspect, to be addicted to any of the following drugs: cocaine, dextromoramide, diamorphine, dipipanone, hydrocodone, hydromorphone, levorphanol, methadone, morphine, opium, oxycodone, pethidine, phenazocine and piritramide. Particulars to be notified are the person's name and address, sex, date of birth, National Insurance number, date of first attendance, and the name or names of the drug or drugs to which the patient is, or is suspected of being, addicted. The information is for statistical purposes and will be treated in strict medical confidence.

The A & E department's main responsibility with these patients will be treating the results of overdoses, hypersensitivity to drugs, and complications and will not be dispensing drugs. Nevertheless we should endeavour to educate those afflicted and direct them to suitable drug abuse centres in the district.

Munchhausen's syndrome

These patients will attend with convincing tales of medical sagas which rival the stories of Baron Munchhausen of Bodenwerder himself. They frequently seek admission with convincing dramatic symptoms which require urgent attention. They are usually well read with a good clinical knowledge of their chosen complaint, and have had considerable experience of hospitals throughout the country. In the present climate, where casualty officers are worried about missing serious diagnoses, these patients often find it easy to get admitted for further investigations. They frequently discharge themselves after a series of tests, many of which are uncomfortable. Some may have multiple scars from surgical procedures. A thorough examination of the patient may show evidence of the multiple investigations they have had before. Sadly, with the rapid turnover of staff (medical, nursing and reception) in A & E Departments, it is increasingly easy for these psychiatric problems to gain the attention they seek. If this diagnosis is considered, psychiatric referral is indicated: but it is at this stage that the patient will discharge himself.

The nameless patient

Many patients are seen in casualty who are lost and cannot remember who they are or from whence they came. Some will be suffering from toxi-confusional states such as alcoholic excess, hypoglycaemia, post-ictal states, drugs, or head injury. They will require full investigation and treatment at this stage so are best admitted. The elderly confused patient should be referred to the psycho-geriatrician for advice, but efforts to trace relatives or abode will need help from the police and social services. Depression (see page 79) may present this way; the psychiatrist can then be of help. Hysterical amnesia may be the result of background emotional and family stress and will need assistance from the police and social services so are best admitted for sorting out after organic disease has been excluded.

Difficult situations

Riot victims

Victims of picketing, street violence and inner city riots; patients may attend with injuries inflicted by the rioters, including the normal cross-section of wounds from blunt or sharp objects familiar to A & E Departments. Crowd control itself produces casualties and occasionally these are seen:

CS gas

This has been used in crowd control overseas, and occasionally canisters have been let off in this country. CS gas causes a burning and prickling irritation of the skin which is followed by an inflammatory reaction but no blistering. There is an immediate effect on the eyes — production of tears and painful blepharospasm. There is also chest pain, coughing and profuse salivation. The effects are usually short in duration, but if the patient has been trapped in a confined area and has received a large dose the symptoms may be more severe. The effects of previous chronic respiratory illness may be exacerbated by these gases so admission is advised. Antispasmodics and oxygen should be started as soon as possible. The eye symptoms can be relieved by washing with saline followed by antihistaminic eyedrops as in the treatment of burns.

Baton rounds

Otherwise known as rubber bullets. These are high mass–low velocity missiles fired from a riot gun. Fifteen cm (six inches) long, four cm (one-and-a-half inches) in diameter, they weigh 140 g (five ounces). A plastic bullet can be fired more accurately at safe areas of the body where they should not cause much damage. However if released at close range, or if children are hit, quite serious injuries can result, particularly if the face and eyes are involved. Severe damage to the eyes is frequently seen. Concussion and cerebral haematomata, contusion of the lung and in the abdomen, intestinal perforation, and liver and spleen injuries may occur. In the young, cardiac contusion can cause ventricular fibrillation and other conduction irregularities, so all chest injuries should have ECG monitoring. Head and abdominal injuries should be admitted for observation and ophthalmic opinion.

Disaster planning

Each NHS hospital with an A & E Department has a plan prepared to deal with disasters. The disaster is related to the hazards of its catchment area — main roads, railway lines and stations, airports, and varied local industries. There may be a wide range of chemical or other potentially dangerous factories in the area. The terrorist threat can produce large numbers of casualties from bomb explosions. Fire is always a risk. Each A & E Department should be organised to cope with a large number of cases which can easily saturate their medical and surgical facilities. Better planning and organisation to disperse casualties over a larger number of hospitals would ease the burdens.

The hospital plan is usually written and should be readily available; newcomers to an A & E Department should make themselves familiar with its contents. The hospital is usually alerted by the ambulance service or police, then there is a phased response depending on the expected number of casualties.

- (i) Green: mobilise the A & E Department.
- (ii) Amber: for a moderate number of casualties, all on-duty staff are mobilised.
- (iii) Red: a major community disaster when off-duty teams need to be called in and twenty-four-hour duty rotas need to be organised.

Staff deployment in the department is best carried out by means of action cards which clearly define the task at different stages of the alert. These are given to the staff on arrival in the department.

Disaster facilities in the hospital need to be reviewed regularly. The reception is in the A & E Department, which should be adequately signposted. The waiting-halls and expansion areas should be identified. The casualty officer's role in this situation is to work in the department he knows best.

Mobile teams are available in most hospitals, and many of these are involved in the British Association of Immediate Care schemes and turn out regularly. These teams need to be well trained and well equipped with adequate protective clothing and insurance.

Medical management

Control of the whole operation is taken by the A & E Consultant, or if not available a nominated appointment such as RSO or RMO. A senior A & E sister or doctor carries out triage which is the sorting of casualties into the categories which determine the priority of treatment:

Category 1: patients require immediate resuscitation and surgery.

Category 2: treatment can be delayed but early surgery will be required.

Category 3: this includes most of the injured and will be mainly lacerations and contusions which require minimum treatment and can be delayed.

The dead must be sent straight to the mortuary for identification later. Triage is a vital process and all categories may alter. Each patient on arrival should be allocated a numbered tag and suitable admission notes which have been pre-prepared. The patient is transferred to the requisite treatment area.

Primary treatment areas

   (a) Resuscitation : advanced life-saving care is carried out in an area where early intervention with airways, endotracheal tubes, intravenous therapy and chest drains can be carried out.

   (b) Those requiring delayed treatment are sent, after registration, to a designated ward for ongoing reassessment and allocation to the theatre list.

   (c) Minor treatment area must be large and adjacent to small theatres/cubicles where wounds can be cleaned, excised and sutured.

Pre-determined guidelines on the surgery of wounds, transfusion fluids, tetanus and antibiotic treatment should be readily available.

Other administrative tasks such as a casualty location board with the patient's name, number, and diagnosis needs to be updated continually by the administrative staff and police liaison group.

Communications with relatives and the press will be organised away from the A & E Department to avoid further congestion.

Social work referrals

Referrals to the social worker should be made as soon as any problem is anticipated. Often it takes time and many telephone calls before the hospital social worker is able to arrange a solution to your patient's problem, particularly in crisis situations where resources are scarce, for example 'part 3' beds. The social worker is employed by the local authority, to whom he/she has statutory responsibilities, and has their full resources available.

Statutory responsibilities

Physical and emotional well-being of:

   (a) children up to 16 years;

   (b) the elderly;

   (c) the mentally infirm;

   (d) pets.

Patients to be referred

    (a) Uncared for children under 16 and dependent relatives.
    (b) Child abuse — any suspicion of deprivation, physical, sexual, emotional or moral danger.
    (c) Vulnerable elderly being discharged home.
    (d) Vulnerable mentally disabled: sectioning of patients under the Mental Health Act 1983 (MHA83) (see 'Psychiatry' page 83).
    (e) The homeless.
    (f) Victims of physical or sexual violence.
    (g) Those needing urgent financial advice.

Services from the local authority for which there is a statutory responsibility

    (a) Old people's home placement (part 3 accommodation).
    (b) Meals on wheels.
    (c) Home help.
    (d) Day centre — for elderly, mentally or physically disabled.
    (e) Telephones for medically vulnerable and physically disabled.
    (f) Sheltered housing.
    (g) Children's homes.
    (h) Lunch club.
    (i) Bus pass for elderly, physically or visually disabled.

The social worker will also provide a counselling service for distressed or anxious patients or relatives. They will help at 'bad news' interviews. They can provide specialist knowledge of welfare rights and other local resources: accommodation, agencies for helping alcoholics, to assist victims of rape, battered women's refuges, charitable and voluntary agencies.

A dedicated social worker in the A & E Department will help in providing a more compassionate and effective service and will relieve you of many difficult problems.

NOTES

MANAGEMENT OF MAJOR TRAUMA
Trauma team call out

Vital signs

Glasgow coma score < 13
Systolic BP < 90
Respiratory rate < 10 >29

CALL TRAUMA TEAM

Anatomical injury and
mechanism of injury

Penetrating injury to trunk head or neck
Two proximal long bone fractures
Burns of > 15% or airway or face
High-energy impact Fall 20 ft
                                   Deceleration >20 m.p.h.
                                   Ejection
                                   Rollover
                                   Death of occupant

CALL TRAUMA TEAM

Lower threshold for
call out

Age ≤ 5 or ≥ 55 years
Cardiac or respiratory disease

REASSESS

WHEN IN DOUBT: CALL THE TRAUMA TEAM OUT

(a) RSO
(b) Anaesthetist
(c) Cardiothoracic Registrar
(d) Orthopaedic Registrar
(e) Intensivist

Multiple injuries in the Accident and Emergency Department

The patient with multiple injuries should be admitted to a well-lit large resuscitation room which has airways, endotracheal tubes, intravenous cannulae with fluids and thoracostomy tubes readily available. (See Table 2.1.)

Note the time on the wall board together with drugs and fluids given. This can be transcribed to the notes when things are quieter.

History. This is obtained by a reliable person from the ambulance driver who brought the patient in, police, and relatives, enabling background detail and pertinent clinical observations to be reported back to those involved in ongoing resuscitation.

Assess the amount of trauma absorbed by the patient: a crush injury, a fall from height, an accident which involves the patient being thrown off motor cycle, or an impact with severe damage to vehicle all imply heavy blows to the patient.

Look. The Mark I eyeball and fingers are essential at this stage — the clinician's eye will never be replaced by elaborate electronic machines. Monitor the patient's level of consciousness carefully: in the early stages of hypovolaemia a slight change in personality occurs, mental aberration and inappropriate reactions indicate disturbances of cerebral blood flow and oxygen. Changes in the level of responsiveness must be watched for allowing for effects of head injury, alcohol and drugs. The hunted look of battle fatigue with dilated pupils, wrinkled forehead, the patient staring 1,000 metres ahead, occurs also in the patient with mild cerebral anoxia who also does not respond typically to painful stimulae. A cold nose with clammy skin may be the vasoconstriction of shock, hypothermia from delay in evacuation or too much cold fluid intravenously. A warm patient with good capillary filling of nail bed is good to see. Watch his movements whilst removing clothing: minor fractures and dislocations may then be spotted which can be embarrassing if missed.

TABLE 2.1
Major trauma

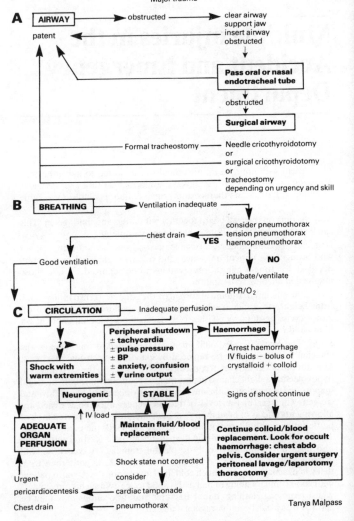

Tanya Malpass

Resuscitation room

A routine for doctors and nurses must be properly organised so that, as the doctor is examining the patients, assisting nurses are removing clothing then recording pulse, blood pressure (BP) and level of consciousness.

(a) Airway

Assess the patient's colour, airway and neck: insert an airway or quickly pass an endotracheal tube if these are disturbed.

(b) Breathing

Assess the breathing pattern, chest movements, flail segment and ventilation and look carefully front and back for stab wounds.

(c) Circulation

A low blood pressure on admission carries a high mortality so urgent fluid replacement is required. Two large-bore intravenous cannulae are inserted with the rapid infusion of a crystalloid such as Hartmann's solution: follow with a colloid volume expander such as Haemaccel, Gelofusine or Dextran 70, then cross-matched blood. In extreme emergencies, blood of the patient's group or group ORh. negative will avoid unnecessary delay, and can be life-saving. Monitor central venous pressure (CVP). (See page 404.)

Head injuries or other disturbances of consciousness require serial observations which are recorded on the Glasgow Coma Chart (see page 179). Check the cervical spine for injury always.

(d) Blood loss

A quick count of all major fractures, injuries and wounds will help estimate the quantity of blood in litres the patient may require. (See Figure 2.1.) Fractures and wounds are obvious in the limbs but large quantities of blood may be in the chest, peritoneum or retroperitoneally with fractures of the spine or pelvis.

Having secured the airway, controlled obvious bleeding from wounds with haemostat and pressure dressings, and supported the circulation with intravenous fluids, look at the patient again to make a more accurate assessment. *Call Trauma Team:* see page 14.

The limbs—fractures require urgent splintage (see page 416) to prevent further soft tissue damage, pain and aggravation of shock. Pneumatic splints or box splints are required for the lower bones of limbs, a Thomas splint with skin traction (see page 416) for fractures of the femur.

Wounds are covered with large sterile pads which are fastened with crepe bandage; if bleeding continues more pads and pressure are applied.

Shock

There is an absolute or relative inadequacy of the circulating blood volume resulting in inadequate tissue perfusion. Causes are: loss of volume; expansion of the vascular capacity; or pump failure. (See Table 2.2.)

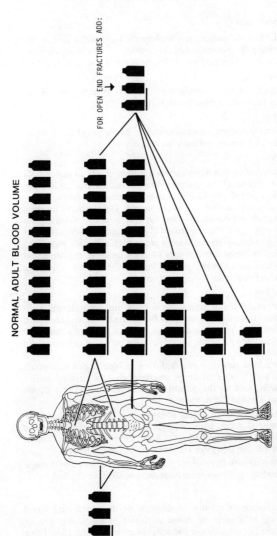

NORMAL ADULT BLOOD VOLUME

FOR OPEN END FRACTURES ADD:

Rough equivalence between site and severity of injury and blood required for replenishment.

Bottles underlined represent the usual order of loss, the whole row the possible need.

With multiple injuries the individual losses have to be added and may considerably exceed a blood volume.

Figure 2.1 *Blood loss in multiple injuries (after Ruscoe Clark & Peter London)*

TABLE 2.2

Findings and blood requirements will vary according to age and fitness of patient, rate of loss of blood and state of continuing losses.

CHART

Blood loss % BV	<750 ml <15%	<750–1500 15–30%	1500–2000 30–40%	>2000 >40%
Pulse	<100	>100	>120	140+
BP, systolic	Normal	Normal	↓	↓
diastolic	Nor ↑	↑	↓	↓
Capillary refill	Nor	Slow ↓	Slow ↓	Undetectable
Respiration	14–20	20–30	30–40	>35
Urine output ml/hr	30+	20–30	5–15	<5
CNS	Anxious or Normal	Anxious	Anxious + Confused	Confused + Lethargic
Blood transfusion	No	Probable	Yes	Urgent

Recognition

Look

Pallor; greyish white; may be cyanosed peripherally; peripheral vascular shut-down; dilated pupils; sighing respiration; venous filling in neck veins. Agitation, anxiety, or confusion due to hypoxia. Profound thirst.

Feel

(a) *Peripheral vasoconstriction*, cold with clammy skin — slow capillary return on finger nail bed; rapid thready pulse; but note that tachycardia does not occur until 750–1000 ml loss and may be absent in young fit patients once peripheral vasoconstriction and compensatory mechanisms have occurred.

(b) *Abdomen:* If distended — aneurysm; intestinal obstruction. Tenderness plus rigidity — perforation; peritonitis; acute pancreatitis.

(c) *Femoral pulses:* Check if absent (aneurysm); check volume loss. Core temperature: query septic shock. Query hypothermia. Flushed, hot, or rashes — query anaphylaxis or drug overdose.

Blood pressure

First sign is an increased diastolic pressure with normal systolic, therefore decreased pulse pressure: decreased systolic pressure may not occur until 1500–2000 ml blood loss.

N.B. Blood loss greater than 2 litres is life-threatening therefore detect shock before BP falls too far.

Auscultation

Listen over chest for fine crepitations.

Cardiovascular system (CVS).

Myocardial contusion may cause arrhythmias; traumatic rupture of valves causes severe heart failure. Muffled heart sounds with distended neck veins and shock refractory to fluid replacement strongly point to cardiac tamponade: x-ray, aspirate or thoracotomy.

Abdomen: query bowel sounds, query bruits from aneurysm.

To recognise shock and start resuscitation are most important. Firm diagnosis may wait a while. At least try to decide whether the cause is more likely to be surgical or medical. Refer at the start of the golden hour.

Investigations

1 Blood for group and cross-match.
2 ECG.
3 X-ray cervical spine, skull, chest, abdo, pelvis — in all patients with major trauma.
4 Acid base/blood gases.
5 Cardiac enzymes if any irregularities on ECG.

Injuries of the trunk

An erect chest x-ray will be of considerable value in abdominal and chest injuries; it should be done before the limb x-rays. If the patient is not fit to sit up, lie him on one side.

Closed abdominal injuries

Carefully examine the pelvic ring and spine. Palpate, then auscultate, the abdomen; repeat this several times, particularly if there is any disturbance of consciousness or restlessness. A soft abdomen may contain a large quantity of blood yet gut sounds are still audible. An urgent laparotomy must be considered if shock is not responding to transfusion with increasing abdominal distension. *Girth measurements alone are unreliable.*

Passage of a catheter should be easy: blood in the urine indicates renal tract damage — then an emergency IVP is essential. Blood at the tip of the penis, a boggy urethra PR with displaced prostate and pelvic rami fractures suggest urethral damage, in which case a urethral catheter should *not* be passed. If the patient cannot pass urine this assists the diagnosis; as the bladder fills suprapubic catheterisation becomes easy. Retrograde urethrography is required.

Peritoneal lavage

Haemoperitoneum may be difficult to diagnose, so peritoneal lavage is required. One litre of warm 0.9 per cent saline is inserted into the abdomen using a standard giving set through a cannula inserted 2 fingers below the umbilicus in the midline, and re-aspirated after 5 minutes by free drainage back into drip bag. Frank blood enables a decision to operate to be made. If not so frank, a red cell count greater than 100,000 should be accepted as positive. If you cannot read *The Telegraph* through the specimen, it is positive. Bile and white-cell counts may also demonstrate pathology. Mini laparoscopy is more accurate.

When the patient is not so acutely ill and a decision is difficult, ask the radiologist for help:

(a) ultrasound; as reliable as lavage.
(b) angiography;
(c) CT scan;
(d) radionucleotide imaging techniques can be of great assistance if available;
(e) the older technique of double contrast enemas may still give us valuable information.

High index of suspicion

Must prevail with patients with lower rib fractures, particularly on the left; seat belt or tyre mark bruising; multiple injuries with evidence of damage to both chest and pelvis.

Retroperitoneal damage to vessels may lead to ischaemia of large bowel and endotoxaemia. Reassess carefully if abdominal bruising presents.

Chest x-ray

This should be done early and, after x-ray of the cervical spine, be the first film requested in a patient with multiple injuries. If the patient's condition allows, an erect or semi-erect film should be taken, otherwise lie him on his side.

What to look for on the chest x-ray

1 Pneumothorax. The lung edge may be seen more clearly by turning the film on its side so that you are looking for a horizontal line rather than a vertical one. Beware of the completely collapsed lung — it is surprisingly easy to miss, especially on a poor-quality film or where there is much surgical emphysema. (See Figure 2.2.)

2 Haemothorax. On an erect film there is usually no problem recognising this, especially if there is an air-fluid level. However, in a supine film the blood may be visible only as a slight overall increase in shadowing. If there is massive haemorrhage, the whole of the hemi-thorax may be radio-opaque. (See Figure 2.3.)

3 Widened upper mediastinum. This may be due to a ruptured aorta or other major vessel damage. (See Figure 2.4.)

4 Shifted mediastinum. This is a sign of a tension pneumothorax. (See Figure 2.5.)

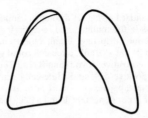

Figure 2.2 *Shallow right apical pneumothorax*

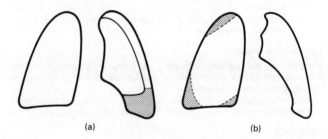

(a)   (b)

Figure 2.3 *Haemothorax*
(a) Left haemopneumothorax
(b) Right haemothorax

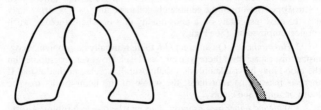

Figure 2.4 *Rupture of aorta*   **Figure 2.5** *Left tension pneumothorax, shifted mediastinum*

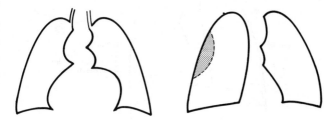

Figure 2.6 *Cardiac tamponade*

Figure 2.7 *Pulmonary contusion*
Usually the overlying ribs are fractured

5 Globular heart. Remember that the film will almost certainly be an antero-posterior (AP) one, not PA, so the heart will tend to look larger than usual. However, a globular enlarged heart, convex left border, right cardio–phrenic angle below 90°, suggests bleeding into the pericardium. (See Figure 2.6.)

6 Fractured ribs. They are not always easy to see, but there is no point in doing oblique films just to try to show fractures. If more than one rib is broken, separated by apparently uninjured ones, the chances are that the in-between ones are also broken. Fractures of the first rib require considerable force and imply severe injury. Fractures of the posterior parts of the ribs require more violence than lateral and anterior parts. Fractures of the 9, 10, 11 left are often associated with rupture of the spleen: on the right side, the liver.

7 Pulmonary contusion. This may show up as patchy homogenous shadowing in the lung fields, often peripheral. (See Figure 2.7.)

8 Ruptured diaphragm. On the left, loops of bowel or the stomach may be visible. Alternatively, and on the right, there may be opacification of all or part of the hemithorax. (See Figure 2.8.)

9 Ruptured aorta. The classical x-ray signs are:
(a) Widened upper mediastinum
(b) Left pleural cap (i.e. a radio-opaque shadow over the apex of the lung due to clot)
(c) Trachea shifted to the right
(d) Left haemothorax (See Figure 2.4.)

10 Surgical emphysema. If massive, this may outline the muscle fibres, particularly of pectoralis major, and cause confusion. Air in the mediastinum suggests oesophageal damage.

11 Fractured sternum. This needs a special lateral view and cannot be seen on a straight PA chest film.

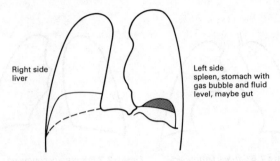

Figure 2.8 *Bilateral traumatic rupture of the diaphragm*

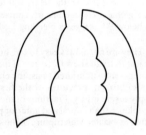

Figure 2.9 *Ruptured aorta — increasing width of mediastinum*

Missile wounds of the abdomen

May result from high- or low-velocity bullets or fragments of exploding bomb. All missile wounds of the abdomen must be explored, not observed; never be confused by the conservative approach often used with closed abdominal injuries. These patients must be operated on soon, so refer to the surgeons quickly.

Diagnosis

1 Ask the patient.
2 Examine abdomen and back carefully to assess direction and line of tract. An entry wound anywhere between the nipples and mid thigh may involve the abdomen. Beware of the solitary penetrating wound of the buttock, it will involve the adjacent pelvis.

3 The belly is painful, rigid and silent; the general condition of the patient may be worse than expected from other injuries. If he is vomiting, distending, and tender PR with a rising pulse rate and poor response to transfusion, he requires early laparotomy.
4 With wounds of the abdominal wall alone, guarding tends to be more localised and shock not so severe. Bowel sounds will appear, tenderness and guarding will subside. If in doubt — explore.
5 Chest x-ray might help; free gas may be seen under the diaphragm; and foreign bodies can be located and bone chips seen.

Pre-operative.

Pass catheter and examine urine for blood.

Stab wounds of the abdomen

The well-stabilised patient with a small penetrating wound anteriorly between the nipple and the pubis can be discussed. There are those who will wait and watch carefully, but stab wounds are frequently deeper than one would suspect. If doubtful arrange for peritoneal lavage or admit for observation (see page 402). Look carefully for signs of peritonism and shock. Stab wounds of the back may not show peritonism; penetration to the retroperitoneal structures may have no obvious signs of damage until, too late, haemorrhage and sepsis manifest themselves. Stab wounds of the back and loin must be properly explored under adequate anaesthesia and theatre conditions. *Refer.*

Trauma to the thorax and lung

A quarter of car fatalities result from chest injury, and in another 25 per cent chest trauma is a factor. (See Table 2.3.)

Simple fractures

Simple fractures of up to 3 ribs are always painful and the symptoms may last for several months; non-steroidal anti-inflammatory agents are helpful. With severe pain consider intercostal nerve block. Watch the elderly — their respiratory reserve is low and pneumonia rate high. Fractures of the first rib, however, are the hallmark of severe trauma and are often associated with vascular injury. Multiple fractures often result in a flail segment with paradoxical movement. (See Figure 2.10.) Measure FEV and blood gases. Fractures of the sternum may be associated with cardiac muscle contusion and cardiac irregularities. In the young with a compressible chest wall a baton round ('rubber bullet') may damage the heart causing cardiac contusion, conduction irregularities or ventricular fibrillation without fracturing ribs or sternum.

Traumatic pneumothorax

Traumatic pneumothorax is seen following lung penetration by fractured ribs: often associated with bleeding, haemothorax and surgical emphysema of chest wall.

TABLE 2.3

Chest injuries: physical signs

Clinical Sign	Open pneumothorax	Flail segment	Tension pneumothorax	Bilateral pneumothorax	Simple pneumothorax	Haemothorax	Lung contusion	Bronchial injury	Fractured ribs	Ruptured diaphragm	Cardiac tamponade	Ruptured aorta	Oesophageal injury
CYANOSIS (despite a clear airway and oxygen)	X	X	X	X	(X)	(X)	X	X	(X)	X	X		
DYSPNOEA	X	X	X	X	(X)	(X)	X	X		X			X
DECREASED CHEST WALL MOVEMENT			X*		X								
PARADOXICAL CHEST WALL MOVEMENT		X											
DISTENDED NECK VEINS			X								X		
SURGICAL EMPHYSEMA			X**	X	X								+
TRACHEAL SHIFT			X		X								
ABSENT OR DECREASED BREATH SOUNDS			X	X	X	X (if massive)						X	
ABSENT OR DECREASED FEMORAL PULSE (relative to the upper limbs)												X	
PERSISTING HYPOTENSION despite adequate transfusion, and with distended neck veins			X								X		

Key: (X) Symptoms more likely to occur in patients with pre-existing respiratory disease
* Hyperinflation
**May be massive
+ Begins in the neck

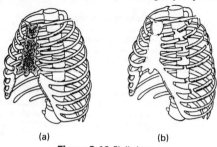

(a)   (b)

Figure 2.10 *Flail chest*
(a) Anterior segments
(b) Lateral segments

The tension pneumothorax must be diagnosed and treated quickly. The patient is dyspnoeic; cyanosed; the affected side of the chest is expanded, does not move; and breath sounds are absent. The trachea and apex beat move away from the affected side. A tube thoracotomy with an underwater seal or Heimlich valve is urgently required. A white hypodermic needle gauge 19 can be inserted whilst preparing the tube. *Do not wait for the chest x-ray if you are confident.* (For insertion of chest drain see page 399.)

Penetrating wound of chest

Penetrating wound of chest causes a haemo-pneumothorax often without a major mediastinal injury, and on the whole the lung expands well. Tube thoracotomy with an underwater seal is often the only treatment required (see page 400). Indications for urgent thoracotomy in the A & E Department are acute deterioration, cardiac tamponade or cardiac arrest. Wounds of the intercostal vessels or heart can cause severe haemorrhage, and if the initial drainage is greater than 1500 ml or continues at a rate greater than 300 ml for an hour — thoracotomy.

Sucking wounds

Sucking wounds from stab or high-velocity missile fragments rapidly cause a tension pneumothorax. The sucking wound is sealed with vaseline gauze and melolin dressing or a temporary suture and the tension pneumothorax relieved by tube thoracotomy with an underwater seal drain. (See page 400.) Eighty-five per cent of simple stab and gunshot wounds of the chest can be managed with a 32F tube thoracotomy.

Cardiac tamponade

Cardiac tamponade: increasing distension of neck veins with elevation of the CVP, a small quiet heart with increasing shock demands urgent action. Distended neck veins and increased CVP may be absent if the patient is also hypovolaemic. Pericardial aspiration through a needle gauge 18

Penetrating chest wounds

15% of penetrating chest wounds have cardiac involvement

GROUP ONE 80%	GROUP TWO 15%	GROUP THREE 5%
Remote stab wound. Blood pressure stable.	Suspicious stab wound. Hypotensive — responds to IV fluids: may deteriorate suddenly.	Significant stab wound. Apparently dead; warm; BP unrecordable; JVP ↑ faint heart sounds; feeble efforts at breathing.

TREATMENT

IV cannula, fluids. CXR, + − chest drain. Observe.	Double IV cannulae, CXR, + − chest drain. Observe in thoracic unit.	*Antero-lateral THORACOTOMY immediately* Relieve tamponade; Internal cardiac massage IV fluids and blood.

IF PATIENT
Fails to respond to
IV fluids;
    and/or
continuing blood loss
(>300 mls for 4 hours);
    and/or
sudden haemodynamic
deterioration;
    and/or
echocardiogram shows
pericardial effusion:
*Left Antero-lateral
THORACOTOMY.*

Below nipple line
look for
abdominal injury

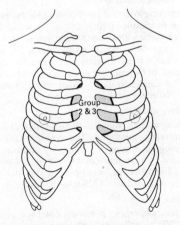

Group
2 & 3

Figure 2.11 *Penetrating wounds of chest (D. Watson)*

inserted to the left of the xiphoid and passed upwards towards the left shoulder and backwards at 45° can be life-saving but urgent left antero-lateral thoracotomy may be essential. Operating facilities should be available in the emergency room — many young lives will be saved this way. (See Figure 2.11.)

Pulmonary contusion

Pulmonary contusion and haematoma may occur with multiple fractures and may progress for 48–72 hrs; x-ray changes occur within 1–6 h, adult respiratory distress syndrome (ARDS) may result from a combination of the effects of contusion, volume overload and fat embolism. Haemato-mata usually resolve but if infected may cavitate. Note that fluid overload will complicate with ARDS later. Give 2 g methyl-prednisolone IV over 20 minutes (30 mg/kg). (See Figure 2.7.)

Traumatic rupture of the diaphragm

Traumatic rupture of the diaphragm is usually on the left side. It is often missed in the early stages as in one third of cases there will be no initial signs. There will be dyspnoea and a mild non-specific abdominal pain. X-ray is diagnostic and will show the gastric air bubbles, multiple air and fluid levels with loss of the left hemi-diaphragmatic shadow; if there is any doubt a gastrografin swallow will confirm — this diagnosis is made with an erect chest x-ray. It should be emphasised that all abdominal injuries benefit from an erect chest x-ray: it will show ribs, subphrenic air, as well as the state of the lungs. (See Figure 2.8.)

Flail chest

The ribs are fractured in 2 places. (See Figure 2.10.) Paradoxical chest movements are easily recognised. The segment of chest wall moves in on inspiration and is seen better tangentially. Turn patient onto affected side. In mild cases monitor blood gases and if these are normal the patient can be watched: relieve pain by intercostal nerve block. Use the Trinkle regime replacing blood volume losses with colloid, preferably blood, and then a low IV electrolyte fluid input for daily requirements. In severe cases with respiratory embarrassment when the pO_2 is less than 8 kPa (60 mm Hg) and the pCO_2 greater than 6 kPa (45 mm) endotracheal tube and IPPR is essential. When the patient is more severely ill, tracheostomy and positive expiratory end pressure (PEEP) with a chest tube and monitoring of blood gases may be required.

Blunt trauma to the heart

Blunt trauma to the heart may produce cardiac arrhythmias often fol-lowed by ARDS and, if refractory, cause death. Intracardiac damage to the valves is not uncommon.

Death after multiple injuries to the chest and lung is often the result of cardiac complications. Close monitoring of ECG changes and cardiac enzyme elevations is essential.

Limit intravenous fluids: patient should be treated as a cardiac infarct.

Late cardiac complications following damage to cardiac vessels, myocardium and valves will occur.

Haemodynamic monitoring using a Swann Ganz Catheter which monitors cardiac output and other essential intrathoracic measurements.

Aortic damage. The early chest x-ray may show mediastinal widening and this must be carefully monitored by repeating the CXR. Damage to the media and intima layers of the thoracic aorta distal to the ligamentum arterosium with the adventitia intact is common. Half survive and reach an A & E Department. If the superior mediastinum on the x-ray is greater than 8 cm, or if the trachea is moved to the right with a left haemothorax, particularly if the first rib is fractured, you must look carefully at the aortic arch. Repeat the film later (see Figure 2.4) and, if any doubt, tomography, angiography, or computerised tomography, and refer.

There is no substitute for experience and frequent eyeballing in the assessment of injury to the trunk so watch all cases carefully and remain in the resuscitation room after the surgical team has arrived.

NOTES

3

Chest problems

Chest pain

The problems in the casualty department are usually:

    1 Is this chest pain cardiac in origin?
    2 If it is, has there been myocardial damage?

Chest pain of cardiac origin?

Classic cardiac chest pain is characteristically a central, crushing chest pain which may radiate to the left arm, occasionally right arm or neck, and be accompanied by sweating, pallor, nausea and shortness of breath. Unfortunately, many cases pose problems because the pain is atypical and signs are absent or confusing. Classical ECG changes of ST elevation or Q waves are often absent at the early stages of myocardial infarction.

    There are no hard-and-fast laws to guide us to the answer, we must treat before confirmatory evidence (serial enzyme results and serial ECGs) arrives, but there are one or two pointers which may be of help:

Pointers towards the possibility of chest pain being cardiac

- Characteristic *site and quality*.
- *Precipitation* by exercise or emotion with relief by rest (generally within 10 minutes). N.B. Pain started regularly by a given level of effort is an important diagnostic feature of angina.
- *Relief by glyceryl trinitrate* (GTN) within 1–3 minutes strongly suggests angina. Failure to relieve pain may mean one of 3 things:

1 The pain is not cardiac in origin
2 The pain is due to myocardial infarction
3 The GTN tablets are out of date

Relief after 5 minutes is likely to be coincidental and not attributed to GTN.

Has there been myocardial damage?

Angina pectoris is chest pain of cardiac origin, causing a disturbance of myocardial function but not associated with myocardial necrosis.

TABLE 3.1 Algorithm for the management of chest pain in A & E

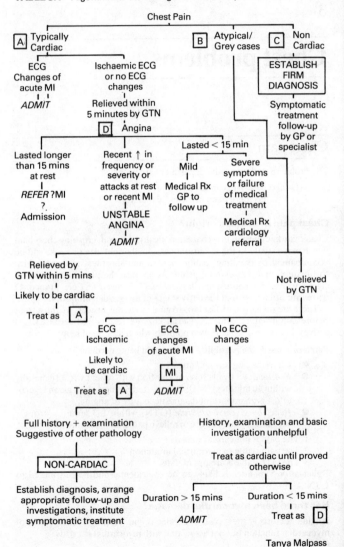

Tanya Malpass

The electrocardiogram (ECG) may show changes of ST depression during the acute attack. Between attacks, though there may be other ECG abnormalities, many patients have a normal ECG. The presence of resting ST segment depression is a poor prognostic sign, as are the presence of other physical signs of heart disease such as hypertension, cardiomegaly or cardiac failure. The initial diagnosis of angina rests on the history.

If the diagnosis of angina can be made easily clinically and its severity is not great, medical treatment may be instituted. Further regular follow-up to assess its effect and the progression of the disease is performed by the GP. If the diagnosis cannot be made with certainty, or if the angina is severe (marked limitation of ordinary activities) referral to a cardiologist and further investigations such as exercise, stress testing, radionucleotide imaging or cardiac catheterisation may be indicated. Patients who do not respond to medical treatment should also be referred.

Indications for urgent admission

1 *Angina at rest lasting longer than 15 minutes and not relieved by GTN is a myocardial infarction (MI) until proven otherwise.*
2 Angina accompanied by ECG changes of ST elevation, even if pain has been very short lived, indicates myocardial infarction.
3 Angina of effort with a recent change in pattern (increasing severity, frequency or onset at rest) is *unstable angina*. These patients should be admitted for intensive medical treatment until stabilised. If not treated, risk of MI is high (40 per cent within 1–3 months) as is mortality (17 per cent within 1–3 months).
4 Recurrent angina early in the post-infarction period carries risks as above and should be treated similarly.

Pitfalls

- A normal ECG does not exclude MI.
- A normal CPK does not exclude MI.
- Pain relieved by GTN is not always cardiac though it is a good diagnostic pointer.
- GTN tablets 'go off'; always check expiry date of tablets in stock or the patient's tablets. Failure of response may be due to this. Sublingual 'spray' is more stable.
- Tenderness in the chest wall may help confirm a diagnosis of costochondritis or musculoskeletal pain but has been reported in cardiac pain.
- Patients with history of other pathology, e.g. peptic ulcer, hiatus hernia, can still have MIs; always listen if the patient says this is a different pain.

TABLE 3.2

Myocardial infarction: changes in waveform

	Onset	Disappearance
1 ST elevation	HOURS (1st few)	24 hrs — days
2 Q waves	HOURS (after ST)	weeks/months/ indefinite
3 T wave inversion	HOURS to days	days to months

ECG returns to normal eventually in 10 per cent of cases.

Site of infarction is indicated by abnormalities in leads:
Inferior   = II, III, AVF. (Right coronary artery.)
Anterior   = I, AVL ± leads V1–6. (Left anterior descending artery.)
Septal   = V1–4.
Lateral   = I, V4–6. (Circumflex arteries.)
Subendocardial infarct does not produce Q waves but ST depression and T wave inversion are seen.

Cardiac enzymes

An initial sample may be taken in A & E Department, but the result should not be awaited. No diagnostic significance should be attached to this result in isolation. Serial results at 12 and 18 hours will help confirm the diagnosis. The characteristic pattern of rise of enzymes is shown in Figure 3.1.

Other baseline blood/concentrations

Full blood count (FBC) electrolytes, glucose, may be taken in A & E Department as a baseline for later.

Figure 3.1 *Serial rise in cardiac enzymes in acute myocardial infarction*

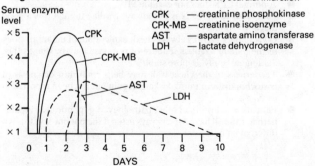

CPK	— creatinine phosphokinase
CPK-MB	— creatinine isoenzyme
AST	— aspartate amino transferase
LDH	— lactate dehydrogenase

TABLE 3.3

Differential diagnosis of cardiac pain

Pericarditis	Oesophageal reflux
Pleurisy	Peptic ulceration
Pulmonary embolus	Costochondritis
Pneumothorax	Musculoskeletal pain
Aortic dissection	Cholecystitis
Pancreatitis	

Cardiac neurosis (this is a very dangerous diagnosis to make in casualty)

Treatment of suspected myocardial infarction

1 First:
- Admit to resuscitation bay — sit patient up.
- Administer high concentration O_2 via face mask.
- Establish IV access — slow infusion of 5 per cent dextrose. (N.B. it is reasonable to take blood for initial investigations at this stage in order to avoid further puncture.)
- Cardiac monitor.
- Take baseline readings — BP, pulse, etc.

2 While establishing above, obtain briefly from patient (or delegate someone to obtain from relatives): duration of symptoms; previous history of cardiac events; and drug history.

3 IV analgesia 5 mg diamorphine and 10 mg metoclopramide (repeat as necessary according to response).

4 Attend to stabilisation of patient, treating anxiety, pain, symptomatic arrhythmias, failure and shock.

5 Transfer at earliest opportunity on a cardiac monitor to coronary care unit (CCU).

6 Consider thrombolytic therapy if no contra-indications. Intravenous thrombolysis has been shown to reduce mortality in acute MI. Early administration, if possible within the first four hours, is advantageous. Choice of agent will reflect local policy. Dosage schedules are shown below.

   (a) *Contra-indications*
      Recent major surgery
      Peptic ulceration
      Subarachnoid haemorrhage
      Recent head injury (even minor)
      Prolonged or traumatic CPR.

   (b) *Precautions*
      Avoid vascular puncture for up to 30 minutes after alteplase

and 6 hours after streptokinase. Avoid repeated use of streptokinase for six months after first exposure.

(c) *Aspirin*
Enhances the benefit of thrombolysis and may be commenced
(150 mg EC tablet) on admission.

(d) *Dosage schedules*
Streptokinase 1 500 000 units in 100 ml saline infused over 60
minutes, or 750 000 units slow IV injection repeated after 30
minutes.
Alteplase (TPA) 10 mg bolus followed by 50 mg over one hour
and 40 mg over two hours. (Total 100 mg over 3 hours.) For
patients under 67 kg use 1.5 mg/kg total, divided as above.
Anistreplase (APSAC) 30 units as slow IV injection over 2–5
minutes.

7 Use intravenous nitrates to control recurrent pain or cardiac failure
which fails to respond to initial measures.

Investigations

ECG

Initial ECG may be taken in A & E Department as a baseline. Treatment
should not be withheld or delayed pending results. *A normal ECG does
not exclude MI.* Serial ECGs in the CCU will help confirm diagnosis. (See
Table 3.2.)

Blood gases. Appreciable cyanosis, confusion, shock, or cardiac failure
require urgent treatment. Blood gas analysis is required as a base line.

Use of oximetry may be valuable in monitoring progress.

Management of acute complications

Cardiac failure (Table 3.4)

Treat on clinical grounds: do not await chest x-ray (CXR). May be
secondary to an arrhythmia which needs treating.

Give O_2, diamorphine, diuretic (IV frusemide, 40 mg). If the patient is
already on large doses of diuretics this dose may be increased.

Intravenous nitrates may be of value in severe failure.

Cardiogenic shock

Relieve pain, treat arrhythmias, administer oxygen

If hypotension is not relieved by the above simple measures it is unlikely
that it can be rectified in A & E. The patient needs urgent intensive
coronary care and should be transferred urgently to CCU on a monitor.
The outlook is poor and treatment is in CCU with diuretics, vasodilators.
inotropes, and, in some cases, intra-aortic balloon pumping. Careful
control of fluid load and measurements of pulmonary capillary wedge
pressures is indicated.

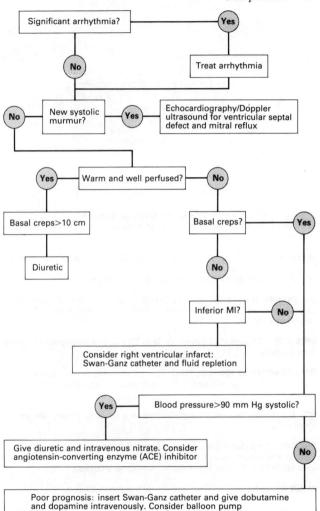

Reproduced with permission of Medical International

TABLE 3.4 Management of cardiac failure after acute myocardial infarction.

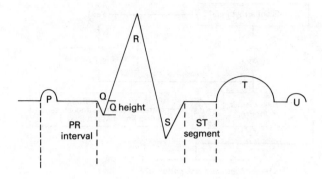

P WAVE bifid in LA hypertrophy (P mitrale); peaked in RA hypertrophy, e.g. cor pulmonale; lost inverted or displaced in nodal rhythm; lost in ventricular rhythms

Q WAVE — may be normal in lead III and V2–6 if <1 mm wide and <¼ of the height of the following R wave, or <2 mm deep.
Abnormal Q indicates infarction or bundle branch block.

PR INTERVAL 0.12–0.2 secs (3–5 mm). Short in Wolf-Parkinson-White: prolonged in first degree heart block: irregular or variable in second or third degree heart block.

QRS 0.08–0.11 secs (1–2.5 mm). Wide in BBB and hypertrophy: abnormal forms in BBB.

ST SEGMENT IS ISOELECTRIC. Convex elevation in myocardial infarction: concave elevation in pericarditis: depression — digitalis toxication, LVH, ischaemia.

ST <0.5 mm depression. <1 mm elevation in limb leads, <2 mm elevation in chest leads.

T WAVE <5 mm tall in limb leads, <10 mm in V leads.
Peaked in hyperkalaemia and early MI.
Inverted in BBB, digitalis, hypertrophy, ischaemia, infarction.

U WAVE can be normal. Seen best V3–4. ↑ in hypokalaemia.

Figure 3.2 *The electrocardiogram (ECG)*

TABLE 3.5

System for reading electrocardiograms (see also Figure 3.2)

---

1 *RATE* — Check paper speed is on 25 mm/sec. Count number of squares between 2 consecutive R waves and divide into 300. (Normal = 60–100. Slower in athletes. Faster in children)

---

2 *RHYTHM* (a) of P waves —⎫ (b) of QRS ⎭	Take the edge of a piece of paper. Mark 3 consecutive peaks. Move paper one peak along and your marks should still exactly coincide if rhythm is regular.
(c) relationship of P to QRS?	
(d) P waves irregular =	1) SVE? 2) Wandering pacemaker? 3) Sick sinus syndrome?
(e) QRS irregular?	1) AF (no P waves) 2) Wenckebach (lengthening PR intervals) 3) Variable heart block? 4) VE (P. waves missing from abnormal beats) 5) SVE (P. waves same rhythm as QRS)
(f) Variable PR interval —	1) Wenckebach (irregular QRS) 2) Complete heart block (regular QRS)

---

3 *ST SEGMENT*
Look for elevation from isoelectric line. Beware of wandering or sloping isoelectric lines and high take-off, e.g. T wave in tachycardias.
Identify in which leads the abnormality occurs:

                    Inferior = II III AVF
                    Anterior = V leads
                    Septal   = VI–4
                    Lateral = I,V4–6

---

4 *QRS*
Look at width, wave form
Look for abnormal Q/R waves
Check voltage inline
Check QRS axis

---

5 *T WAVES*
Look for inverted T waves — as a general rule the T wave should point in the same direction as main QRS complex.

---

6 *LOOK FOR PATTERNS WHICH YOU MAY HAVE MISSED*
e.g. pulmonary embolus, digitalis toxicity, etc.

Abbreviations
Auricular fibrillation AF
Supraventricular extrasystoles SVE
Ventricular extra systole VE

Arrhythmias

Treat the patient, not the ECG

Arrhythmias that are not impairing cardiac function and are unlikely to deteriorate to a more serious rhythm should not be treated.

Treat in A & E Department arrhythmias which are causing, or threaten to cause, any of the following:

(a) Severe chest pain that has not been relieved by the diamorphine.
(b) Severe shortness of breath.
(c) Confusion, decrease in level of consciousness.
(d) Severe hypotension/circulatory collapse/cardiac failure.

See Table 3.6 for guidance on treatment of arrhythmias.

TABLE 3.6
Treatment and recognition of arrhythmias

	Recognition	*Treatment*
Sinus tachycardia	Regular P waves regular QRS; rate greater than 100/min normal complexes unless aberrantly conducted; rate usually less than 150/min (except in children).	Usually symptomatic of underlying condition e.g. hypovolaemia, fever, anxiety, pain. Therefore treat underlying cause.
Supraventricular tachycardia (SVT)	Regular P waves (may be obscured by previous complex) regular QRS — normal complexes *but* often aberrantly conducted. Atrial rate 140–240 Ventricular rate depends upon degree of block. Often 2:1 may be 1:1 (at slower ventricular rate).	Carotid massage –> Sinus Rhythm or slows rate by A–V block. If haemodynamically stable transfer and treat on CCU by DC Shock. or Verapamil or disopyramide or β blocker.
Atrial flutter	No p wave. F waves 300 per min QRS regular (often 150 per minute) exhibiting 2:1 or 3:1 block or occasionally variable block giving rise to irregular QRS.	Usually haemodynamically stable, therefore do not require treatment in A & E department. Carotid massage causes slowing of the rate. (May convert IV amiodarone; low energy DC shock; atrial override pacing. IV verapamil will control rate.)

TABLE 3.6—*contd.*

Atrial fibrillation (AF) 	No P waves fibrillation waves; irregular QRS with normal complexes unless aberrantly conducted.	No treatment in A & E Department. Treat severe CCF (may be cause or effect of AF). When stable consider digitalisation/ diuretics. Consider: Thyrotoxicosis, Emboli.
Ventricular tachycardia (VT)	Greater than 3 VpBs in succession with the same form and separated by a fixed interval. No P-waves (rarely A—V dissociation enables P waves to be seen but these bear no relation to QRS and are very difficult to see because of QRS complexes). Rate usually 140–200 per minute.	Treat if: greater than 10 seconds' duration, repetitive associated with haemodynamic consequences. DC cardioversion if associated with profound hypotension. Lignocaine if patient is conscious or less unstable. If this fails try disopyramide or amiodarone (centrally) if all else fails.
SVEs	Ectopic complexes preceded by P wave. P may differ from normal and QRS may be normal aberrantly conducted.	No treatment required.
Ventricular extrasystoles (VEs)	No preceding P wave complexes always abnormal.	Rarely require treatment in A & E. Treatment if R or T has been witnessed as a precursor of potentially haemodynamically unstable rhythm or if patient has had treatment for VT or VF.
Sinus bradycardia 	regular P waves regular QRS } constant relationship rate less than 60 per minute	Very common in acute MI and usually benign. Rarely requires treatment in A & E. If hypotensive give atropine.

TABLE 3.6—*contd.*

1st-degree heart block	PR greater than 5 mm.	No treatment required.
Complete heart block (3rd degree) (CHB)	Regular P waves Regular QRS P and QRS rates totally unrelated.	Treat in A & E only if very slow and symptomatic Atropine up to 2 mg bolus. Isoprenaline 2 mg in 500 ml, 15–60 dpm. (Cardiac pacing may be indicated depending on aetiology.)
2nd-degree heart block (A) *Mobitz type I — Wenckebach*	P waves regular. QRS irregular. Progressive lengthening of PR interval culminating in a dropped beat.	No treatment necessary in A & E Department. Refer.
Mobitz type II (B)	Intermittent failure of conduction dropped beats. May be regular, e.g. 2:1, 3:1 or variable. P waves regular, QRS regular (unless variable).	No treatment necessary in A & E Department. Refer.
Idioventricular rhythm	No P waves, regular abnormal QRS. May be very slow or normal (accelerated) rate.	Treat if very slow and symptomatic as for complete heart block.
Nodal rhythm	Normal regular QRS but no P waves. May be slow fast or normal rate.	Treatment: usually requires no treatment.
Ventricular fibrillation (VF)	Totally erratic discharge No P waves No QRS	*CARDIAC ARREST* CPR

TABLE 3.6—*contd.*

Asystole	Straight line.	*CARDIAC ARREST* CPR

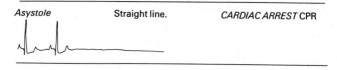

SVT OR VT?
RBBB pattern is usually SVT.
'Fusion beats'
'Capture beats' } rare but said to be pathognomic of VT
QRS greater than 3½ squares should be diagnosed as VT.
If a.v. dissociation can be discerned diagnose VT.
QRS exactly like sinus rhythm — diagnose SVT.

TABLE 3.7

Other recognisable ECG patterns and significance

1 LBBB V5 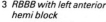	QRS > 3 mm M shape over V5 6 deep slurred S in VI absence of normal QR in LV leads.	No treatment required in A & E. Usually associated with ischaemic heart disease.
2 RBBB V1	QRS > 3 mm M shape over V1 deep-slurred S in V6 small QR in V6	No treatment in A & E. May be associated with ischaemia, ASD or idiopathic fibrosis. May be congenital.
3 *RBBB with left anterior hemi block* Left Axis Deviation 	recognition (RBBB with axis < −30)	Treatment indicative of more serious heart disease. May progress in the future to Complete Heart Block and therefore should not be ignored. Therefore *refer*.

TABLE 3.7—*contd.*

4 *ST Depression* >0.5 mm in all leads.

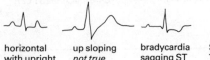 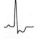

horizontal	up sloping	bradycardia	ST depression
with upright	*not true*	sagging ST	T wave inversion
T *Ischaemia*	*depression*	short QT	Tall complex
	often occurs	T wave often	slight widening
	with ↑ rate.	flat	QRS. *Ventricular*
		digoxin	*hypertrophy.*
		toxicity.	

5 *ST Elevation* > 1 mm in limb leads: > 2 mm in chest leads.

convex upwards
T ↑ or ↓
localised
reciprocal depression
in opposite leads
Myocardial infarction

concave top
T *wave usually* upright
generalised
pericarditis.

high take-off
*spurious elevation
increased rate in
normal ECG.*

6 *SI. QIII. T. III*

I   II   III

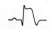

Deep S lead I
deep Q in lead III
inverted T in lead III

Right ventricular strain
Without other changes of acute MI
may be indicative of pulmonary
embolus but can be normal variant,
especially with short stature.

TABLE 3.8

Cardiac Drugs

Drug	Indications	Adult dosage
Amiodarone	1 Wolfe Parkinson White syndrome	Orally
(cordorone)	2 Supraventricular and ventricular	IV up to 5 mg/kg
Not in AV blocks	tachyarrhythmias which have proved refractory to other treatment.	over 20 minutes — 2 hours via central line.

TABLE 3.8—*contd.*

Flecainide	restricted in use to life thractory SV arrhythmias.	up to 2 mg/kg IV over 10 min
Atropine	Bradycardia Asystole	Up to 1 mg in bradycardia. Repeat if necessary. 2 m in asystole.
Disopyramide (rythmodan)	Ventricular arrhythmias especially if lignocaine fails.	Bolus 2 mg per kg 150 mg slowly. Infusion 400 μg/kg hr. Maximum of 300 mg hr.
Lignocaine (xylocard) Not in heart block and all degrees AV block	Ventricular arrhythmias resistant V.F. *1st choice*	100 mg bolus 4 mg/min infusion titrating downward (2 g in 500 ml 20 dpm titrating downwards).
Mexiletine (mexitil) Not in heart block	Ventricular arrhythmias resistant to lignocaine.	bolus 250 mg over 5–10 minutes. 250 mg/hour infusion for 1st hour, 125 mg/hour infusion for 2 hours. Then 500 mcg/minute.
Verapamil (cordilox) Not within 8 hours if on beta blocker Not in heart block	Supraventricular arrhythmias *1st choice*	5 mg IV bonus repeated after 5–10 minutes if necessary. Infusion 5–10 mg/hour. Maximum 100 mg/24 hour.
Propranolol Not within 30 minutes of IV verapamil and then with caution Not in bronchospasm	Supraventricular arrhythmias.	1 mg/min IV up to 10 mg
Isoprenaline (saventrine)	Heart Block severe bradycardia.	0.5–10 μg/minute (1000 μg in 500 ml fluid − > 0.5 μg/min = 5 dpm)

Respiratory problems

The breathless patient — diagnostic problems

The breathless patient may be unable to give a history, but if available the following pointers are helpful:

1 Onset

The mode of onset, sudden or gradual, will help differentiate between a precipitate event such as pulmonary embolus, pneumothorax, myocardial infarction (MI) with pulmonary oedema, or the more gradual exacerbation of chronic obstructive bronchitis or asthmatic attack. Acute asthmatic attacks often follow loss of control with episodes getting steadily worse.

2 Chest pain

May indicate MI, embolus or pneumothorax, or may follow trauma (see Table 3.1, page 32).

3 Medical history (MH)

A history of bronchitis, asthma, or angina may help, or a history of orthopnoea or paroxysmal nocturnal breathlessness leading up to the acute episode may give clues.

4 Drug history

This not only may give clues regarding medical history but is also vital when considering treatment.

There have been reports of severe bronchospasm, with some deaths, associated with beta blocker or non-steroidal anti-inflammatory drug (NSAID) treatment.

5 Sputum

Green infective as in bronchitis or pneumonia, clear as in cardiac failure, frothy and pink as in acute pulmonary oedema, or containing fresh haemoptysis as in pulmonary embolus (PE) neoplasms or tuberculosis.

6 Patterns of breathlessness

For example, on exertion, nocturnal, or precipitate with associated factors such as allergy, or diurnal variations as in asthma.

Exercise intolerance

Exercise intolerance is an indicator of severity, especially in asthma, so enquire about limitations of life-style.

These pointers, along with physical findings, should allow a working diagnosis to be made.

Important physical findings

Wheeze

If expiratory, indicative of airway obstruction; if inspiratory, indicative of stridor (upper airway obstructions).

Inspiratory crackles

    (i) Late as in pulmonary oedema or fibrosing alveolitis.
    (ii) Early and louder in pneumonia, bronchiectasis or chronic obstructive bronchitis.

Peripheral oedema

Indicative of right ventricular (RV) failure and often a pointer to CCF as a cause of breathlessness, but beware of chronic bronchitis with corpulmonale.

Raised jugulovenous pressure

Again indicative of RV failure. If found in the absence of crackles suspect pulmonary embolus, but check for tricuspid regurgitation or if intermittent heart block.

Cardiac enlargement

Indicative of cardiac failure.

Hyperinflated chest

Indicative of airway obstructions and emphysema.

Cyanosis

Hypoxia — a poor sign, especially if not controlled with the inspired O_2.

Peripheral perfusion

Decreased in CCF, often decreased in asthma — warm periphery and bounding pulses in respiratory failure associated with carbon dioxide retention. (Check inspired O_2.)

Respiratory failure

Definition

PaO_2 is less than 8 kPa (60 mm Hg) in a resting patient at sea level breathing air.

Type I respiratory failure — low PO_2 normal PCO_2

May occur in chronic bronchitis/emphysema/asthma/pneumonia/pulmonary oedema/pneumothorax/pulmonary chest injury/poisonings with respiratory depression.

Treatment

Administer a high concentration of O_2 and start treatment of underlying pathology. IPPR may be indicated in severe cases.

Type II respiratory failure

Definition: Low PO_2 and raised PCO_2 (>6 kPa 45 mm Hg).

May occur in chronic bronchitis/emphysema; severe asthma; severe respiratory depression, e.g. drug overdose; hypoventilation due to muscular disorder.

Treatment

Administer:

(a) Low concentration of O_2 (<28 per cent)
(b) Bronchodilators
(c) Respiratory stimulants (e.g. doxapram). Ventilation may be indicated but in chronic cases should be instituted with caution because of dependence on CO_2 drive and difficulty in withdrawal of ventilatory support later.

Danger signs

Hypoxia not corrected by $\uparrow$ FIO_2
Rising PCO_2
Acidosis
Diminished conscious level/confusion.

Treatment — general principles

- Sit the patient up.
- *Do not sedate.*
- *Avoid opiates* — unless you are *confident* that this is due to acute pulmonary oedema alone, in which case diamorphine 5–10 mg IV stat is indicated.
- *Oxygen via face mask.* Inspired O_2 concentration of 40–50 per cent unless you suspect respiratory failure with CO_2 retention. (When in doubt it is best to administer 28 per cent O_2 and establish the base line with urgent blood gas tests.)
- *Steroids.* Hydrocortisone 200 mg IV. Has synergistic action with Beta 2 stimulants. Prednisolone 40 mg orally has been shown to be as effective.
- *Bronchodilators.* Selective Beta 2 adrenoceptor stimulants (e.g. salbutamol) may be administered effectively via nebuliser: nebuliser solution 0.5 per cent 1 ml (5 mg) over 10 mins followed by 5 mgs 15–30 minutes after response. This often terminates acute bronchospasm quickly but is likely to have less beneficial effect in the chronic bronchitic.

Nebulised Ipratropium bromide has been advocated in acute

asthma for additional bronchodilator effect (0.5 mg (2 ml) with saline). (See Figure 3.4.) Aminophylline has a bronchodilator effect and also may be helpful in left ventricular failure (LVF) because of its mild positive inotropic effect. It should always be administered *very slowly* (250 mg over 5–15 minutes period) and with care, because it produces tachycardia which can be counter-productive.

- *Diuretics.* Frusemide 40–80 mg IV is indicated in cardiac failure.
- *Opiates.* Contraindicated in respiratory failure or any degree of asthma or bronchial obstruction. Beneficial in acute pulmonary oedema. Do not give if in any doubt. If respiratory failure results from opiates an IV line with naloxone (200 μg IV, repeated at 2–3-minute intervals).
- *Respiratory stimulants.* Indicated in some cases of acute respiratory failure associated with CO_2 retention with COAD in order to avoid ventilation where patients are unable to tolerate low-inspired-concentration (24 per cent) oxygen without becoming drowsy. Doxapram 0.5–4 mg IV continuous infusion per minute. Avoid in patients with status asthmaticus, CAD, thyrotoxicosis or severe hypertension.
- *Ventilation.* Always consider early in acute asthma if hypoxia persists despite O_2 therapy.
  Establish base line with urgent PO_2 and PCO_2.

Severe acute asthma

Asthma can and still does kill young adults. It should never be treated lightly.

The mortality rate from acute attacks of asthma has risen steadily, particularly in the younger age group. The acute severe attack often follows poor control for several weeks with attacks getting steadily worse. Monitoring with the peak flow meter can show a morning pattern with levels of 60 l/m rising to 200 l/m in the afternoon during this period. Bronchoconstriction with plugging of the bronchioles leads to severe hypoxaemia and consequent risk to the brain cells and myocardium.

The history may show the patient has had a preceding respiratory or viral infection, or exposure to allergens before the onset of the acute attack. Patients with persistent breathlessness, not relieved by high dose $\beta2$ bronchodilators, restlessness, exhaustion, tachy- or bradycardia and low-peak expiratory flow rate need urgent treatment with full resuscitation facilities available.

There is a marked diurnal variation in peak expiratory flow rate (PEFR) which is an adverse prognostic factor in asthma. Patients presenting at night need prompt treatment with inhaled and oral therapy to reduce the fall in lung function and mortality.

Management of acute severe asthma

The severity of an attack of acute severe asthma is often underestimated by patients, their relatives and their doctors. This is largely because of failure to make objective measurements. If not recognised and not treated appropriately such attacks can be fatal.

Aims of management

The aims of management are:
1 to prevent death
2 to restore the patient's clinical condition and lung function to best levels as soon as possible
3 to maintain optimal function and prevent early relapse.

Recognition and assessment of acute severe asthma

1. Potentially life-threatening features

The presence of any of the following indicates a severe attack:

    (a) increasing wheeze and breathlessness so that the patient is unable to complete sentences in one breath or get up from a chair or bed

    (b) respiratory rate $\geqslant$25 breaths/minute

    (c) heart rate persistently $\geqslant$110 beats/minute

    (d) PEAK EXPIRATORY FLOW (PEF)* <40% of predicted normal or of best obtainable if known (<200 l/minute where best obtainable value not known)

    (e) inspiratory fall in systolic blood pressure $\geqslant$10 mmHg

2. Imminently life-threatening features

The presence of any of the following indicates a very severe attack:

    (a) a silent chest on auscultation

    (b) cyanosis

    (c) bradycardia

    (d) exhaustion, confusion or unconsciousness.

3. Arterial blood gas markers of severity

Arterial blood gases should always be measured in patients with acute severe asthma admitted to hospital. The following are markers of a very severe (or life-threatening) attack:

    (a) A normal or high arterial carbon dioxide tension ($PaCO_2$) in a breathless asthmatic patient

    (b) Severe hypoxia: arterial oxygen tension (PaO_2) <8 kPa (60 mmHg) irrespective of oxygen therapy.

    (c) A low pH.

There are no other investigations that are needed for immediate management.

Note on assessment of severity

Patients with a SEVERE (i.e. life threatening) attack often do not have distressing symptoms and they do not necessarily have all of the abnormalities in signs and measurements outlined above, but the presence of any of these should alert the doctor.

Peak Expiratory Flow

Ideally the results of PEF measurements are most easily interpreted when expressed as a percentage of the predicted normal value or of the previous best obtainable value on optimal treatment. In patients in whom neither of these is known decisions have to be taken based on the absolute level recorded remembering that normal values vary with age, sex and height (older people, females and shorter people having a lower normal range). Values expressed as a percentage of the predicted normal are not useful in patients with chronically impaired lung function. Bearing in mind these qualifications, the guidelines express PEF as a percentage of predicted normal or of best. Absolute values are shown in parentheses to suggest the levels at which action should be taken in instances in which previous best values are not known.

Immediate management

Begin treatment at once with:

1. Oxygen

Use the highest concentration available and set a high flow. CO_2 retention is not aggravated by oxygen therapy in acute severe asthma; thus masks delivering 24% or 28% are not appropriate.

2. High dose inhaled β_2-agonist

Give inhaled β_2-agonist (e.g. salbutamol 2.5–5 mg, terbutaline 5–10 mg)

This may be nebulised with oxygen (hospital and ambulance), nebulised with an air compressor (general practice) or, if both are unavailable, the β_2-agonist may be given by multiple actuations of a metered dose inhaler into a large spacer device (2–5 mg, i.e. 20–50 puffs, 5 puffs at a time).

3. High dose systemic steroids

Give prednisolone 40–60 mg and/or intravenous hydrocortisone 200 mg immediately.

4. Intravenous bronchodilators

If obviously life-threatening features are present, give intravenous aminophylline (250 mg over 30 minutes) or β_2-agonist (e.g. salbutamol 200 micrograms or terbutaline 250 micrograms over 10 minutes). A β_2-agonist is preferred if the patient is already taking oral theophylline.

Criteria for emergency referral to hospital

1 Any life-threatening features.
2 Any features of a severe attack which persist after initial treatment.
3 PEF 15–30 minutes after nebulisation <40% of predicted or of best (<200 L/min).
4 A lower threshold for admission is appropriate in patients:
   (a) seen in the afternoon or evening rather than earlier in the day;
   (b) with recent onset of nocturnal or deteriorating symptoms;
   (c) with previous severe attacks — especially where the onset was rapid;
   (d) where there is concern over their assessment of severity of symptoms;
   (e) where there is concern over social circumstances and/or relatives' ability to respond appropriately.

Use of these guidelines will probably lead to more patients with attacks of asthma being admitted to hospital. Patients not admitted continue to need close supervision over following few days.

Subsequent management

1. Continuing treatment

   (a) Ensure that a nurse or doctor stays with the patient for at least 15 minutes and certainly until clear improvement is seen to occur.
   (b) Continue oxygen.
   (c) Continue high dose steroids: prednisolone orally 40–60 mg daily (or intravenous hydrocortisone 200 mg six hourly in patients who are very seriously ill or vomiting).
   (d) If improving, continue nebulised β2-agonist 4-hourly.
   (e) If no better or worse after 15–30 minutes, repeat nebulisation and add ipratropium bromide 0.5 mg to nebuliser solution.
   (f) If progress still unsatisfactory, consider aminophylline or parenteral β2-agonist.
       (i) Aminophylline infusion
            If weight is unknown, approximate doses depend on patient's size:

small	1000 mg/24 hours
medium	1250 mg/24 hours
large	1500 mg/24 hours
	(0.5–0.9 mg/kg/hour)

            No loading dose is required unless the patient's condition is deteriorating. Lower doses may be needed in patients with liver disease or heart failure and in patients taking cimetidine, ciprofloxacin or erythromycin. Higher doses are appropriate in smokers.

      (ii) Salbutamol or terbutaline infusion
12.5 micrograms/minute (3–20 micrograms/minute). The infusion rate should be adjusted according to PEF and heart rate responses.

2. *Further investigations in hospital*

    (a) Arrange chest radiograph, to reveal pneumothorax, consolidation or pulmonary oedema.

    (b) Arrange: measurement of plasma electrolytes and urea, a blood count and, in older patients, an ECG.

3. *Monitoring treatment*

    (a) Repeat PEF 15–30 mins after starting treatment and as required. Measure and record PEF before and after nebulised or inhaled β2-agonist (at least four times daily) throughout admission.

    (b) Repeat blood gases within 2 hours of starting treatment if

       (i) initial PaO2 < 8 kPa (60 mmHg) unless oxygen saturation measured subsequently is over 90%.

      (ii) initial PaCO2 was normal or raised.

     (iii) patient deteriorates

       ... and again if patient has not improved at 4–6 hours.

    (c) Measure and record heart rate.

    (d) Measure serum theophylline concentration if aminophylline is continued for more than 24 hours (aim for 10–20 micrograms/ml).

    (e) Measure serum potassium and blood glucose.

4. *Unhelpful treatment*

(a) Sedatives are absolutely contraindicated outside the intensive care unit.

(b) Antibiotics are not indicated unless there is evidence of a bacterial infection.

(c) Percussive physiotherapy is contraindicated.

Indications for intensive care

Patients with features of life-threatening asthma require intensive monitoring by experienced staff. Where there are no beds available on a properly staffed medical ward, this may only be available on an Intensive Care Unit (ICU). Patients with the following features always require intensive care:

1 hypoxia indicated by $PaO_2 < 8$ kPa (60 mmHg) despite 60% inspired O_2.

2 hypercapnia indicated by $PaCO_2 > 6$ kPa: (45 mmHg).

3 onset of exhaustion.

4 confusion or drowsiness.
5 unconsciousness.
6 respiratory arrest.

Indications for intermittent positive pressure ventilation (IPPV)

Not all patients admitted to the ICU need ventilating, but those with worsening hypoxia or hypercapnia, drowsiness or unconsciousness and those who have had a respiratory arrest require IPPV.

Emergency self-admission service

A list of patients with severe unstable asthma should be kept in the A & E Department; they should be given full facilities for ambulance and priority treatment.

All cases requiring treatment in A & E should be observed for some time after treatment has worked and only the mildest cases can be discharged from the department.

1. Features of acute severe attack present

Recognise, assess and manage the severe attack as outlined above and call medical registrar/SHO to admit the patient.

If the patient is unconscious or confused:

- call the anaesthetist at the same time and arrange admission to ICU.
- ensure uninterrupted high flow oxygen administration.
- do not attempt intubation until the most expert available doctor (ideally anaesthetist) is present.

2. No features of acute severe attack

If there are no clinical markers of a severe attack, measure PEF and proceed as below. N.B. if PEF <40% of predicted or of best, treat as severe.

- Give inhaled or nebulised $\beta2$-agonist (see above for doses).
- Thirty minutes after $\beta2$-agonist, repeat PEF measurement

Bronchitis

Chronic bronchitis is defined as a daily cough with sputum for at least 3 months of the year for more than 2 years, but the most significant factor is air flow obstruction.

An acute exacerbation of chronic bronchitis can present to A & E with acute shortness of breath and without a clear past medical history; the differential diagnosis is usually between acute LVF or bronchospasm. The symptoms and signs can often be remarkably similar, though in chronic

1. Features of acute severe attack present

Recognise, assess and manage the severe attack as outlined above and call medical registrar/SHO to admit the patient.

If the patient is unconscious or confused:

- call the anaesthetist at the same time and arrange admission to I.C.U.

- ensure uninterrupted high flow oxygen administration

- do not attempt intubation until the most expert available doctor (ideally anaesthetist) is present.

2. No features of acute severe attack

If there are no clinical markers of a severe attack, measure PEF and proceed as below. NB if PEF<40% of predicted or of best, treat as severe.

- Give inhaled or nebulised β2-agonist (see above for doses).

- Thirty minutes after β2-agonist, repeat PEF measurement.

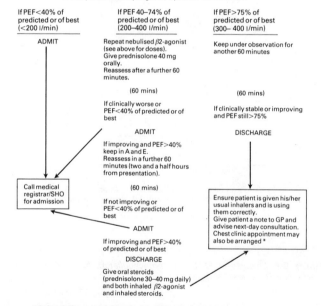

If PEF<40% of predicted or of best (<200 l/min)

ADMIT

If PEF 40–74% of predicted or of best (200–400 l/min)

Repeat nebulised β2-agonist (see above for doses). Give prednisolone 40 mg orally. Reassess after a further 60 minutes.

(60 mins)

If clinically worse or PEF<40% of predicted or of best

ADMIT

If improving and PEF>40% keep in A and E. Reassess in a further 60 minutes (two and a half hours from presentation).

(60 mins)

If not improving or PEF<40% of predicted or of best

ADMIT

If improving and PEF>40% of predicted or of best

DISCHARGE

Give oral steroids (prednisolone 30–40 mg daily) and both inhaled β2-agonist and inhaled steroids.

If PEF>75% of predicted or of best (300– 400 l/min)

Keep under observation for another 60 minutes

(60 mins)

If clinically stable or improving and PEF still>75%

DISCHARGE

Call medical registrar/SHO for admission

Ensure patient is given his/her usual inhalers and is using them correctly. Give patient a note to GP and advise next-day consultation. Chest clinic appointment may also be arranged *

* Before discharge determine why the patient attended A & E with asthma. Such patients usually need extra care in their follow-up. Ideally contact patient's GP's surgery by telephone as soon as possible during surgery hours.

Figure 3.3 *Guidelines for the management of asthma in adults. This statement by the British Thoracic Society, the Research Unit of the Royal College of Physicians of London, the Kings Fund Centre and the National Asthma Campaign has been used with permission.*

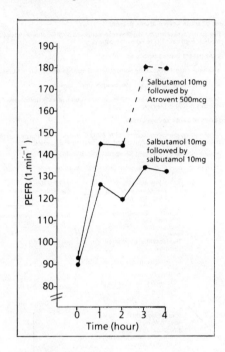

Changes in peak expiratory flow rate (mean ± SEM) after administration of nebulized salbutamol and ipratropium bromide. Response to the two nebulizations are indicated by ——— for salbutamol and ---- for ipratropium bromide.[1]

Figure 3.4 *Changes in PEFR with bronchodilators (M. J. Ward, J. T. Macfarlane, D. Davies, 1985)*

bronchitis the chest is often much looser with a productive cough, green or yellow sputum, and coarse early inspiratory crackles as well as wheeze.

    (a) pulmonary oedema — late inspiratory crackles
    (b) COB — early inspiratory crackles

There is generally a history of smoking. Depending on the degree of associated emphysema there may be a barrel chest with bullae and hyper-flated lungs visible on x-ray. Chest x-ray (CXR) may also show chronic changes of fibrosis, bronchiectasis and infective changes, but in some cases is entirely normal. The patient is more likely to exhibit signs of CO_2 retention, i.e. warm periphery, bounding pulses, drowsiness or confusion, as well as central cyanosis.

Treatment

- Sit the patient up
- Administer $O_2 < 28$ per cent via face mask and take blood gases
- Inhale $\beta2$ stimulants
- Aminophylline 250 mg very slowly IV (over 10–20 minutes)
- IV infusion N. saline plus aminophylline titrated against response
- Admit for intensive physiotherapy and antibiotics
- *Do not sedate*

N.B. Look for:

    (a) evidence of respiratory failure — physical signs/blood gases
    (b) CXR — look for evidence of LVF, infection or pneumothorax
    (c) Reversibility of airways obstruction (measure PEFR before and after bronchodilator); response to bronchodilators is likely to be poor in chronic bronchitis.

Ventilation should be avoided if possible because patients are difficult to wean off ventilator, especially if their bronchitis is of long standing with evidence of respiratory failure.

Other causes of acute breathlessness

Pulmonary embolus (PE)

History — travel; three months on pill; recent hospital admission.

    The symptoms are of pleuritic chest pain. Sudden onset is accompanied in severe cases with tachycardia and hypotension. The jugular venous pressure is increased with distension of the neck veins. Respiratory rate is increased; there may be cyanosis.

    The history is usually of a sudden onset of pain, but patients can present with collapse and breathlessness alone.

    Cyanosis may be noticeable only in a large PE and there may be no signs of a deep vein thrombosis.

    Haemoptysis is characteristic but often absent.

ECG

May be normal or show signs of RV strain — right axis deviation. RBBB, RV hypertrophy, sinus tachycardia, S1 with inverted T wave and Q wave in lead III is characteristic but may be normal, especially in patients of short stature. (See Figure 3.5.)

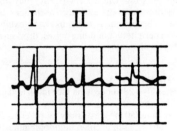

Figure 3.5 *ECG changes in PE*

CXR

May show linear or wedge-shaped shadows with peripheral emboli. The oligaemia of a massive PE is difficult to pick up and the CXR may look normal. A small basal effusion is common in late stage. (See Figure 3.6.)

Perfusion lung scan

Should be requested, following admission and anticoagulation, to confirm diagnosis. However, in co-existent lung disease this can be difficult to interpret, unless associated ventilation lung scan is available in a few days.

Treatment

– O_2 40–50 per cent
– Analgesia
– Admit for anticoagulation with heparin or thrombolysis

Pneumothorax

Spontaneous pneumothorax characteristically occurs in young adults — often males of slender build. The history is of sudden breathlessness with pleuritic chest pain which may be central or lateral. Physical signs are often subtle, hyperresonance, cyanosis and decreased air entry are found.

CXR — should be taken erect and if not clear a film taken in expiration will help demonstrate a small pneumothorax. The pneumothorax is easier to see if the film is placed on its side. (See Figure 3.7.)

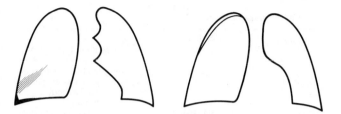

Figure 3.6 *Pulmonary embolus. Triangular infarcted segment: small effusion often seen*

Figure 3.7 *Shallow right apical pneumothorax*

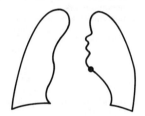

Figure 3.8 *Inhaled foreign body,* ● = *FB*

Treatment

O₂ via face mask.

Intercostal drainage and underwater seal if greater than 1/3 of lung volume, or if respiratory function impaired. (N.B. — very much smaller pneumothoraces will need drainage in patients with chronic chest disease.)

Inhaled foreign body

If an inhaled foreign body is suspected an x-ray in expiration should be done. This will show a hyperinflated area of lung: these cases should be referred to the ENT or thoracic surgeons. (See Figure 3.8.)

TABLE 3.9

Causes of shortness of breath

Airway obstruction	— Asthma	
	— Bronchitis	— acute ⎱ bronchial
		— chronic ⎰ obstruction
	— Stridor	— glottal obstruction, eg:
		— infection (epiglottitis)
		— foreign body
		— tumour
Alveolar	— Pleural	— consolidation, collapse
	— congestive cardiac failure — congestion	
	effusion(s)	
Restrictive	— Pulmonary fibrosis —	
	Abnormalities of chest wall; thoracic	
	spine; painful chest injuries.	
	— emphysema — hyperinflation, bullae,	
	pneumothorax	
	— pneumothorax — traumatic ⎱ collapse	
	— spontaneous ⎰ of lung tissue	
Vascular	a) pulmonary oedema — LV failure	
	aspiration ⎱ toxic materials	
	inhalation ⎰ vomit	
	Septicaemia	
	ARDS	
	drugs	
	b) pulmonary embolus (massive) — alveolar	
	hypoperfusion	
Haematological	— acute — including acute hypovolaemic	
	anaemia shock — gastrointestinal bleed	
Metabolic	— chronic — acidosis ('air hunger')	
	eg: diabetic keto-acidosis	
	salicylate poisoning	
	chronic renal failure	
Neurological		
Cerebral	— Raised intra-cranial pressure	
	— trauma	
	— tumour	
	— infective	
	— haemorrhage	
	— Infarction — Stroke	
	Guillain Barré	
	Myasthenia gravis	
	Poliomyelitis	
Psychogenic	— Voluntary alveolar hyperventilation due	
	to anxiety or pain. This is often	
	accompanied by tingling of fingers or	
	mouth as frank tetany (due to fall in	
	CO_2 leading to alkalosis).	

4

Atopic diseases, allergies and anaphylaxis

Atopy includes allergic rhinitis, asthma, urticaria, eczema and vernal conjunctivitis. These disorders are all associated with reaginic (IgE) antibody in the serum. There are pathophysiological causes which are IgE-independent and may stimulate mast cells directly or act through complement.

Anaphylaxis results from antigen-induced, IgE mediated release of chemical mediators that act on smooth muscle and vascular permeability in a previously sensitised patient. Anaphylactic reactions are uncommon but the speed of onset is important and the outcome fatal if no action is taken. Anaphylaxis does not occur with increased frequency in atopic individuals but may be more severe and bronchospasm occurs often. Two common examples of this type of hypersensitivity reaction are anaphylaxis due to stinging insects and drugs.

Anaphylactoid (non-IgE mediated) reactions are treated the same way but the cause of mediator release is different.

Examples:
- (a) reactions to iodinated contrast material (alternative complement pathway)
- (b) reactions to aspirin and other non-steroidal anti-inflammatories (alteration in prostaglandin synthesis).

Urticaria and angioedema

Urticaria appears as pruritic, circumscribed and elevated erythematous areas of cutaneous oedema (hives). When the oedema extends further into the dermis and extensive erythematous areas with diffuse borders arise, this is known as angioedema. Angioedema most commonly affects the face or portion of an extremity. Individual lesions may appear abruptly but they are seldom pruritic and usually persist less than 24 hours. Cutaneous lesions lasting more than 4–6 weeks are termed chronic.

Hypersensitivity reactions

1 Idiopathic

80–90 per cent of chronic urticaria-angioedema. Physical and emotional factors have been claimed as causes but this is by no means certain.

2 IgE-dependent

  (a) in atopic individuals a history of urticaria-angioedema is often elicited but the atopy is rarely the cause of the cutaneous lesions.

  (b) specific antigens include food (eggs, seafood, nuts, beans, chocolate), pollens and hymenoptera (honey bees, wasps, hornets and ants) venoms.

  (c) Physical urticaria occurs after a variety of stimuli: dermographism occurs in 2–5 per cent of the normal population; pressure urticaria develops under shoulder straps and belts; cold-induced urticaria/cold allergy—cutaneous lesions develop after exposure to cold; chilblains, syncope, hypotension and wheezing occur when swimming in cold water but are easily reversible on gentle rewarming; light urticaria; cholinergic urticaria — developing after warm bath, exercise or episode of pyrexia; and contact urticaria — for example with stinging nettles.

3 Complement — mediated

This includes hereditary angioedema and serum sickness. Hereditary angioedema is autosomal dominant and inherited. It is characterised by functional absence of C1 esterase inhibitor with recurrent oedema of skin, upper respiratory and gastrointestinal tract. *Swelling of the upper respiratory tract may involve the larynx with danger of asphyxiation. Prompt action is necessary. Patients should always carry an emergency kit containing sub-cutaneous adrenalin injection.*

4 Direct mast-cell-releasing agent

Opiates, curare and radio contrast media may precipitate urticaria-angioedema or even anaphylaxis.

5 Agents that alter arachidonic acid metabolism

Aspirin intolerance may account for 20–50 per cent of patients with chronic urticaria. Patients with asthma, particularly those with nasal polyps, in the middle decades of life, are at increased risk. Patients are also intolerant of other non-steroidal anti-inflammatories and azo-dyes notably tartrazine. The reaction may vary from urticaria, angioedema to bronchospasm, hypotension and even death.

Treatment

The best treatment of urticaria-angioedema is avoidance. Recurrent episodes are treated by prophylactic antihistamines (Anti-H agents). Glucocorticoids play no role in long-term management. The treatment of hereditary angioedema can be divided into acute episode (see anaphylaxis) pre-operative prophylaxis and long-term prevention of spontaneous attack. Determine the cause of urticaria-angioedema sensitisation by skin testing. In some cases desensitising vaccines are used. However they should be administered only by an experienced practitioner who has full cardio-respiratory resuscitation facilities close at hand in case of anaphylaxis. After administration of vaccines, the patient should be kept under observation for at least 2 hours.

Anaphylaxis

Systematic anaphylaxis is an immediate hypersensitivity reaction. The release of mediator, either through IgE or not (anaphylactoid), results in an action on smooth muscle and vascular permeability. Antigens that cause anaphylaxis are generally large polypeptides or proteins (venoms, pollens, foods, horse and rabbit serum) although small molecules capable of combining as haptens (e.g. penicillin) may also be responsible. Clinical findings in anaphylaxis range from urticaria, pruritus, flushing angioedema to bronchospasm, laryngeal oedema, hypotension, arrhythmia and death. The severe hypoxia and hypotension may lead to secondary changes e.g. myocardial or cerebral infarction. There is no universal pattern. However, individuals tend to repeat their own characteristic response. The most common manifestations are cutaneous. Rarely other symptoms are associated with anaphylaxis and include gastrointestinal (vomiting, nausea and diarrhoea) and CNS symptoms. Reactions usually begin within seconds or minutes of exposure to antigen. Death may be due to asphyxiation following laryngeal oedema or severe bronchospasm, or circulatory failure secondary to dilation of the splanchnic vascular bed.

Treatment

Establish an airway and maintain breathing. Intubation or even trache-ostomy may be needed in severe glottic oedema.
- *Hypoxaemia: administer high percentage oxygen.*
- *Hypovolaemia: rapid intravenous normal saline and colloid — a CVP line may be necessary.*
- *Intramuscular injection of 0.5–1.0 ml of 1:1000 solution of adrenalin.*
- *Bronchospasm may be improved with inhaled salbutamol from a nebuliser or IV aminophyllin (check that asthmatics are not on theophylline).*

Intravenous glucocorticoids exert effect hours after administration: action is uncertain — 200 mg of IV hydrocortisone are usually given. Intravenous antihistamines (10 mg IV chlorpheniramine) are of use but only in less severe cases, as in anaphylactic urticaria. ITU care and inotropic support with dopamine may be necessary in more severe cases.

Anaphylaxis due to stinging insects

These reactions are caused by allergic sensitisation, not toxic chemicals in the venoms. Repeated injections of venom as in bee-keepers or venom immunotherapy (desensitising vaccines) alters serum antibody from IgE to IgG and renders immunity. Loss of immunity may occur in bee-keepers taking a non-steroidal anti-inflammatory drug.

Allergic reaction to insect stings may be systemic or local. Systemic symptoms have a rapid onset, within 2–3 minutes, with classic manifestations of anaphylaxis. Local reactions are slow in onset and occur with or without concomitant early systemic reaction. The area of induration increases in size over 24–48 hours and resolves over several days. Red streaks resembling lymphangitis may be observed. *Treatment of local reactions:* immobilisation, elevation, analgesia, removal of barbed stingers which remain in the skin after the sting and anti-Hi agents. The treatment of anaphylaxis has been described. Non-immunised patients with histories of systemic reactions to stings, with a positive skin test, should keep emergency self-treatment kits with tourniquets and subcutaneous adrenalin. (Ready loaded adrenalin syringe: Mini-Jet with 0.5 ml of a 1:1000 solution.) The danger periods are April–September for bees and June–October for wasps.

Reactions to drugs

Type A
Reactions are due to overdose or undue sensitivity of the patient to the drug's action resulting in excessive pharmacological action of drug e.g. undue respiratory depression produced by morphine.

Type B
Reactions are unrelated to the drug's pharmacological action and are usually unpredictable. Drug allergies are included in this group. The most important are IgE mediated anaphylactic reactions. Penicillin and other B-lactum antibiotics (cephalosporin) are responsible for more of these than any other drug.

Always ask the patient whether he is sensitive to the drug about to be given. If the patient has a history of sensitivity then another drug should be chosen remembering that cross-reactivity between certain groups of drugs exist (e.g. cephalosporin and penicillins). Family history even of a twin with sensitisation is irrelevant. Rapid desensitisation under medical supervision with resuscitation facilities may be attempted if there is an absolute need to give that particular drug. Refer.

Anaphylactic reactions: treatment as above.

Hay fever

An allergic disorder with bouts of sneezing, profuse watery nasal discharge, irritation and watering of the eyes. It is due to sensitivity to grass and tree pollen and occurs between April and August.

Treatment of hay fever has improved since the introduction of anti-Hi agents which are free of sedative and anti-cholinergic effects. Terfenadine is a popular drug with a rapid onset and offset of action. If may be used prophylactically 60 mg twice daily. Ceterizine 10 mg daily also has a low potential for drowiness.

Astemizole has a slow onset and long action and the dose is 10 mg *once daily*. The CSM is aware of cases of ventricular tachycardia following astemizole overdose and would like to receive any other reports of cardiotoxicity. Monitor ECG in cases of suspected astemizole overdose so that appropriate anti-arrhythmic treatment can be given if necessary.

The main effect of H antagonist is on the sneezing, rhinorrhoea and conjunctivitis with little impact on nasal obstruction. Additional use of nasally inhaled steroids (beclomethasone dipropionate or sodium cromoglycate) may be valuable.

Immunotherapy with specific and purified allergen extracts is widely advocated but must be given in controlled conditions where ability and equipment to treat anaphylactic reactions exist.

NOTES

5

The acute abdomen

Diagnosis of acute abdominal conditions rests almost entirely on clinical and radiological features. Haematological and biochemical tests are helpful, but rarely diagnostic. Usually the diagnosis can be made on history alone. The important facts that must be ascertained are detailed below. If you are in any doubt about the nature of severe abdominal pain it is safest to ask for advice. Assume that any patient with an acute abdomen is a candidate for surgery and therefore keep him or her starved.

Analgesia is not a treatment for abdominal pain: it should not normally be given until a diagnosis and a plan of treatment has been made.

History

1 Pain

(a) Nature

What sort of pain is it? Is it sharp and stabbing or a dull ache? Is it constantly present or colicky? Is it getting worse?

(b) Period

How long has the pain been present? Is it recurrent?

(c) Site

What is the present site of pain? Has this changed? Does it radiate anywhere else?

(d) Associated features

Does the pain make the patient feel nauseated or faint, or does it induce vomiting?

(e) Aggravating or relieving factors

What, if anything, makes the pain worse, or less severe. Does posture make any difference? Does diet influence or even precipitate the pain? Is there any association with bowel action, micturition or menstruation (see below)? Do any drugs make a difference?

2 Vomiting

(a) Nature of vomit

Is it food? If so, is it recent or old? Is it altered? Is it bile stained or pure bile? Is it foul or faecal? Is there any blood present? Is this fresh or altered? Altered blood is usually described as 'coffee grounds', but this can often be confused with faecal vomiting.

(b) Associated factors

Is vomiting associated with pain, or drugs or with bowel action?

3 Bowel actions

(a) Normal bowel habit

The variation in 'normal' is extremely wide. Determine the patient's normal habit.

(b) Recent changes

Is the patient constipated? Define this in terms of frequency of bowel action and in nature of stool. If there is a history of diarrhoea, determine the colour and consistency. (Exclude melaena or steatorrhoea). Is there any blood passed with the stools? Is it fresh bright red blood or dark old blood? Is it mixed in with the motions or just on the surface? Is there any associated mucus?

4 Genito-urinary

Does the patient compain of dysuria? Is this a true burning at the urethral orifice or is it abdominal or loin pain precipitated by micturition? Is there any haematuria? Is this old or fresh, at the beginning or end of micturition or throughout the stream? Do not forget that pneumaturia is a symptom of vesico-colic fistula. Always take a full gynaecological history. Ask about menstrual periods, vaginal bleeding and vaginal discharge.

5 General

Has the patient had a fever, rigors or been sweating? What drugs has he or she been taking? Is there any relevant family history. Has he or she had any recent illness or been abroad? Is there any relevant past medical history, e.g. inflammatory bowel disease or previous surgery.

Examination

As in all clinical examination, examination of the abdomen must follow a pattern. Do not forget other areas, however, such as the hands, chest and lymph nodes.

1 Observations

Check pulse, blood pressure and temperature (if there is any doubt about the validity of the temperature reading, repeat it, leaving the thermometer in or replacing it until it has stopped rising).

2 Inspection

(a) General Note Distress, anaemia or pallor, jaundice or cyanosis. Does the patient have a foetor?

(b) Abdomen Look at the whole abdomen (including below the inguinal

ligament) and the scrotum. Note any scars, other skin changes or obvious masses. Is the abdomen distended? Is there visible peristalsis? Most importantly in the acute abdomen — is the patient relaxed and breathing with abdominal muscles or holding the whole abdomen tense and rigid?

3 Palpation

(a) Gentle Feel for areas of tenderness or large masses and examine the hernial orifices and scrotum.

(b) Deep Attempt to palpate organs and ascertain the presence of guarding. Rebound tenderness can be ascertained both by pressing in and letting go or, more elegantly and more kindly, by gentle percussion.

4 Percussion

This defines areas of dullness or hyper-resonance.

5 Auscultation

(a) Bowel Sounds Note whether these are normal or absent. They may be increased in the presence of acute obstruction. Bowel sounds are described as 'tinkling' in distended obstructed bowel.

(b) Other Sounds Bruits may be audible.

6 Rectal examination

(a) External Note the nature of the perianal skin. Are there any external fistulae? Is there an abscess or a perianal haematoma? Are there external or thrombosed piles?

(b) Internal Is there any tenderness? Is this superficial, causing sphincter spasm, or deep? Are there any palpable masses either in the rectal wall or palpable through the wall. Remember to feel the cervix in women and the prostate gland in men. What does the rectal mucosa feel like?

(c) Faeces Is the rectum full or empty? If stool is present, is it normal? Is there melaena or steatorrhoea? If there is any blood, is it fresh or altered? Is there any mucus?

7 Vaginal examination

Is this necessary? If so, see page 127.

Acute appendicitis

History

The pain is usually steady. It begins centrally and shifts to the right iliac fossa after a few hours. The patient is usually anorexic and may be nauseated or vomiting. There may also be increased abdominal pain on micturition.

Examination

The patient is usually flushed with a mild pyrexia (often approximately 37.5°C) and a tachycardia. There may be foetor. There is tenderness in the right iliac fossa with localised guarding and rebound tenderness. A mass in this area is a sign of an appendix mass or abscess. Rectal examination may reveal tenderness to the right.

Differential diagnosis

Urinary tract infection, tubal pregnancy, salpingitis, torsion or ruptured ovarian cyst, mesenteric adenitis, Crohns Disease.

Investigation

Full blood count may show leucocytosis.
Mid stream urine (MSU) microscopy showing micro organisms suggests UTI. Red and white cells may also be found in appendicitis with bladder involvement.
X-rays Unhelpful.
Treatment Refer to surgical team.

Cholecystitis

History

Constant right upper quadrant pain which may be associated with vomiting. There may be right shoulder tip pain.

Examination

Pyrexia, tachycardia, occasionally mild jaundice.

Abdomen

Tender RUQ with localised guarding and rebound tenderness. Occasionally there is a palpable mass. Look for the two signs:
Murphy's sign — halt in deep inspiration with deep palpation in RUQ.
Boas' sign — hyperaesthesia over the tip of the right scapula (rarely present). PR is usually normal.

Differential diagnosis

Acute peptic ulcer, acute pancreatitis, high retrocaecal appendix, right lower lobe pneumonia.

Investigations

FBC leucocytosis may be present.
Plain abdominal X-ray — 10% gall stones visible.
Abdominal ultrasound — investigation of choice, but rarely available in casualty.

Treatment

For severe pain and vomiting — analgesia (if no doubt) and IV fluids.
For mild pain — clear fluids only (check with surgical team).

Cholelithiasis

History

Colicky upper abdominal pain. Associated with diet — usually fatty foods.

Examination

Pyrexia is rare. Tachycardia is associated with pain.

Abdomen

Tender RUQ with occasional voluntary guarding. No rebound tenderness. No Murphy's or Boas' sign.

Investigations

As for cholecystitis.

Ureteric (renal) colic

History

Severe dull pain extending from loin to groin and possibly radiating to the scrotum. The site of pain may shift.

Examination

The patient may be writhing or curled up in pain. There may be a tachycardia.

Abdomen

Tender in renal angle with a soft abdomen and no guarding.

Investigation

Urine testing — The presence of red cells is consistent with the diagnosis.
Plain X-ray — 90% of calculi are radio-opaque but often difficult to see.
IVP is investigation of choice, if facilities allow.
MSU — microscopy to exclude infection.

Differential diagnosis

Pyelonephritis — exquisitely tender area in renal angle. Pyrexia, infected urine.

Treatment

Analgesia. Surgical or urological referral.

Acute peptic ulcer

History

Duodenal ulcer

Pain is classically worse between meals, eased by antacids and eating. Pain may come on between 2 and 3am — eased by milk. This may result in weight increase.

Gastric ulcer

Pain may be made worse by food and may be eased by vomiting. In the long term this results in weight loss.

Gastritis

Usually precipitated by event such as eating curry or a heavy drinking session. It may be associated with vomiting.

Examination

Impossible to separate clinically. Tenderness in epigastrium with or without guarding. Occasionally there may be rebound tenderness if there is an acute anterior ulcer.

Differential diagnosis

Cholecystitis, perforated ulcer, pancreatitis.

Investigation

FBC — little help.
Amylase — excludes pancreatitis.
X-rays — if pain is extremely severe, plain abdominal films or CXR will help to exclude perforation.
Barium meal or gastroscopy if available, investigation of choice.

Treatment

Acute ulcer — Bedrest, antacids, stop smoking. It is better to delay H2 blockers or Omeprozole until a firm diagnosis has been made. It is therefore worth referral to a gastroenterologist or surgeon.
Gastritis — antacids, reassurance.

Acute pancreatitis

History

Severe pain. May begin in epigastrium, spreading to the whole abdomen, and radiating through to back. Pain may be associated with vomiting. Determine history of alcohol intake.

Examination

May be pale and sweaty and possibly mildly icteric.

Abdomen

Mild tender in epigastrium.
Severe rigid abdomen and generalised guarding. Bowel sounds may be absent.
Grey-Turner's sign — discoloration in flanks.
Cullen's sign — discoloration around umbilicus.
Epigastric mass suggests pseudocyst formation.

Investigation

FBC occasional leycocytosis.
Amylase usually, but not invariably raised.
X-rays plain abdominal X-rays exclude peptic perforation and may show a 'sentinel loop' of small bowel around the pancreas.
Calcium may be low in severe cases.
Glucose may be elevated.
Blood gasses $\downarrow$ $_pO_2$ $\uparrow$ $_pCO_2$ in severe cases.
Ultrasound if available, this may demonstrate gallstones, a swollen pancreas or complications of pancreatitis (pseudocyst or abscess).

Differential diagnosis

Mild cholecystitis, peptic ulcer, acute gastritis.
Severe myocardial infarction, perforated peptic ulcer, peritonitis, ruptured aortic aneurysm, mesenteric artery thrombosis, ruptured ectopic pregnancy in young females.

Treatment

Intravenous fluids, NG tube, Surgical referral.

Perforated ulcer

History

Sudden onset of severe abdominal pain. There is often no predisposing pain, although there may be a history of peptic ulceration.

Examination

Pale and sweaty. May be hypotensive with tachycardia.

Abdomen

Rigid and usually silent (although bowel sounds do not exclude a perforation).

Investigation

X-rays — free gas seen on erect films — best on erect chest X-ray.

Differential diagnosis

See pancreatitis (*Amylase* — usually normal).

Treatment

Intravenous fluids, NG tube, (analgesia), surgical referral.

Acute diverticular disease

History

Slow onset LIF pain. May be associated with change in bowel habit.

Examination

Pyrexial, tachycardia.

Abdomen

'Left sided appendicitis'. Tender with guarding and rebound tenderness in LIF. Occasional mass. pR tenderness to left, with mass sometimes palpable.

Investigation

FBC — leucocytosis
X-rays — usually unhelpful, but small bowel 'sentinel loops' may be seen.

Treatment

Depending on severity, IV or oral fluids. Surgical referral.

Acute bowel obstruction

History

Nausea and vomiting, abdominal distension. There may be colicky pain. Complete constipation and lack of flatus suggests large bowel obstruction.

Examination

Distress, dehydration or tachycardia may be present.

Abdomen

Distended and tympanic with occasional visible peristalsis. Bowel sounds may be increased, high pitched or tinkling. NB check for strangulated herniae. pR empty rectum is indicative of large bowel obstruction.

Investigation

FBC — high haemoglobin and PCV suggests dehydration. Leucocytosis associated with infection or compromised bowel.
Biochemistry — high urea from dehydration.
X-rays (CXR, erect and supine abdominal views) will show dilated small or large bowel.

Treatment

IV infusion, NG tube if vomiting. Refer to surgical team.

Peritonitis

History

Any of the above conditions may predispose. Thus it may be purulent, faecal or ischaemic in origin.

Examination

Severe pain, tachycardia, and usually pyrexia. May be dehydrated or shocked.

Abdomen

Generalised tenderness with guarding and rebound. Absent bowel sounds. pR general tenderness.

Investigation

FBC — leucocytosis.
Amylase — may be raised in bowel ischaemia and necrosis as well as pancreatitis.
X-rays — free gas, dilated bowel, sentinel loops, etc. may give a clue to cause.
Urea and electrolytes — show state of hydration.

Differential diagnosis

See pancreatitis.

Treatment

IV infusion. Immediate surgical referral.

Ruptured aortic aneurysm

History

Although the presentation may be one of increasing back pain, it may also be one of generalised abdominal pain of sudden onset.

Examination

Pale and sweaty. Tachycardia and low blood pressure.

Abdomen

Occasional bruising in flanks. Pulsating mass is sometimes palpable. Occasional shifting dullness from free blood.

Investigation

X-rays $-\frac{}{\bullet}$ if any doubt, calcified aneurysm sac may be seen. If the patient is stable, *ultrasound* may determine the size of the aneurysm.
As for pancreatitis/peritonitis if there is real doubt.

Treatment

Intravenous infusion with a wide bore cannula. Cross match blood. Urgent surgical referral. If the patient is severely shocked, a 'G Suit' (pneumatic compression suit), if available in the department, may be lifesaving.

Ruptured ectopic pregnancy

History

Sudden onset abdominal pain and a lack of periods. Pregnancy may have already been confirmed. See page 130.

Examination

Shocked — pale and sweaty; tachycardia and low blood pressure.

Abdomen

General tenderness and rebound.

Investigation

Pregnancy test, if in doubt.

Treatment

Intravenous infusion with a widebore cannula. Cross match blood. Urgent gynaecological or surgical referral.

Torsion of testis

History

Testicular pain in any male (especially under the age of 21) without a history of dysuria, haematuria or trauma.

Examination

Pyrexia in late torsion or infection. Tender over testis and cord. pR tender in prostatitis.

Investigation

Mid stream urine culture.

Differential diagnosis

Epididymo-orchitis. Torsion of Hydatid of Morgagni (embryological remnant).

Treatment

First Aid — twisting medially may help, but surgical referral is essential in young age group. In all cases, however it is *TORSION UNTIL PROVEN OTHERWISE*.

Gastro-intestinal bleeding

Haematemasis Bright red, fresh blood; 'coffee grounds' altered blood.
Melaena Black, tarry, bulky, offensive stool.

History

Occasional known peptic ulcer/liver disease. Ask specifically about drugs — steroids, NSAIDs — and alcohol.

Examination

Tachycardia (beware disguising effects of β blockers), hypotension, jaundice, spider naevi, etc.

Abdomen

Epigastric tenderness may signify peptic ulcer.
LIF tenderness and fresh malaena may signify diverticular bleeding.

Investigation

Endoscopy Investigation of choice.
FBC (baseline investigation. NB The Hb value DOES NOT bear any relation to the amount of blood lost acutely).
Plain Abdominal X-Rays No value.

Differential diagnosis

Iron therapy (green tinge to stool after PR examination).

Treatment

Intravenous infusion with a wide bore cannula. Cross match blood. Urgent medical or surgical referral, depending on hospital protocol.

Functional abdominal pain

Functional abdominal pain can be just as severe and disabling as organic pain and may cause a major disturbance in the life of the patient. In about 5 per cent of patients with functional abdominal pain, their symptoms are refractory to all standard therapy. It is a characteristic of the disease that any new treatment, and especially an operation, produces benefit *for a time*. This is particularly true in the child with recurrent abdominal pain. The single most important aspect of management is to recognise these patients early and to resist the temptation to undertake extensive and repeated investigations.

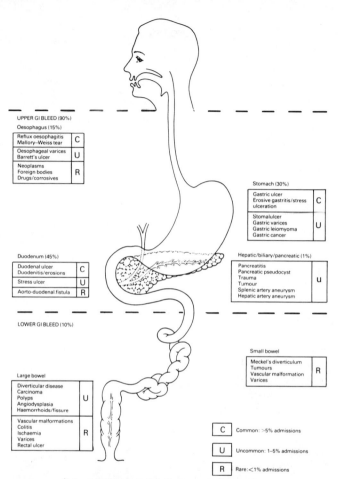

Figure 5.1 *Causes of acute blood loss from the gastrointestinal tract.*

Haematemesis — bright red, fresh blood – 'coffee grounds' altered blood
Malaena — black, tarry, bulky, offensive stool
History — Occasional known peptic ulcer/liver disease. Drugs — steroids, NSAIDs
Examination — Tachycardia (beware disguising effects of β blockers)
Hypotension
Jaundice, spider naevi etc.
Abdomen — Occasional epigastric tenderness – peptic ulcer. LIF tenderness — diverticular disease. Ascites — liver disease. PR — malaena
Differential diagnosis — Iron stool (green tinge). Swallowed epistaxis
Treatment — Crossmatch blood, wide bore IV cannula + fluid. Urgent medical/surgical referral.

NOTES

6

Psychiatric illness

Psychiatric Illness

There is a wide range of behaviour within the limits of normality, and this range can often be affected by illness, trauma, alcohol, and other drugs. The return to the community on medication of many patients who previously had lived in mental hospitals now presents further problems in A & E. Many are unable to fend for themselves, they lose touch with their doctors and medication and join the homeless, rootless, inadequate, and chronic alcoholics so that all degrees of mental illness will be seen in A & E Departments. They will attend both for primary medical care and psychiatric treatment. Under the Mental Health Act 1983 A & E is a public place. Some hospitals, with a psychiatrist on the staff, are recognised as a place of safety, so will be used by the police using Section 136 of the Act.

For many patients there is little one can do, but it is important that, difficult though it may be, they receive full medical care and attention so that the complications of illness and trauma are not missed.

Remember when taking the history that you list the symptoms and complaints in the patient's terms and describe his feelings and sensations — sad, confused, exhausted — rather than depression, which is a diagnosis. When the examination is complete you should use the description of the mental state in medical terms. The Casualty Officer's principal task is to detect the illness, define the symptoms and signs of illness and assess the risks of possible self-harm or suicide.

The common conditions seen in A & E are depression, anxiety, self-harm, psychotic illness such as acute and chronic schizophrenia, violence and alcoholism.

Depression

There are several sets of symptoms:

- Depressed feelings of hopelessness, helplessness, pessimism, gloom, irritability, and low mood.
- Physiological or biological symptoms of anorexia, constipation, weight loss, insomnia, early morning wakening.
- Symptoms of anxiety, feeling nervous or anxious, panic attacks with hyperventilation, sweating, and tachycardia.

- Miscellaneous symptoms, obsessional ruminations — thoughts going round and round in their heads, hypochondriacal symptoms such as abdominal pain and headaches, etc.
- Abnormal ideas and delusions which are false but completely believed in, such as 'my bowels are rotting' and ideas which are often depressed or guilty in content.
- Thoughts of, plans for, or attempts at, suicide.

On examination

Patients may be dishevelled, self neglected, and thin. They may appear sad, gloomy, anxious, distressed or tearful. Their speech may be slow (retarded), or fast (pressure). They may have little to say — poverty of expression — they describe depressive ideas or delusions. Often they do not realise they are ill.

Treatment

Psychotic symptoms such as delusions and auditory hallucinations merit discussion with a psychiatrist. Suicidal thoughts need assessment as below. Severe low mood or anxiety may need medication and urgent appointment in the OPD. Less disturbed patients with good support, such as a caring spouse, could be referred to their GP.

Acute anxiety and reactions

The patient, his friends, family, or doctor may have noticed changes in his thinking or feeling which are causing difficulties. It is possible by talking, but particularly by listening, to the patient without rush to find the root cause of many of these problems. The following examples should illustrate this:

A A man is feeling anxious and sleeping poorly one week after losing his job. The offer of a job would quickly resolve his symptoms.

B A woman feeling anxious and sleeping poorly after losing her job one week ago, but she describes other symptoms which have been present six months, such as constipation, early morning wakening and suicidal feelings. In fact she lost her job because she was irritable and couldn't concentrate at work. She seems quite unwell and a job won't help. As she hadn't realised it had been going on so long she blamed her illness on losing her job. At this stage she needs admission and medication.

C The third person lost his job today and is shaking, shouting and upset. When he is a bit calmer he tells you his marriage is in trouble, his daughter smokes cannabis, and he is in debt. You can easily see why he is overwhelmed. He comes to A & E because his wife threw him out and he is homeless. The social worker rings his sister who takes him home, so that his symptoms last only a few hours.

These three patients all used similar words to describe their feelings, but by asking more questions their problems became clearer and the solutions emerged.

A   A normal reaction to a temporary or permanent loss. Listening is therapeutic.

B   An illness causing multiple symptoms and signs and affecting the second patient's daily life required more positive treatment with medication.

C   Decompensation occurred after a further crisis on a background of many problems; the straw that broke the camel's back. Calming him down, then advising on the problem on hand is crisis intervention.

D   In some cases the normal reactions to the crisis could go on and become an illness. In other words the normal reaction to the feelings caused by events become bigger problems in time.

Having identified the problem, several agencies are available to assist in therapy. The family, voluntary organisations, social services, GP or psychiatric services can all be involved, depending on the severity of the illness. It is important to appreciate that a patient, like the depressed woman, has several problems, maybe both an illness and loss of job, so therefore needs several kinds of help. A quick response with sympathy and action at the time of crisis is necessary, be it of reassurance, referral or intervention. It is not unusual to make a psychiatric diagnosis and not refer to a psychiatrist. For example, if you decide chest pain results from muscle tension secondary to an anxiety which causes a panic attack, reassurance is often enough. Although this is often a symptom of early depressive illness further review by the GP might be advisable.

Overdose/deliberate self-harm

The vast majority of overdose, self-harm cases seen in A & E are not true suicide attempts. They may be termed 'cries for help', 'para suicide', 'attention seekers', or any number of other misnomers. Unfortunately, however, the likelihood of success is not directly related to the seriousness of the attempt. Many 'cries for help' actually succeed where others fail. Also there is a high incidence of recurrent attempts following an unsuccessful suicide gesture and the more often the attempt is repeated the more likely the patient is to succeed eventually.

Important factors in the history

- Precipitating events
- Social and family history

- History of depression
- Past psychiatric illness
- Medications, especially antidepressants
- Sedatives
- Past medical history and recent physical illness

All these factors may be important in planning treatment and follow-up, both medically and socially.

The following are essential in assessing current suicidal risk.

- Situation and timing of the event, mode of discovery, attempts to conceal
- Age of patient
- Intent of patient
- Feelings after the event and future intentions
- Depression, feelings of hopelessness, etc.
- How does the patient see the future?

A formal assessment of psychiatric and mental state is not really possible in the acute A & E situation, but it should be borne in mind that suicide attempts in a patient who appears to be psychotic are very serious indeed and urgent psychiatric help should be sought. Nowadays with pressure on beds in some hospitals patients are not always assessed by psychiatrists following an episode of deliberate self-harm. It is even more important therefore to assess carefully and note down all relevant history and findings. Providing this is done with care by someone knowledgeable and practised in the assessment of such patients, the follow-up and treatment can be managed in many cases by a physician, social workers, and GP, with help from psychiatric community or OP services as appropriate, and acute psychiatric referral reserved for difficult or uncertain cases.

Psychoses

Mental disorders in which impairment of mental function has developed to a degree that interferes grossly with insight, ability to meet ordinary demands of life, or to maintain adequate contact with reality. It is not an exact or well-defined term.

Organic

(a) Senile and pre-senile organic, psychotic conditions
(b) Alcoholic psychoses
(c) Drug psychoses

Functional

(a) Transient psychotic reactions
(b) Schizophrenic psychoses
(c) Affective psychoses
(d) Paranoid states
(e) Psychoses with origin specific to childhood

Psychotic illness is a difficult subject. With these patients one needs to observe for inconsistencies, strange comments and unusual moods or reactions to procedures or interviews.

1 You must listen not only to what is said but the manner of saying it. The words may jumble and make no sense (thought disorder).

2 The sentence may make sense but the subject is unbelievable — e.g. 'the people in the flat above are pouring gas on me' (delusions — fixed, false beliefs). May be misinterpretation of physical symptoms! 'Rat in my chest' = MI!

3 They may experience interference with their thoughts (thought broadcast, blocking, deprivation, insertion) i.e. other people are tampering with their thoughts.

4 The patient may hear and see things that no one else does (hallucinations).

5 He may be depressed, elated or perplexed.

6 The patient may talk about the treatment he has been receiving:
   (a) 'my injection' from the community psychiatric nurse (depot anti-psychotics given every two to three weeks in schizophrenia),
   (b) electricity (ECT, depressive illness).

7 Note. Physical illness often mimics the psychiatric symptoms of a previous psychiatric illness. Hence acute confusion in an old hypomanic patient may appear to be a relapse of hypomania when first seen.

Psychotic illnesses are affective either where the mood is mainly disturbed, or schizophreniform with problems in thinking or behaviour.

The causes may be drug (or alcohol) intoxification or withdrawal; or part of major illnesses such as schizophrenia or manic depressive psychosis.

The cause may be confused with acute confusional states, with problems of orientation and level of consciousness predominating.

Psychotic symptoms generally merit discussion with a psychiatrist, where there may be need to consider the use of the provisions of the Mental Health Act 1983.

Use of the Mental Health Act

There are occasions when a patient does not want to be admitted for treatment but it is considered necessary for the sake of themselves or others. Under the Mental Health Act 1983 the basic principle is that if someone has a mental illness affecting their decisions, and if because of this they are a risk, a danger to themselves (suicide, self-neglect, dehydration) or to other people, they can be detained against their will.

Sections 2, 3, 4, 5 and 136 are relevant to A & E.

Patients should be admitted under sections 2 and 3. Both orders require an approved psychiatrist who has MRCPsych; and the patient's GP (a doctor with prior knowledge) to see the patient. They ask and recommend

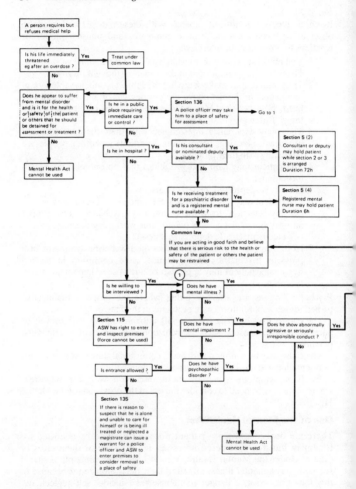

Acknowledgement: M. Bristow, B. Harris.

Figure 6.1 *Compulsory detention in hospital under the Mental Health Act 1983 (Martin Briscoe and Brian Harris)*

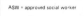

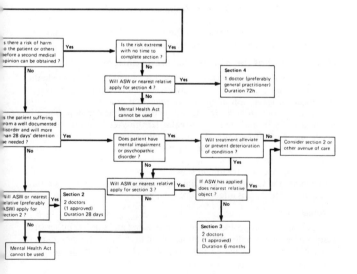

ASW = approved social worker

Is there a risk of harm to the patient or others before a second medical opinion can be obtained ?

Is the risk extreme with no time to complete section ?

Will ASW or nearest relative apply for section 4 ?

Mental Health Act cannot be used

Section 4
1 doctor (preferably general practitioner)
Duration 72h

Is the patient suffering from a well documented disorder and will more than 28 days' detention be needed ?

Does patient have mental impairment or psychopathic disorder ?

Will treatment alleviate or prevent deterioration of condition ?

Consider section 2 or other avenue of care

Will ASW or nearest relative (preferably ASW) apply for section 2 ?

Section 2
2 doctors
(1 approved)
Duration 28 days

Will ASW or nearest relative apply for section 3 ?

If ASW has applied does nearest relative object ?

Mental Health Act cannot be used

Section 3
2 doctors
(1 approved)
Duration 6 months

admission to a social worker who sees the patient, who then agrees or not to admission. There may be a delay in finding these people, and if the patient whom you believe to be at risk insists on leaving, he may be held in good faith, or under Section 4. Good faith implies your decision is to act in the patient's best interests in an emergency. You need to be able to say why you thought there was an immediate risk; why you thought they might be ill and why there was not an alternative, including 'section'. This should be well documented as you could be sued for assault. Also you could be sued for negligence if you allow a depressed and suicidal person to go and kill himself.

Section 4 allows emergency admission, and any registered doctor can recommend emergency admission to a social worker. Again you need to justify not organising admission under Section 2. It is advisable, if the situation allows, to contact a psychiatrist, the patient's GP, and social worker before either acting in good faith or organising Section 4.

Section 136 is used by the police to bring someone from a public place to a Place of Safety, at the hospital, to see a psychiatrist and a social worker. The police should remain with the patient until the two assessments are complete.

Interpretations of the Mental Health Act vary and hospitals have different policies depending on local resources of staff and accommodation. Sections 2 and 3 allow treatment — the others don't though you may have to act in good faith or in an emergency under Section 4.

Management of the acutely disturbed patient

The doctor has power and authority over his patient. He decides whether the patient can go home, tells his employers that he is really ill, even tells the police to leave him alone. Sometimes that power is denied — the patient does not want to know and refuses to accept the decision. It may be because he is ill and then the Mental Health Act is appropriate and necessary. Not infrequently the confrontation becomes heated between anxious doctors and the frightened patient. These situations can escalate until a psychiatrist is called. Usually he will send everyone away, explain the importance of the treatment slowly in words the patient understands, and contact the family if that is the cause of the worry. He is, therefore, trying to institute crisis intervention.

Medication

The patient and his problem have been assessed and this has either been resolved by the Casualty officer, referring to his GP, a voluntary body, or the psychiatrist. Some medication may be required in the meantime.

There are essentially two situations:

    1 Symptom relief until psychiatry or GP appointment.

Useful drugs are low-dose diazepam, chlorpromazine or thioridazine. These can be used for severe anxiety but do have side effects — particularly the latter two. Refer BNF. Limit treatment and refer to GP with letter to supervise further management. Dependance may develop with medico–legal consequences.

2 Acute sedation of a highly disturbed and ill patient.

This is a controversial area and any procedures will usually be carried out under good faith or the Mental Health Act. The idea is to act swiftly and calmly without any atmosphere of threats or violence. The decision has been made that further discussion is of no use and the risk of injury to the patient, other patients, or staff is too high.

Under the direction of the doctor a number of people, at most about six, should approach together. Each person is told which limb he or she is to hold so that the act is organised and not an assault. One person is made responsible for protecting the head and one person to hold each limb, by the forearm or calf, firmly and without causing any discomfort. The patient should be on a bed or mattress, and must be comfortable although restrained. The leader is the only one to talk and this is mainly to the patient explaining what is happening. He *must explain calmly* and kindly why he is doing it — because of the patient's illness.

Nurses and doctors must be present, including a woman if it is a female patient.

The area should be *as private as possible* as this is a medical procedure. It is better *not to involve members of the family* in restraining the patient.

Intravenous sedation may be achieved with haloperidol or droperidol but this can be risky and should be done only in extreme emergencies and preferably with a psychiatrist present. (Refer BNF.)

Diazepam can be used but may disinhibit a disturbed patient further. It is unsafe in Casualty when the patient's alcohol intake is unknown.

Intramuscular anti-psychotics take about twenty minutes to work; take advice on dosage from BNF or psychiatrists. Generally haloperidol is preferred in acute situations, being less hypotensive. After sedation the patient must be intensively nursed, exactly as post-anaesthetic. Any patient transferred later must be transferred with a qualified nurse and resuscitation equipment immediately available. Note time and dose administered. Haloperidol: 10 mg IM, wait 15–30 min; 10 mg stat again. Repeat until sedation achieved.

Re-examination of the patient and any necessary investigations should be carried out to exclude chest infections, extradural or sub-arachnoid haemorrhages, or alcohol or drug withdrawal. Note in latter case neuroleptics. ↓ fit threshold. Use hemineverin or diazepam.

Referral

Having identified the most serious or immediate aspects of the situation it is necessary to decide who can best help and when, and whether a wait is safe and reasonable.

(a) psychotic symptoms — immediate psychiatric opinion

    (b) neurotic symptoms —
        (i) immediate psychiatric opinion or
        (ii) delayed psychiatric opinion or
        (iii) GP referral
    (c) financial, housing, marital problems —
        (i) social services or
        (ii) psychiatric services or
        (iii) marriage guidance
    (d) anorexia, alcoholism, drug abusc —
        (i) physicians/psychiatrists
        (ii) Alcoholics Anonymous
        (iii) Narcotics Anonymous

Note Hemineverin outpatient detoxification must be supervised. This can be dangerous and CSM suggests should not be done. May lead to abuse, dependence or even death with alcohol.

NOTES

7

Eye problems

Eye Problems

A wide range of eye problems present in A & E but most of these are minor. Always record visual acuity and presence or absence of cardinal signs. Serious lesions need to be recognised and referred at an early stage to prevent complications.

History

Ask particularly about pain, photophobia, discharge, and effect on vision. Clarify the nature of any injury: get a full account including use of hammer and chisel, exposure to sunlight lamp, or arc-welding.

Previous history of eye disorders or allergy is noted.

Examination

Visual acuity is measured monocularly with distance spectacles from a Snellen chart and recorded. Test the visual fields using the finger method.

Examine the bony orbit, eyelids, conjunctiva, cornea, iris, and pupil reflex with good pencil torch or slitlamp. Use an ophthalmoscope for the posterior pole and retina. Flourescein is inserted to demonstrate corneal abrasions. Test tension with fingers. If unable to examine completely, e.g. children, marked swelling: *refer*.

Cardinal signs which are significant

- Corneal haze or loss of brightness may be due to impending infection or raised intraocular pressure
- Inequality of pupil: especially if related to loss of visual acuity
- Redness of eye around periphery of cornea is highly significant
- Loss of translucency of the media which obscures the fundus

Conjunctivitis, both simple and allergic, superficial foreign bodies (FB) and abrasions can easily be treated in A & E but penetrating FB, keratitis, iris, and acute glaucoma must be referred immediately. At this stage consult the diagnostic table on page 96.

Conjunctivitis

The cause is usually bacterial, or sometimes viral, but in spring allergy to pollen is common. The patient complains of a gritty prickly feeling, discomfort not pain, watering and often queries a foreign body as the cause of his symptoms. If bacterial, because of a muco-purulent discharge, the eyelashes are often stuck together on waking in the morning.

Note the pattern of redness. There is widespread injection of the conjunctiva, in two thirds of cases unilateral only. Allergic conjunctivitis is usually bilateral with tarsal plate involvement, is seasonal and accompanies hayfever.

Treatment

    (a) Advise on hygiene; not sharing towels.

    (b) Irrigate eyes if profuse discharge.

    (c) Antibiotic eyedrops, chloramphenicol, hourly for 48 hours then 4 hourly for 48 hours; fusidic bd. Do not pad the eye.

    (d) Allergic lesions respond to sodium cromoglycate eye drops 4 times daily.

Other causes of red eye

Keratitis

History resembles conjunctivitis but may be secondary to FB.

Vision may be reduced and pain is more marked.

Examination: the injection is around the cornea (circumcorneal) which may be stained and look hazy. *Refer.*

Iritis

History of deep ache with photophobia and slight weeping. Irritation may be intense. Systemic effects, nausea and vomiting, may be present. Vision may be blurred and visual acuity is often reduced. The pupil is constricted, often irregular, and there is circumcorneal injection with pain and photophobia; pus cells are seen in the anterior chamber (hypopyon). May be associated with ankylosing spondylitis, inflammatory bowel disease or sarcoidosis. *Refer.*

Acute glaucoma

History

Severe pain is the rule; occurs in people over 55.

Examination

Visual acuity is reduced; circumcorneal injection around a hazy cornea; hard eyeball. The pupil is fixed, usually semi dilated and may be oval.

Treatment

Pilocarpine 4 per cent eyedrops every 5 minutes for one hour then continue drops 2 hourly to constrict pupil and relieve drainage angle. *Refer to ophthalmologist as this is an emergency.* If a delay is foreseen start Acetozolamide (Diamox) 250 mg IM and 250 mg IV, then 250 mgs orally qid.

Give adequate analgesia and apply an eye pad.

Cornea

Foreign bodies

Foreign bodies are often associated with corneal abrasions. (See Figure 7.1.) Patient complains of pain, gritty FB, watering, blurring of vision, and photophobia.

X-ray orbit if there is a history of working with metal chisels, grinding, drilling: or glass, at work or RTA.

Lie patient on couch. Anaesthetise the eye with amethocaine 1 per cent eyedrops to get full co-operation. Look under both eyelids and wipe off any loose FB with cottonbud. (See Figure 7.2.)

Patient fixes gaze on an object above, use small sterile hypodermic needle to remove FB. Remember that a corneal abrasion is left. Always apply an eyepad if the eye has been anaesthetised. If the FB is deep or rust staining is present *refer*.

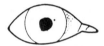

Figure 7.1 *Corneal foreign body*

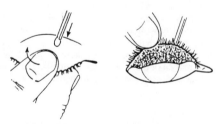

Figure 7.2 *Eversion of eyelid (subtarsal foreign body)*

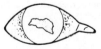

Figure 7.3 *Corneal abrasion*

Corneal abrasions (See Figure 7.3.)

Follow 'finger in eye' injuries, often from baby. They are usually extremely painful but superficial. Anaesthetise eye to examine, stain with fluorescein to see size of lesion. Antibiotic cream is inserted and an eyepad applied. (See Figure 7.4.)

Corneal abrasions are usually associated with an FB or injury but may be recurrent or indolent — *Refer*.

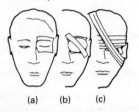

(a)   (b)   (c)

Figure 7.4 *Correct procedure to apply eye pads*
(a) Tulle gras
(b) Cotton wool pad, elastoplast
(c) Bandage

Blunt injuries

Usually caused by blow from fist or boot and patient has a black eye. Assessment of blunt injury must be systematic and recorded. Visual acuity: use Snellen chart.

Note if diplopia is present, particularly on looking up:

(a) this may be transient due to bruising of ocular muscles;
(b) but if constant, and more serious, a blowout fracture of the orbital floor may entrap the ocular muscles. Enophthalmos and infraorbital nerve anaesthesia must be excluded.

Subconjunctival haemorrhage — no posterior margin suggests fracture of the anterior cranial fossa, especially if there is an orbital haematoma confined to the margin of the orbit (often bilateral). The blood is purplish and haemorrhage does not move with conjunctiva.

Corneal laceration (See Figure 7.5)

Is always present with a penetrating FB. The iris may be caught in the wound causing an irregular pupil. The orbit must always be x-rayed if an FB is suspected.

Scleral tear — 2–3 mm from corneo-scleral junction with uveal pigment in wound and vitreous humour. (See Figure 7.6.)

Iris tear — hyphaema and dilated irregular pupil. (See Figure 7.7.)

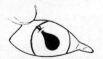

Figure 7.5 *Corneal laceration*

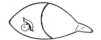

Figure 7.6 *Scleral rupture*

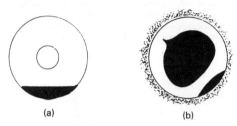

(a)   (b)

Figure 7.7 *Iris tear*
(a) Hyphaema
(b) Dilated irregular pupil

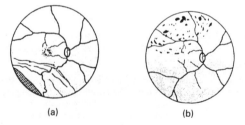

(a)   (b)

Figure 7.8 *Retinal tear*
(a) Macular oedema and retinal detachment
(b) Commotio retinae

Retina (a) oedema — lost red reflex/looks white, with loss of acuity; (b) detachment — lost red reflex/looks grey, decreased acuity; (c) rupture — lost red reflex, lost acuity. (See figure 7.8.)
Refer — if any of these stigmata: decreased visual acuity; flashing lights, floaters; if unable to look under lids due to swelling.

Advise patient that these symptoms may occur later and that he should return quickly if they do.

Subconjunctival haemorrhage is not uncommon without trauma in the older age group; most resolve spontaneously in 10 to 14 days, so reassure patient. If recurrent: check BP, do FBC, ESR and clotting times.

Arc eye (Figure 7.9)

A superficial keratitis which follows over-exposure to ultraviolet light from welding, sun-lamps or sun-beds, when patients have not worn goggles. There is acute pain with reflex epiphora and blepharospasm. Insert amethocaine 1 per cent eyedrops before examining. Treatment: cyclopentolate 1 per cent eye drops stat; chloramphenicol eye ointment; or fusidic bd; tullegras and eyepad; analgesics. Review daily.

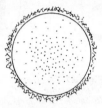

Figure 7.9 *Arc eye*

Burns

Eyelids are often involved in superficial and sun burns. If not full thickness burns of lids (see page 234) treat eye as above and eyelid by exposure.

Chemical spillage

Whether acid or alkali does not matter: irrigate the eye immediately with copious amounts of normal saline. Most units have a bag hanging ready; if not use tap. If a limeburn irrigate with IV glucose solution and carefully examine under both lids to make sure that all fragments have been removed. *Always refer*: but not until all the chemical has been washed out. Apply chloramphenicol eye ointment; cyclopentolate 1 per cent eyedrops every 4 hours and rest the eye under an eyepad and review next morning.

Red eyelids

Stye (Figure 7.10).

Is a staphylococcus aureus folliculitis of an eyelash and often the infection is in a chronic carrier. Treat with hot bathing and topical chloramphenicol or fusidic eye ointment. General health measures should be taken.

Chalazion

Is a granuloma of a tarsal gland on the conjunctival side of the eyelid: *Refer*. If actually infected hot spoon baths (HSB).

Figure 7.10 *Stye*

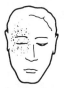

Figure 7.11 *Herpes zoster ophthalmicus*

Herpes zoster ophthalmicus (Figure 7.11)

Involvement of the ophthalmic division of the trigeminal nerve causes a typical herpetiform rash of eyelids, forehead, scalp and side of nose. The vesicular rash is preceded by pain which may be severe and persistent. Complications to the eye may be keratitis, iritis, or glaucoma. Treat the eye with chloramphenicol or fusidic eye ointments plus mydiatric drops twice daily. *Refer.* Calamine lotion will soothe and dry the skin lesions. Systemic acyclovir is also recommended but must be given early as soon as the diagnosis is made.

Herpes simplex keratitis (Figure 7.12)

Sufferers from herpes labialis may have dendritic ulcers as a complication. Typical symptoms and signs of keratitis occur; fluorescein staining shows

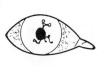
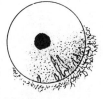

Figure 7.12 *Herpes simplex keratitis*
(a) Dendritic ulcer
(b) Keratitis

Figures 7.8 to 7.12 reproduced from 'Ocular Emergencies' by Andrew B. Richards, courtesy of Smith & Nephew.

the typical branching (dendritic) ulcers. *Do not use steroid eye ointment for fear of perforation.* Idoxuridine eyedrops or acyclovir eye ointment should be started. *Refer.*

Contact lenses

These must not be worn while eye conditions are being treated.

Differential diagnosis

(See Table 7.1.)

TABLE 7.1

Differential diagnosis

	Conjunctivitis	Keratitis	Iritis	Acute Glaucoma
HISTORY				
Trauma	Occasionally chemical	Occasionally FB or abrasion	Rare	Rare reflex
Pain	Grittiness	Mild	Mild to severe, deep, ocular	Severe, deep, ocular, radiates
Photophobia	+ −	+ +	+ + +	
Discharge	Purulent bacterial, watery viral	As conjunctivitis	Slight weeping	No
SIGNS				
Vision	Normal	N → → if central cornea involved → secondary iritis	→	→ → preceded by mistiness or halo
Injection	Generalised	Ciliary, often mixed	Ciliary	Ciliary, maybe mixed
Cornea	Clear, no staining	Localised haze. Staining areas	Clear. Look for KP	Hazy. Epithelial Oedema
Iris	Normal	Hazy. Detail behind	Small	Semi dilated
Pupil	Active	Maybe sluggish	Fixed.	Fixed.
			Maybe irregular	Vertically oval
Tension	Normal	Usually normal	Maybe normal, low or high	Always very hard

8

Ear, nose and throat problems

Ear, nose and throat problems

Patients with ENT problems are best examined in a separate cubicle where suitable ENT instruments and essential medicaments can be kept and checked daily. This place should be in the main part of the department as the condition of some patients may change rapidly and help may be required quickly.

Ear

The history should include onset, duration and recurrence of the principal symptoms:

- pain — earache, headache, onset, nature, radiation, relief, sleep?
- discharge — nature, amount ↑ or ↓, associated with pain?
- hearing loss?
- vertigo — imbalance, rotation?
- tinnitus
- facial nerve weakness — sudden or progressive?
- general — headcold, trauma, weakness as seen in motor neurone disease
- dental history?

Pain

Pain may be referred but is usually associated with an infection of the outer or middle ear:

- Furuncles, diffuse otitis externa (OE), impacted wax or FB, acute viral myringitis, bullosa haemorrhagica are all possibilities. In children particularly, acute otitis media (OM) should be suspected.

  A sudden onset of pain in adults with chronic suppurative otitis media (CSOM) is a forewarning of the onset of complications;

with a decrease in discharge the patient should be referred for an urgent opinion.

● Trauma may be local from a pencil, paperclip or hairgrip, or be part of a severe head injury, blast or barotrauma.

● Otalgia is commonly referred from many sites in the head and neck such as the parotid gland, tonsils or temporo-mandibular joint. Involvement of dental branches of the trigeminal nerve is probably the most common but the early ganglionic stage of herpes zoster may be encountered. (Similarly, the ganglion of the facial nerve, lying in the middle ear, may be involved.) Less frequently the pain may be referred from the glossopharyngeal or vagal nerves. Sometimes pain in the ear is found with cervical disc degeneration, cervical spondylosis or musculoligamentous strain from a whiplash injury, involving the 2nd or 3rd cervical intervertebral joints.

● Malignancy of the posterior tongue, fauces or pharynx must be considered if other causes have been eliminated.

Discharge

Onset, amount, periodicity, character and smell together with the combination of symptoms and signs, should be noted. The external meatus is cleaned prior to inspecting the drum. A purulent discharge is usually infective but may accompany an FB. If bloody consider a viral cause or acute otitis media. Pain followed by mucopurulent discharge is usually from OM or furunculosis; itching with a serous discharge with diffuse OE. Watery discharge accompanies eczema or contact dermatitis. A clear watery leak of CSF, with a positive reaction to a glucose test, may be a sequel to a fracture. Rarely mycotic infection can be diagnosed by a black seedlike discharge. Treat an infection, if resistant then take bacteriological swab for sensitivity.

Hearing loss

Patients frequently attend A & E asking for advice, usually requesting ear syringing. Wax is a common cause of deafness but not the only one. Otosclerosis, of gradual onset, may be present, as is deafness following otitis media (OM). Serous OM (glue ear) is a problem of childhood. Blockage of the eustachian tube following a headcold or barotrauma is another frequent cause.

Trauma to the drum or ossicles occurs in bomb explosions and must be suspected in all victims.

Foreign bodies are often found embedded in wax and all details about insertion have been forgotten.

It is not possible to treat anything but the simple causes of deafness in A & E so these patients must be referred.

TABLE 8.1

Causes of deafness

Conductive hearing loss:
    (i) obstruction of canal: wax or FB;
   (ii) perforation: infection or trauma;
  (iii) discontinuity of ossicular chain; head injury or blast; infection.
  (iv) fixation of ossicular chain; otosclerosis;
   (v) inadequate eustachian tube; glue ear.

Sensori-neural:
    (i) sudden and unilateral: trauma, viral infections, acoustic neuroma.
      Refer.

Facial nerve palsy

Early Bell's palsy can be diagnosed easily because of bilateral cortical representation: the muscle weakness involves the lower part of the face only.

Vertigo

75 per cent are:
    (i) Ménière's disease;
   (ii) benign paroxysmal positional vertigo;
  (iii) sudden vestibular failure; or
  (iv) vascular disturbances.

Usually occurs in older patients: often there is a history of atherosclerosis, cervical spondylosis, headcold or ototoxic drugs.

Individual disorders

Impacted wax

Can cause pain, deafness, or vertigo. Softening with glycerine and sodium bicarbonate eardrops thrice daily is advisable before removing the wax with a small hook. Syringing must not be done if there is a history of perforation of the drum. The drum must be inspected after cleansing is completed.

Foreign bodies

It is dangerous to attempt to remove beads from a child's short wide external meatus because of the danger of damaging the drum and middle ear. If an ENT surgeon cannot be found: anaesthetise (general) the child *and use a hook to get behind the bead.*

    Cotton wool, paper, matches should be easy to remove: insects and flies need warm olive oil poured into the ear first.

Do not syringe vegetable matter.

Always observe for secondary otitis externa (OE) after removal.

Otitis externa

Eczema responds to aluminium acetate eardrops applied on a 1 cm gauze ribbon wick. Alternatively use ichthammol and glycerine or hydro-cortisone eardrops.

Purulent discharge should be cleaned out thoroughly using a cotton-wool bud; send a swab for C & S. The drum is inspected to see whether there is a perforation from otitis media (OM). A wick impregnated with antiseptic (Vioform) and hydrocortisone is inserted. The correct anti-biotic eardrops may be inserted with a wick, but, to avoid the risk of fungal infection, not for more than a week.

Fungal infections are common in hot moist climates with patients who swim often. The external meatus should be cleaned and kept dry, use nystatin locally.

For severe infections use systemic antibiotics or antifungal agents.

Furunculosis

The pinna is swollen with tender, red swelling in the cartilaginous part of meatus and lymphadenitis; this is an infection of the pilo-sebaceous glands which rarely needs incision. A local wick, of aluminium acetate or mag-nesium sulphate, is inserted and systemic antibiotics are prescribed.

Acute otitis media

Infections of the middle ear are often associated with infection of the upper respiratory tract, obstruction of the eustachian tube and large adenoids; they are more common in children than adults. Pain is common early in the child but occurs later in adults. The patient is ill, with pyrexia, and has a conductive hearing loss. Tenderness over the mastoid suggests early mastoiditis, a complication to be aborted by prompt and effective antibiotic therapy. The eardrum loses its normal sheen and light reflex, and becomes inflamed, the colour passing from pink to red. The drum bulges posteriorly accompanied by increasing pain, then perforates with relief of pain. Treatment is by systemic antibiotics: phenoxymethyl-penicillin orally following an initial intramuscular dose of benzylpenicillin or amoxycillin if under 5 years. Oral analgesics are given regularly.

Serous otitis media

Glue ear frequently follows eustachian tube obstruction and is a cause of recurrent mild earache and deafness in children. There is fluid in the middle ear and the drum is dull on inspection. Treat with anti-congestants and *refer*.

Myringitis bullosa haemorrhagica

Is a collection of bloody vesicles over the drum and external meatus. It is of viral origin and accompanied by a respiratory tract infection. Treat pain with analgesics, keep ear dry and *refer*.

Chronic suppurative otitis media (CSOM)

Is a complication resulting from failure to cure the acute stage. There are two types:

    (a) tubotympanic — central perforation
    (b) attico-antral — marginal perforation

Recurrent flare-ups with otalgia, discharge, deafness and, often, vertigo bring the patient to A & E seeking a cure. There is little to do other than clean the meatus, swab for C & S and *refer* all cases. However the dangerous time is when the discharge ceases, pain becomes more severe and early signs of intracranial complications may be missed. *These patients need urgent admission for CT scan and treatment.*

Ménière's disease

Is seen most often in males aged 35–65 years. Paroxysmal attacks of vertigo, preceded by tinnitus, are often accompanied by vomiting and sensorineural deafness. Often there is no obvious pathology. It may accompany vertebrobasilar insufficiency from atherosclerosis or cervical spondylosis. Treat symptomatically with promethazine, prochlorperazine or betahistine. Patients with severe symptoms may need to lie down in a darkened room and be given prochlorperazine rectally or IM if vomiting. Refer for investigation.

Eustachian tube blockage

Occurs frequently with headcolds, hayfever, and adenoids. When flying or diving there is the risk of barotrauma to the middle ear because of the inability to equalise pressures. There is pain and some deafness. The patient needs nasal and systemic decongestants such as brompheniramine maleate or chlorpheniramine maleate: during the acute stage advise yawning, swallowing, or suckling for babies.

Acute deafness

All patients seen with bomb or blast injuries should have their hearing tested and the drum examined: tearing of the drum and dislocation of the ossicles is not uncommon. *Acute neuronal deafness is an ENT emergency*.

Bell's palsy

Results from oedema of the sheath of the facial nerve in the bony canal. It is unilateral and of sudden onset. Treatment: hypomellose eye drops. Eye pad at night. Consider steroids only if palsy complete, sudden onset, painful — *refer*.

Herpes zoster

Herpes zoster involving the geniculate ganglion is accompanied by pain and the typical herpetiform rash around the ear.

The pain may be quite severe and non-steroidal anti-inflammatory agents will give relief. The rash should be treated with calamine lotion. Refer; acyclovir treatment may be required.

The nose

Epistaxis

The commonest causes are trauma and infection. In the older patient associated hypertension, arteriosclerosis, a bleeding disorder, or use of anticoagulants, and less frequently neoplasia, may be responsible. To examine the nose one needs a good headlamp and a Thudicum nasal speculum. A good A & E tool is the auroscope with the largest speculum. To relieve any nasal congestion and to anaesthetise the nose use cocaine nasal spray. Little's area of the nasal septum is then easily seen. (See Figure 8.1.)

X-rays

In cases involving injury to the nose with severe epistaxis, x-rays of the nasal bone and occipito-mental views to show the maxillary sinus are required.

Control of epistaxis

80 per cent of the bleeding occurs from Little's area of the anterior nasal septum behind the muco-cutaneous junction. This is often caused by minor trauma such as picking the nose, particularly if there is a nasal infection or headcold. Stop the bleeding by making the patient lean forward over a bowl while compressing his nose. A cocaine and adrenaline spray follows, and if this is not successful, then the nose requires packing with gauze impregnated with BIPP. This packing should be left in over-night and the patient reviewed the following day. The area can then be caurterised with silver nitrate. Then treat with naseptrin antiseptic cream for one week.

Allergic rhinitis

Common in spring or in houses with housemites: watery discharge, sneezing and, on examination, a pale swollen mucosa. Eustachian tube blockage may occur.

Treatment

By using antihistamine decongestant nose drops such as Otrovine-Antistin or sodium cromoglycate in the short term. If symptoms persist refer for sensitivity tests.

Acute sinusitis

Headcolds causing congestion of the nasal mucosa may cause blockage of the sinuses opening into the nose. Secondary infections soon occur. The pain is related to the site of the sinus:

(a) maxillary, occurring in the cheek;
(b) ethmoid, occurring behind the eye;
(c) frontal, occurring in the supraorbital region.

Treatment is with systemic antibiotics and decongestant nasal drops.

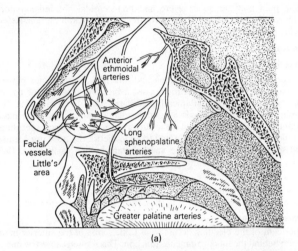

(a)

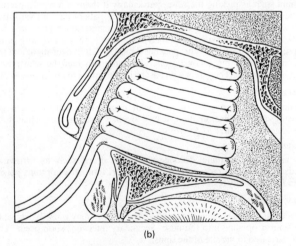

(b)

Figure 8.1 *Epistaxis*
(a) Arterial supply of Little's area
(b) Technique of packing nose

Foreign bodies

These commonly occur in children or mentally impaired adults. Often they have been there for a long time and there is a foul-smelling discharge. The nose should be cleaned gently, making sure that the FB is not displaced backwards. Those in the anterior part of the nose can be removed easily. Where the FB is in the posterior part it is better to admit the patient so that it can be removed with protection of the air passages by the anaesthetist.

Pharynx

Foreign bodies

These often injure the pharynx or upper oesophagus and, if sharp, may scratch the mucosa, causing symptoms. Small sharp FBs catch in the lower pole of the tonsils. FBs in the oesophagus impact just below the crico-pharyngeus. Twopenny coins (25 mm) will stick in most young children. The solitary false tooth often is swallowed inadvertently. X-ray the neck and the chest; if the denture is not radio-opaque, a swallow of gastro-graffin will outline it. A barium swallow is not advised because of sub-sequent problems if an anaesthetic is required. It is important to take a good history and to find out exactly what object was swallowed and when. Anaesthetise the mouth and pharynx with an anaesthetic spray when using a good light and mirror it should be possible to see the tonsil, the base of the tongue, the valleculae and piriform fossa. If the foreign body is not seen here the post-cricoid region of the hypo-pharynx is inspected using a laryngeal mirror. If the x-ray shows the FB or if symptoms persist in the hypopharynx or the oesophagus, the patient should be referred for oesophagoscopy.

Larynx

Obstruction

If stridor occurs on inspiration obstruction is likely to be in the larynx or above. If in expiration, it is bronchial: biphasic stridor suggests tracheal or subglottic obstruction. If the patient is apyrexial, the cause of the stridor may be foreign body or trauma. The laryngeal obstruction may be seen in restaurants where large pieces of meat may stick in the hypopharynx. They can be treated by using the Heimlich manoeuvre. (See Figure 8.2.) Disappearance of stridor indicates the foreign body may be in the right bronchus. Chest x-ray will show a hyperinflated segment of lung. *Refer*.

Acute laryngotracheal bronchitis

The patient, age 6 months to 4 years, has an elevated temperature and a painful cough. He needs fluids, antibiotics, humidification and, if there are signs of respiratory obstruction, give 100 mgs of intravenous cortisone and intubate the patient with an ENT surgeon present.

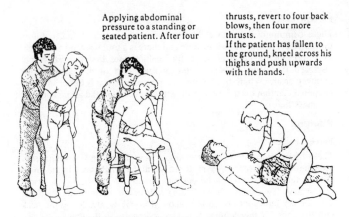

Applying abdominal pressure to a standing or seated patient. After four thrusts, revert to four back blows, then four more thrusts.
If the patient has fallen to the ground, kneel across his thighs and push upwards with the hands.

Reproduced with permission of the Consumers' Association.

Figure 8.2 *Heimlich's manoeuvre*

Acute epiglottitis

Laryngitis and epiglottitis are much more severe in children.

Dysphagia and inspiratory stridor require treatment by humidification, antibiotics, fluids and careful observation. In cases where the obstruction is acute, perform endotracheal intubation. If not possible, a mini-tracheostomy or crico-thyrotomy with a wide-bore needle 19G, or cannula, should be done immediately. (See Figure 8.3.)

Tracheostomy is more difficult and needs some surgical expertise. *If you are worried about a patient or child's breathing, and hear laryngeal stridor, this would be the time to call an anaesthetist and ENT surgeon to do an intubation and give the patient humidified oxygen, steroids and antibiotics.*

Trauma

Trauma to the larynx may occur from a seat belt in a road traffic accident or from sports such as basketball and karate. Intubation or rarely, if stridor is heard, tracheostomy may be required.

Salivary gland swelling

These frequently appear in the A & E department. Causes are mumps, lymph nodes, calculi, or tumour.

Mumps is associated with a general malaise and pyrexia. The swelling is painful and of acute onset.

IF IMMEDIATE RISK OF CHOKING
(simple emergency airway before expert tracheostomy is available)

Indications: Trauma
Epiglottitis
Angioneurotic oedema
Foreign body

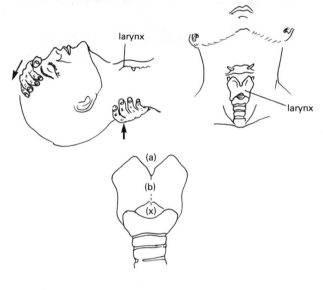

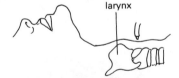

Figure 8.3 *Crico-thyrotomy*
  * *Lie patient flat on back*
  * *Tilt head well back*
    —*place one hand under neck*
    —*place other hand on forehead*
    —*tilt head well back as shown by arrows*
  * *Find the 'Adam's Apple'*
  * *Find notch of upper edge (a)*
  * *Run finger down ridge (approx. 2 cm) (b)*
  * *Find dip at (x)*
  * *Insert large-bore cannula at (x) at 45°*

A calculus commonly occurs in the submandibular gland and the pain and swelling are associated with food. The classic test is lemon on the tip of the tongue. The calculus is often palpable in the floor of the mouth, and will show up on x-ray and sialography.

The mixed parotid tumour is slow-growing and may involve the facial nerve.

NOTES

9

Dermatology

Cutaneous infections and infestations

Bacterial infections

Impetigo

Superficial infection due to staphylococcus auerus, or β haemolytic streptococcus; often occurs in children, and is highly contagious.

Presents with vesicles, which pustulate to give honey-coloured crust. Usually occurs on the face. May be single or multiple.

Treatment:

    (a) Systematic antibiotics, usually erythromycin or flucloxacillin

    (b) Saline soaking to remove the crust

    (c) Topical antibiotic, e.g. fucidin or mupirocin.

Erysipelas

Superficial skin infection with streptococcus pyogenes and occasionally staph aureus. Usually an obvious port of entry.

Presents as red, brawny, oedematous, sharply demarcated eruption. Pustules may be present at advancing margin. Patient may be systemically ill. Leg most common site affected.

Treatment:

    (a) Systemic antibiotic, e.g. penicillin V. *Refer*

Cellulitis

Deep infection of the dermis, indistinct border of erythema tender, swollen, may blister, usually constitutional illness and lymphadenopathy.

Treatment:

    (a) Systemic antibiotics ampicillin and flucloxacillin, and if a limb is affected tubigrip bandage and elevation. *Refer*

Viral infections

Warts and verrucae

Treatment:

    (a) Salicylic acid paint or ointment

    (b) Liquid nitrogen

    (c) Podophyllin on genital warts (N.B. not if pregnant)

Molluscum contagiosum

This is an infection with pox virus, usually affects children. Common sites are face and neck, presents as small smooth reddish papule with a central umbilicus. Single or multiple.

Treatment:

    (a) Puncture the lesion with a curette and apply phenol
    (b) Liquid nitrogen

Herpes simplex

Can be:

- a primary infection
- recurrent (cold sores)
- herpetic whitlow
- genital herpes simplex
- Kaposi's varicelliform eruption eczema herpeticum.

Treatment:

    (a) Topical antiseptic
    (b) Idoxuridine
    (c) Acyclovir: topical or systemic.

Herpes zoster

Treatment:

    (a) Acyclovir
    (b) Analgesic and antibiotics if infected: topical antiseptic
    (c) Post-herpetic neuralgia treat with carbamazepine

Pityriasis rosea

Occurs in young adults as self-limiting disorder.

Starts with a herald patch usually on trunk and 5–15 days later develops oval pink patches with fine scales in Christmas tree distribution across the trunk.

Treatment: (usually none required)

    (a) Antipruritics (N.B.: differential diagnosis is secondary syphilis, therefore check VDRL if does not resolve).

Fungal infections

Dermatophyte

   1 Tinea pedis (athlete's foot) — usually starts as macerated skin between the 4th and 5th toes; may spread to dorsum and sole of foot
   2 Tinea unguium — this is an infection of the nails, and it starts distally with the nail plate becoming thick and roughened
   3 Tinea corporis — the trunk, face or limbs can be affected with circular scaly erythematous lesions with central healing

4 Tinea cruris — well-demarcated erythema and scaling in the groin with central healing

5 Tinea capitis — circular bald patches with erythema scaling and brittle hairs. Only in children.

Diagnosis: Examine skin scrapings and nail clippings. Wood's light examination.

Treatment:

(a) Clotrimazole or miconazole ointment

(b) T. capitis or T. unguium may require griseofulvin.

Candidiasis

1 Mucosal — oral or vaginal — angular stomatitis, is often due to candidiasis

2 Cutaneous — often in moist skin folds (intertrigo) or in nappy rash

Diagnosis: Swab

Treatment: Nystatin or imidazole.

Pityriasis versicolor

Usually presents in young adults with pale brown, pink, hyper or hypo pigmented scaly macular lesion on the trunk. Signs are usually more noticeable after tanning when the lesions remain pale.

Treatment:

(a) Sodium trisulphate paint for 6 weeks

(b) Clotrimazole cream

Cutaneous infestations

Scabies

Common sites — finger webs and sides of fingers, flexor aspect to the wrists, breasts, genitalia, and trunk. Presents as pruritic excoriated papules with linear burrow which may become secondarily infected.

Treatment: malathione, gamma benzene hexachloride.

Pediculosis (lice)

1 Pediculosis capitis

2 Pediculosis corporis

3 Pediculosis pubis

They generally all present with pruritus and diagnosis can be made by seeing the lice with naked eye. For P. corporis, lice are noted on clothes.

Treatment:

(a) *Pediculosis capitis and corporis* can be treated with 0.5 per cent malathion lotion

(b) *Pediculosis pubis* can be treated with 1 per cent gamma benzene hexachloride

The pilo-sebaceous unit

Acne

This usually presents in adolescents but may rarely have other causes:

1 Chemicals, e.g. halogenated hydrocarbon
2 Drugs, e.g. steroids, phenytoin, iodides.

Presents with comedones, papules, pustules, cysts, and scars.

Treatment:

(a) Benzoyl peroxide
(b) Antibiotics, e.g. oxytetracycline 1 gm/day or erythromycin 1 gm/day for 4 months initially
(c) Roaccutane — a vitamin A derivative prescribed on a named patient basis only by a consultant dermatologist. *Refer.*

Rosacea

Diffuse facial erythema with inflamed papules and pustules exacerbated by sun or heat. Alcohol may cause flushing.

Treatment:

(a) Topical 1% hydrocortisone cream or lotion
(b) Antibiotics, e.g. oxytetracycline 1 gm/day.

Perioral dermatitis

Erythema papules and pustules around the mouth and nose. Usually occur in young women. Probably due to using steroid cream on the face.

Treatment:

(a) Avoidance of steroids and treat as for rosacea.

Urticaria, angioedema and vasculitis

Urticaria

An itchy, papular erythematous eruption often with central pallor (wheal and flare).

Types

1 *Acute* — type I allergic reaction.

Causes — food — avocado, prawns — drugs, e.g. penicillin.

Treatment:

(a) Antihistamines
(b) Often resolves in a few weeks — needs *referral* if it persists

2 *Chronic* — An acute reaction which fails to resolve in a few months.

Causes — drugs, e.g. aspirin — dyes and preservatives, e.g. tartrazine.

Treatment: Antihistamines. Needs dermatological *referral*.

3 *Physical*

(i) Dermographism
(ii) Pressure
(iii) Cold
(iv) Sun (solar urticaria)

Treatment: Antihistamines.

> 4 *Cholinergic:* Crops of small itchy wheals after sweating, whether due to heat, exertion, emotion or spicy foods.

Treatment: Antihistamines

Angioedema

Variant of urticaria. Swelling affecting the lips and periorbital tissues. Can have hereditary cause — C1 esterase inhibitor deficiency.

Treatment: Antihistamines (the first dose should be IV); may need intravenous hydrocortisone if the reaction is severe: needs dermatological *referral*.

Vasculitis

> (a) *Polyarteritis nodosa*

Skin manifestations include livedo reticularis, subcutaneous nodules, purpura, punched-out ulcers, and gangrenous lesions.

Treatment: Immediate dermatological *referral*.

> (b) *Erythema nodosum*

Painful, palpable, red, oval patches usually on shins. Lesions resolve in 2–6 weeks fading through the colours of a bruise.

Causes:

- Streptococcal throat infection
- Drugs, e.g. sulphonamides
- Sarcoid
- Viral and chlamydial infections
- TB
- Pregnancy or contraceptive pill

Treatment: Needs *referral* for full investigations.

> (c) *Pyoderma gangrenosum*

A rare condition. Large ulcerating lesions appear suddenly. These normally start as tender nodules which break down to form ulcers, which often become infected. Often associated with inflammatory bowel disease.

Treatment: Needs dermatological *referral*.

Blistering eruptions

Blistering can occur in many disorders and may reflect the severity of inflammatory or in some cases may be due to autoimmune disorders.

Pemphigus

Usually affects people in middle age and Jews in particular. Occasionally fatal if untreated and needs immediate referral. Presents as widespread blisters which rupture easily. Mucous membranes are often involved. It is often painful although not usually itchy. *Refer*.

Diagnosis

Skin biopsy and immunofluorescent staining.

Treatment:

High dose steroids; azathioprine may be added as a steroid sparing agent, and if so regular haemoglobin and platelet counts must be done.

Pemphigoid

Usually occurs in the elderly and presents with large tense bullae on an urticated erythematous base. Mucosal involvement is rare and it may be quite itchy.

It often runs a more benign course than pemphigus, and is usually self-limiting.

Diagnosis

As for pemphigus.

Treatment:

Steroids, usually in lower doses than pemphigus. *Refer*.

Dermatitis herpetiformis

Occurs in the 30–40 age group; is more common in males than females, and is associated with gluten-sensitive enteropathy. It presents with intensely itchy crops of blisters which are quickly excoriated to leave erythematous papules which may scar.

Common sites — scalp, scapular area, elbows, shins, sacrum.

Diagnosis

As above

Jejunal biopsy may be required. *Refer*.

Treatment

(a) Dapsone
(b) Sulphapyridine
(c) Topical steroids

Epidermolysis bullosa

See Paediatric Dermatology (see page 150).

Erythema multiforme

Causes

(a) Infections — herpes simplex, mycoplasma, mumps
(b) Drugs — oral contraceptives
(c) Connective tissue disorders
(d) Pregnancy
(e) Idiopathic

Common sites affected are the hands and feet. Present with target lesions with central pallor.

Severe form with mucosal involvement is the Stevens Johnson syndrome.

Treatment
Refer.

Acute eczema and pompholyx

Herpes simplex

Herpes zoster

Porphyria cutanea tarda

Insect bites and scabies

Impetigo

Psoriasis

2 per cent of the population.

Predisposing factors

1 Genetic — HLA B7, B17, CW6.
2 Environmental — streptococcal infections, drugs, e.g. beta blockers, trauma — Koebner phenomena, and stress.

Patterns

Chronic plaque psoriasis (psoriasis vulgaris)

Well-demarcated raised red patches with silvery scale on knee, elbows, scalp. Not usually itchy.

Nails may have pits, an onycholysis, or subungual hyperkeratosis.

Arthropathy
  (a) Distal interphalangeal joints
  (b) Ankylosing spondylitis and sacro-ileitis
  (c) Small joints (like rheumatoid arthritis)
  (d) Destructive
  (e) Mono- or oligo arthritis (large joints).

Guttate

Showers of lesions on the throat, usually young people. Precipitated by streptococcal throat infections. May affect face.

Flexural

May loose the scale and diagnosis may be difficult.

Pustular psoriasis

Palms and soles small yellow sterile pustules.

Erythroderma

Greater than 90 per cent of the body covered. Patients often ill. Often leads to circulatory problems. *Refer*.

Treatment

Topical treatments

Emollients e.g. emulsifying ointment, are very useful, they can be added to the bath water daily and used to moisturise the skin.

Dithranol used in a base of Lassar's paste, or yellow soft paraffin, or as dithro cream. Concentrations of 0.1 per cent to 4 per cent. Applied once a day to the plaques only (may burn normal skin and stain clothing and skin brown). At home can also do a short contact treatment where patients apply the Dithranol for half an hour and remove it: use once a day.

Tar. Crude coal tar in concentrations 1–20 per cent plus is applied once daily to the plaque. May be combined with salicylic acid which acts as a keratolytic agent if the psoriasis is particularly thick and scaly.

Tar solution (as 20 per cent LPC) is also used daily in bath (as part of the Goekerman regime).

Combinations of tar and steroid, e.g. Tarcortin cream (0.5 per cent hydrocortisone and 5 per cent tar solution) can be used twice daily and useful for flexures where dithranol or tar are difficult to use.

If psoriasis is very active and unstable quarter strength of betnovate and 5–10 per cent LPC in combination is useful.

Topical steroids in low dosages, e.g. quarter strength betnovate ointment twice a day can be used when the psoriasis is particularly angry, painful, and itchy, but should be used only for short periods: topical steroids are not a long-term treatment for psoriasis.

UV light

UVB is used daily in hospital in combination with tar or dithranol topical preparation and can also be used on outpatient basis 2–3 times per week at the physiotherapy department at the local hospital.

UVA used in combination with psoralan (PUVA). Needs hospital supervision.

Systemic cytotoxics

All need hospital supervision:

    1 Methotrexate
    2 Etretinate
    3 Cyclosporin A

Eczema/dermatitis

Endogenous

    1 Atopic eczema
    2 Seborrhoeic dermatitis
    3 Discoid eczema
    4 Varicose eczema
    5 Pompholyx
    6 Nodular prurigo
    7 Lichen simplex

Exogenous

1 Primary irritant contact dermatitis
2 Allergic contact dermatitis

Endogenous

Atopic eczema

Usually starts in childhood often associated with hayfever and asthma. Tends to run in families. Flexural but may be generalised. Erythema, some scaling, much itching which may lead to excoriation and lichenification.

Exacerbations often caused by infection with staphylococcus aureus, there may be no pus seen but the eczema becomes painful and may weep and crust. The patient may be pyrexial and unwell.

Remember: Kaposi's varicelliform eruption after exposure to herpes simplex.

Treatment

Emollients, emulsifying ointment or aqueous cream in the bath as a soap substitute, and moisturiser.

Topical steroids

(a) *Body:* betnovate ointment which can be diluted to half or quarter strength twice a day.
(b) *Face:* 2.5 per cent hydrocortisone ointment, 1 per cent is less severe, twice a day.
(c) *Scalp:* genisol shampoo once a day and synalar gel or betnovate scalp application once a day.

Antihistamines to stop the itching, e.g. atarax 25–100 mg qds or 50–100 mg at night. If this causes drowsiness give Triludan as an alternative.

Antibiotics — to treat staphylococcal aureus skin infection. Antibiotic of choice is flucloxacillin; if allergic to this give erythromycin.

General measures, e.g. hoovering the bed weekly, dusting, avoiding wool or nylon clothing.

Seborrhoeic dermatitis

Usually middle-aged men or infants.
Erythema and scaling affecting the scalp, eyebrows, nasolabial folds, ears, sternum, interscapular area, groins, and axillae. (N.B. Axillae may be bright red, moist, and macerated — intertrigo often becomes secondarily infected with candida.)

Treatment

Antiseptic shampoo, e.g. cetrimide

Salicylic acid preparations 1–5 per cent in aqueous cream

Coaltar preparations 1–2 per cent in zinc paste

Broad-spectrum antifungal cream, e.g. ketoconazole

Topical steroids

Discoid eczema

Usually middle-aged adults, males more commonly affected than females. Well-demarcated symmetrical disk of erythema and scaling commonly affecting extensor surfaces of limbs.

Treatment

Emolients

Steroid creams, e.g. betnovate, either in full strength, half, or quarter strength, and in combination with coaltar, e.g. quarter betnovate and 5–10 per cent LPC.

Antibiotics if infected

Varicose eczema

Dermatitis of the lower legs usually associated with venous insufficiency or venous ulceration.

Treatment

Emollients

Treat varicose veins — elevate limbs and apply pressure.

Occlusive bandages, e.g. tar bands or visco bands with compression one-way stretch Dixon Wright bandages.

Topical or steroid creams should be avoided as continued use may lead to steroid atrophy — see varicose ulcer page 280.

Pompholyx

Vesicular eczema affecting the palms of the hands, often occurs in atopic patients and may become secondarily infected.

Treatment

Strong topical steroid, e.g. betnovate, under occlusion in a plastic bag at night. When settled, reduce topical steroid strength and stop occlusions.

Antibiotics for secondary infections, e.g. flucloxacillin.

Nodular prurigo

Multiple itchy excoriated papules and nodules on limbs and trunk. Often resistant to treatment.

Treatment

Occlusion prevents itching, e.g. calaband cream bandages.

Betnovate

Antihistamines

Antibiotics if secondarily infected, e.g. flucloxacillin.

Lichen simplex (neurodermatitis)

More common in females than males, caused by continued rubbing and scratching of a localised area of itchy skin which leads to lichenification.

Treatment

Topical steroid cream and occlusive bandages, e.g. tarbands or icthabands.

Antihistamines

Exogenous

Primary irritant contact dermatitis

A primary irritant will cause dermatitis in anyone if applied in a sufficient concentration for a sufficient length of time, e.g. a strong acid or alkali will cause an acute dermatitis whereas continued exposure to detergent will cause a chronic hand dermatitis, e.g. in housewives.

Acute reactions produce an erythematous vesicular eruption which is painful and itchy.

A chronic irritant dermatitis presents as erythema, with dry and fissured areas susceptible to secondary infection.

Treatment

Acute

Topical steroid — full-strength betnovate ointment bd.

Antibiotics — flucloxacillin (often gets infected especially if it is weeping).

Antihistamine to stop itch.

Emollient

Change detergents and wear gloves.

Chronic

Emollients, e.g. emulsifying ointment.

Topical steroids, e.g. full strength or half strength betnovate ointment twice a day usually under occlusion in plastic bag at night especially for hands or feet.

Fissures may become infected — treatment $KMnO_4$ soaks.

Avoidance of factors causing the dermatitis, e.g. by wearing cotton/rubber gloves while washing up or while at work.

Allergic contact dermatitis

Due to delayed hypersensitivity (Type IV reaction) to an allergen.
Site of eruption often an important pointer to the diagnosis e.g. beneath watch strap.

Common sensitisers are nickel, rubber, dyes, plastics, preservatives in ointments and cosmetics, plants (e.g. primulas or chrysanthemums), drugs, e.g. topical antibiotics.
Diagnosis — patch testing by dermatologist.

Treatment
Avoidance of known sensitiser
Topical steroids
Emollients

Cutaneous manifestations of systemic disease

Sarcoidosis
Blue red subcutaneous nodules, lupus pernio

Porphyria
Photosensitivity, skin fragility, blister formation, hypertrichosis, pigmentation, scarring

Hyperlipidaemia
Xanthomata (tendons, tuberous, planar and eruptive) and xanthelasma

Neurofibromatosis
Multiple cutaneous neurofibromata, axillary freckling and café au lait spots

Tuberose sclerosis
Adenoma sebaceum, shagreen patches, ashleaf macules, periungual fibromata

Pellagra (nicotinic acid deficiency)
'Dermatitis, diarrhoea and dementia'

Scurvy
Bleeding gums, purpura, poor wound healing, perifollicular haemorrhage

Cutaneous manifestations of endocrine disease

Diabetes — necrobiosis lipoidica. This occurs on the shins and presents as shiny atrophic red or yellow plaques with telangiectasia over the surface. There is a tendency for them to ulcerate and they are often very difficult to manage. The severity of necrobiosis is not related to the severity of the diabetes mellitus and is not affected by the degree of diabetic control.

Hypothyroidism — Diffuse hair loss, coarse hair, broken hair, puffy oedema, xeroderma, pruritus, pretibial myxoedema.

Hyperthyroidism — Hyperhidrosis, fine hair and hair loss, pruritus.

Cushing's syndrome — Acne, hirsutism, cutaneous striae, buffalo hump, obesity, ecchymoses.

Acromegaly — Soft tissue hypertrophy, seborrhoea.

Addison's disease — Increased cutaneous pigmentation, especially intra oral mucosa and palmar creases.

Cutaneous manifestations of gastrointestinal disease

Gluten-sensitive enteropathy — dermatis herpetiformis

Malabsorption and zinc deficiency state — flexural eczematous eruptions

Defective zinc absorption — acrodermatitis enteropathica

Small intestinal polyps — Peutz-Jegher's syndrome

Large intestinal polyps — Gardner's syndrome

Ulcerative colitis — Pyoderma gangrenosum

Crohn's disease — perineal ulceration or skin tags

Cutaneous manifestations of systemic malignancy

Acanthosis nigricans. Presents with hyperpigmentation and hyper-keratosis and skin tags, most marked in the body flexures, neck, and may be associated with gastro intestinal malignancies.

Dermatomyositis. May be associated with an occult malignancy involving any body site and may precede the development of the malignancy. Presents with classical heliotrope rash and photosensitivity.

Necrolytic migratory erythema. This presents with a painful tongue, super-ficial erosions and blisters on the face, buttock, thighs, and abdomen. The malignancy is generally a glucagon-secreting tumour of the pancreas. Removal of the tumour may result in clearance of the skin lesions.

Acquired ichthyosis. The development of dry scaly skin may herald the development of Hodgkins disease, non-Hodgkins lymphoma, or a solid tumour.

Connective tissue disorders

Lupus erythematosus

This disease occurs in 3 distinct varieties: the systemic form, chronic discoid lupus erythematosus — a purely dermatological disorder, and subacute cutaneous LE.

(a) *Chronic discoid*

(Lupus erythematosus). This occurs more commonly in females and tends to present in early spring and summer; it affects the face, scalp, neck, and hands and presents with multiple raised red scaly well-demarcated plaques. These may progress to become ulcerated and leave scars, pig-mentary changes, and telangiectasia. Lesions in the scalp leave a permanent scarring alopecia.

Diagnosis: Skin biopsy and immunofluorescence testing.

Treatment: Needs dermatological referral. Treatment includes sun screens, topical steroids, and anti-malarials.

(b) *Systemic lupus erythematosus*

The skin manifestations of this disorder include the characteristic butterfly rash over the cheeks and nose, diffuse erythema of the palms, and a patchy non-scarring alopecia.

Treatment: Includes topical steroids, sun barrier creams, and systemic steroids.

Between 1 and 5 per cent of patients with chronic discoid lupus erythematosus may go on to develop systemic lupus erythematosus.

Scleroderma

As with lupus erythematosus there is a cutaneous form (morphoea) and a systemic form (progressive systemic sclerosis).

(a) *Morphoea*

Usually presents in young or middle aged adults, more common in women. It presents with firm white or violaceous patches of smooth shiny skin on any body site, commonly the trunk or upper arm. In developing lesions there is usually a well-marked red or violaceous peripheral edge.

Treatment: No specific treatment.

(b) *Progressive systemic sclerosis*

Dermatological manifestations of this disorder include those changes seen in the C.R.E.S.T. syndrome.

Treatment: General medical referral.

Lichen sclerosus et atrophicus

This is an atrophic condition, commonly of the vulva, scattered patches of the disease may also be found on trunk and limbs. It presents with white atrophic glazed areas of the skin which may progress to extreme atrophy and shrinkage of genital tissue and may ulcerate and cause pain and pruritus, although it may be asymptomatic. May affect the penis in the male, balanitis sclerosis obliterans. Extragenital lesions are most common around the neck and upper back.

Treatment: Steroids. Topical steroids, creams, or topical oestrogens. Long-term follow-up is required as severe cases may become malignant.

Dermatomyositis

Has two forms: one affecting children, the other affecting adults. In the adult form there is an association between the disease and systemic malignancy. Skin manifestations include heliotrope rash around the eyes and photo-sensitive macular erythema on the dorsum of the hand and finger.

The associated proximal muscle weakness is variable.

Diagnosis: Raised CPK, EMG, and muscle biopsy. Investigations to include systemic malignancy.

Treatment: Prednisolone or azathioprine.
    Refer

Drug eruptions

These are very common and it is important with any eruption to take a thorough drug history.

Common patterns include

1 *Toxic erythema*. A widespread erythematous morbili-form eruption occurs. More common on the trunk, less so the extremities. Often associated with malaise fever and lympha-denopathy, e.g. antibiotic, barbiturates, antirheumatics.

2 *Erythema multiforme and Stevens Johnson*, e.g. sulphonamides, antibiotics, antirheumatics.

3 *Erythema nodosum*, e.g. sulphonamides, oral contraceptives.

4 *Erythroderma*, e.g. antibiotics, barbiturates.

5 *Vasculitis and pruritus*, e.g. phenytoin, indomethacin.

6 *Psoriasform*, e.g. β blockers and lithium.

7 *Blistering*, e.g. allopurinol, phenylbutazone, sulphonamides.

8 *Photosensitivity*, e.g. tetracycline, phenothiazine, gold.

9 *Alopecia*, e.g. warfarin, antithyroid and cytotoxics.

10 *Acne*, e.g. phenytoin, glucocorticords.

11 *SLE-like syndromes*, e.g. hydrallazine, penicillin, sulphonamide.

12 *Exfoliative dermatitis*, e.g. gold, isoniazid, phenylbutazone.

13 *Toxic epidermal necrolysis*. This is often drug-induced in adults and is similar to staphylococcal scalded skin syndrome seen in young children which is due to an epidermolytic toxin produced by certain staphyloccocci.

Disorder presents with blistered or denuded areas of skin which may resemble a burn. May be localised or widespread.

Treatment:

(a) Withdrawal of the drug

(b) Antihistamines

(c) If very severe — *refer*.

Adverse reaction to topical application

Allergic contact dermatitis is a common sequela of topical antibiotics, and once sensitised the patient will react subsequently to systemic as well as topical applications of the drug.

Adverse effects to topical steroids

1 Thin and fragile skin

2 Bruising

3 Telangiectasia

4 Striae

Choice of topical steroid is important and the weakest effective topical steroid should be used whenever possible. In children weaker preparations should be used in general, but also in adults in certain areas of the body such as face.

Relative strengths of steroids

Very strong — Dermovate

Strong — Betnovate, Propaderm

Medium — Locoid, Eumovate
Weak — Hydrocortisone

Tumours and naevi

Malignant lesions

Predisposing factors

1 UV radiation and X-rays
2 Chemicals, e.g. arsenic
3 Scars
4 Genetic — xeroderma pigmentosa
— Gorlins

Squamous cell carcinoma (SCC)

Flat plaque or papule surface may be ulcerated or keratotic. Usually on sun-exposed skin. May metastasize. Bowen's (intra-epidermal carcinoma) presents as persistent erythematous scaly plaque.

Treatment: Urgent dermatological *referral* for excision.

Basal cell carcinoma (BCC)

90 per cent are on the face. An early lesion may present as a pearly pink papule with telangiectasia over the surface. A late lesion may present as an ulcer with a rolled edge.

Treatment: Surgical, cryotherapy or radiotherapy. *Referral* to dermatologists.

Malignant melanoma

These arise in pre-existing melanoma or *de novo*. Signs of malignant change in a naevus include

● enlargement
● irregular borders
● change in colour
● bleeding or ulceration
● itch
● inflammation

Treatment: Urgent *referral* to dermatologists.

Benign lesions

2 *Seborrhoeic wart*

This presents as a flat or raised brown or black keratotic papule.

Treatment: Curettage or excision.

2 *Squamous papilloma and cutaneous horn*

This may resemble a wart or become more enlarged to form a horn.

Treatment: Curettage or excision.

3 *Keratoacanthoma*

It grows rapidly over a period of about 6 weeks to produce a large indurated dome-shaped papule with a central crater filled with a keratinous plug. Spontaneously involute but leaves large irregular scar. Easily confused with SCC.

4 *Pyogenic granuloma*

This is a soft red fleshy tumour which bleeds profusely if traumatised. Finger is a common site and they rise in response to reactive change from a needle or thorn prick.

Treatment: Can be excised, silver nitrate stick or frozen with CO_2.

5 *Histiocytoma*

Firm pigmented or skin-coloured nodule which is usually on the lower leg. These are often left alone but can be excised.

Naevi

1 Melanocytic (moles) — these may present as pink, brown, black, flat, or raised, hairy or hairless, rough or smooth, moles and there is no treatment unless malignancy is suspected.
2 Vascular naevi — see Paediatric Dermatology (page 150).

NOTES

10

Gynaecology

General introduction

The gynaecological patient has special requirements. She should be treated in an area in casualty which offers privacy.

History

Take a detailed history of the presenting complaint.
Ask specifically about:

1 Date of last menstrual period and was it normal.
2 Menstrual cycle.
3 Irregular and postcoital bleeding.
4 Vaginal discharge.
5 Contraception, ? any chance of pregnancy.
6 Obstetric/gynaecological history.

Examination

A general physical examination should be performed. Adequate explanation should be given to the patient prior to pelvic examination and a male doctor should always be chaperoned.

If microbiological or cytological investigations are to be performed, speculum examination should precede digital examination.

Examine women with care and respect in warmth and a good light. Prepare equipment before you start. Take time to explain what you will do before you begin, and warm (not heat) the speculum. Tell the woman she is in control and that you will stop if it hurts — then it is much less likely to.

Do not perform vaginal examinations (PV) in women who've never had intercourse. Never perform them unnecessarily.

Don't touch ulcers or discharge without gloves on.

If you remove a coil, record the type and check that it is complete. Send coil to microbiology for culture.

Pelvic masses are notoriously difficult to localise accurately, even by experts. If you find one, refer to gynaecologist for ultrasound scan (USS). An ovarian cyst, especially in an older woman, may be indistinguishable from fibroids.

If there is any chance of pregnancy prescribe with caution and consult the BNF.

Vaginal bleeding

The normal cycle

The normal menstrual cycle varies between 21 and 35 days. Bleeding may be light, moderate, or heavy but the patient will usually know what is normal for her.

Irregular cycles are the norm in some women, e.g. women with polycystic ovaries, so it is important to listen to the woman's history.

Post-partum it can take up to 6 months to re-establish regular cycles.

Abnormal vaginal bleeding

This may occur in the non-pregnant or pregnant woman.

In non-pregnant women

Oligomenorrhoea — this is defined as the occurrence of menses on only five or fewer occasions per year.

Secondary amenorrhoea — the absence of menses for six months (or greater than six times the previous cycle intervals in a woman who has menstruated before).

Menorrhagia — heavy menses — can be regular *or* irregular.

Intermenstrual bleeding — this is bleeding between the periods.

Post-menopausal bleeding — bleeding after *1 year* of amenorrhoea after the menopause.

Dysfunctional uterine bleeding — this is abnormal bleeding from the genital tract in the absence of any organic disorder.

Common causes of abnormal bleeding

This may be due to pathology of the genital tract or may be dysfunctional. Most cases can be managed by referral to gynaecology outpatients unless the bleeding is so heavy as to warrant admission. Most of the following conditions do not require emergency treatment:

Causes:

Uterine:	Fibroids
	Carcinoma of endometrium
	Endometrial polyps
Cervical:	Erosion
	Polyp
	Carcinoma
Dysfunctional bleeding:	Pill related
	Perimenopausal

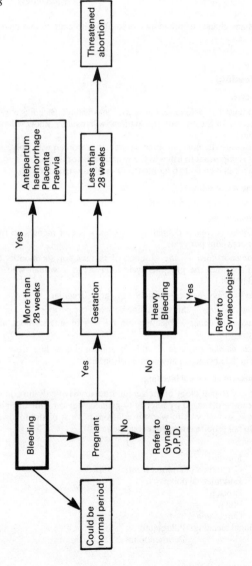

Figure 10.1 *Diagnosis of vaginal bleeding (Ann Milstein)*

In the pregnant woman:

Abortion is defined as the spontaneous or induced termination of a pregnancy before 28 weeks' gestation:

1 Threatened abortion
2 Inevitable/incomplete abortion
3 Missed abortion
4 Ectopic pregnancy

Threatened abortion

History: Light spotting/bleeding early on in pregnancy.
No pain.

Examination: no tenderness.
Uterus enlarged to a size compatible with gestation.
Os closed.

Investigations: None.

Treatment: Bedrest.
No sexual intercourse.
Advise patient to go home but return if bleeding increases or she develops pain. Consider admission if the pregnancy is high risk or precious.

Inevitable/incomplete abortion

History: Heavy bleeding with or without clots or products passed.
Associated with crampy abdominal pain.

Examination: Tender lower abdomen. Os usually open, with/without visible products.

Investigations: Hb if much blood lost.
Group blood and save (check Rh factor if unknown).

Treatment: Evacuation of retained products of conception (ERPC).
May need referral for further investigations if abortions are recurrent.

Missed abortion

History: Confirmed pregnancy initially; later symptoms of pregnancy regress. Vaginal bleeding.

Examination: Fundal height lower than expected for dates.

Investigations: Ultrasound scan confirms presence of sac but no foetal heart present.

Treatment: ERPC.

In all the above cases, Anti D (250 IU) should be given IM if the patient is Rhesus negative.

Ectopic pregnancy

History: This can be difficult to diagnose. There is a variety of presentations from minimal symptoms to sudden collapse. Pain classically precedes irregular vaginal bleeding and may have shoulder tip radiation. Nausea/vomiting, faintness or dizziness may occur.

Irregular bleeding may be the only clue.
Past history of tubal surgery/PID/IUCD.

Examination: Lower abdominal/right or left iliac fossae tenderness and a palpable mass.
Tender in one fornix.
Uterus is normal size or slightly enlarged.
Cervix is closed — with or without cervical excitation.
Breasts may be tender.

Investigations:

- Ultrasound scan — if this reveals an intrauterine pregnancy it is very rare to have an ectopic as well.
- Pregnancy test — can be a help if positive — (if negative does not exclude diagnosis.)
- βHCG estimation may be available (RAMP). Clearview.

Differentiate from:

1 Appendicitis.
2 Torsion of an ovarian cyst.
3 PID.
4 Threatened abortion.
5 Other causes of acute abdomen.

If diagnosis of pregnancy is confirmed, cross-match 2 units of blood and refer.
Give Anti D if the patient is Rhesus negative.

Management of ectopic pregnancy

If the history and clinical findings alone are suggestive of an ectopic pregnancy, laparoscopy (followed by laparotomy if necessary) must be performed.

Antepartum haemorrhage

Over 28 weeks take history and blood for cross-match, put in IV line, never do a vaginal examination. Refer to gynae SHO. Anticipate sudden and heavy bleeding.

Pain

Gynaecological causes of the acute abdomen

Pelvic inflammatory disease (PID)

This is a common condition, although uncommon in pregnancy. It may be acute or chronic.
It may be caused by chlamydia which is difficult to culture.

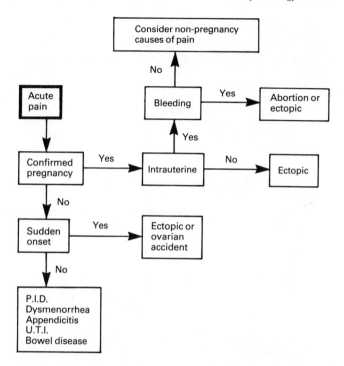

Figure 10.2 *Diagnosis of lower abdominal pain*

History: May be associated with
- recent termination or delivery
- recent invasive procedure, e.g. Hystero-Salpingogram
- intrauterine contraceptive device (IUCD) insertion
- new sexual partner

Patient usually complains of discharge, lower abdominal pain, dyspareunia or irregular bleeding.

Examination: Fever (up to 39.5°C), rigors (acute).

Abdominal tenderness — right and left iliac fossae with or without peritonism.

Tenderness in both fornices.

Cervical excitation and uterine tenderness.

Vaginal discharge.

Adnexial masses may be present if there is a pyosalpinx.

Investigations: Endocervical initially for general culture and then chlamydia swab.

Endocervical/urethral swabs if gonococcus suspected.

Management: Should give:
   (a) ampicillin 3.5 g and probenecid 1 gm.
   (b) Doxycycline 200 mg stat then 100 mg bd for 14 days (erythromycin 500 mg qds for 14 days if there is any possibility of pregnancy).
   (c) Metronidazole 400 mg tds for 7 days.

Referral to genito-urinary medicine (GUM) clinic for follow up after antibiotics are completed. Partner *must* go to GUM clinic.

Chronic PID

Presents with low-grade fever, menorrhagia, deep dyspareunia, discharge, pelvic tenderness and/or a mass. PID initially requires antibiotics and bedrest.

Take swabs:
   (i) black endocervical and HVS.
   (ii) chlamydia — use special swabs if available. Wipe off cervical mucus first to get to cells. Swab at squamo-columna junction — remember where it is if there is erosion(ectopy).

Consider using the opportunity to take cervical smear for cytology.

Remove IUCD (by steady traction of the threads): you may need local infiltration of lignocaine or inhaled analgesia. *Anchor cervix* — no anaesthesia necessary.

Give analgesic tablets and antibiotics. Metronidazole 400 mg tds 10 days and Doxycycline 200 mg once on first day then 100 mg once a day for 14 days. In pregnancy erythromycin 500 mg four times a day (but this is ineffective against mycoplasma hominis).

Remember effect of antibiotics on oral contraceptives; advise use of additional contraception (and prescribe it) for fourteen days. Remember also that diarrhoea caused by antibiotics will affect absorption of the contraceptive pill.

Treat sexual partner(s). Advise self-referral to GUM clinic — this is essential — as soon as possible. Follow up in fourteen days with swab results.

NB. *Gonorrhoea* is best treated at GUM clinic, or give ampicillin, then start a course of tetracycline and send an urgent black swab.

Chlamydia

Causes the infection that blocks up tubes; chlamydia infects tubes, causing infertility and a great deal of pain, investigation, distress and expense. Swab for it carefully and have a high index of suspicion in women under 25, single, recent change of sexual partner, on oral contraception, who present with vaginal discharge, cervicitis or erosion.

Trichomonas vaginitis

Often association with other sexually transmitted diseases (STDs), even if not initially found 10 per cent also have gonorrhoea. So all should be referred to GUM clinic.

Accident to ovarian cyst/torsion of pedunculated fibroid

There may be a history of known ovarian cyst or fibroids.

Other causes of pain

- 1°dysmenorrhoea — this is defined as painful for which no organic or psychological cause can be found.
- 2°dysmenorrhoea — this is painful periods for which an organic or psychological cause is found.

The causes of 2° dysmenorrhoea are usually either PID or endometriosis.

- Early pregnancy complications, e.g. abortion.

Vaginal discharge

This can be physiological or pathological. There is an increase in normal vaginal discharge in certain physiological conditions.

Physiological

- Normal cycle
- Pregnancy
- Normal variation

Pathological

- Infective (common)
- Neoplastic
- 2° to foreign body

If the partner also presents with a discharge the couple should be advised to attend the genito-urinary medicine clinic.

Common conditions

Candida (Thrush)

History: Is she taking the contraceptive pill?
Diabetes mellitus?

Examination: Cheesy white pruritic discharge and vulval excoriation.

Investigation: HVS.

Treatment: Clotrimazole pessary 500 mg × 1 at night. Prescribe clotrimazole cream topical bd for 14 days.

Trichomonas vaginalis

History: Offensive discharge.

Examination: Frothy green vaginal discharge.

Investigation: Endocervical swab.

Treatment: Metronidazole 400 mg twice a day for 5 days: both partners *referral* to a genito-urinary medical clinic.

Gardnerella vaginalis

Examination: Yellowy white discharge.
HVS reveals 'clue' cells.

Treatment: Metronidazole 400 mg twice a day for 5 days.

Gonorrhoea

Always take an endocervical swab when treating for PID.
A Bartholin's abscess can be caused by gonococcus.
If cultures are positive, *refer* to a genito-urinary medicine clinic.

Miscellaneous

Bartholin's cyst/abscess

The Bartholin's glands lie posteriorly in the labia minora.
An abscess may be of gonococcal origin.

Abscesses need incision and drainage under general anaesthesia. (*Refer.*)

Cysts are referred to gynaecology OPD.

Foreign bodies in the vagina

These can present with a foul-smelling discharge. Lost tampons are often a case. They are most easily removed with fingers rather than instruments. Entonox can be helpful if the patient is finding it difficult to relax.

Always think of non-accidental injury in children with vaginal discharge.

Sexual abuse

Young women and children are asking for help more and more, thus giving an apparent massive increase in the incidence of sexual abuse, particularly of minors. Covert presentations include overdose/suicide attempts, abdominal pain, vaginal discharge and occasional pregnancy. Always ask overtly. Refer immediately to social worker.

Rape

If possible a female doctor should see the woman, especially a gynaecology SHO/registrar in preference to the casualty officer.

Confine examination to the absolutely necessary. If a police surgeon is to see the woman, she will be obliged to examine more fully, so you don't need to. However, shock, intra-abdominal injuries, lacerations, may need to be treated as early as possible. Respect the woman's right not to report to the police if she chooses (see page 258). X-rays and specialist opinions — if urgent — are best sought while at hospital. Remember tetanus, post-coital contraception and prophylactic antibiotics.

Do not leave the woman alone, or unclothed.

Liaise with Rape Crisis Centre etc. who will advise you and send someone to help if necessary.

Offer follow-up with same doctor — especially if woman is not being seen somewhere else.

Advise and give details of GUM clinic — make appointment if possible. Keep detailed records with diagrams in all cases. Many women are able to report the crime only later on.

Sexually transmitted diseases (STDs)

STDs are best treated at a GUM centre. The opening times of the nearby ones should be available at the reception desk. Men and women are seen at separate clinics. Patient can self refer. Send everyone with unusual ulcers/non-specific urethritis and requests for HIV antibody testing. All authorities strongly recommend expert pretest counselling.

Obstetrics

Generally: refer to the obstetrician but frequently the patient is in advanced labour and cannot wait for midwife or to travel to the labour ward. A system for calling the midwife and a place suitable for delivery should always be available.

Normal delivery

History

- Has the patient had antenatal care? If so she will have a co-operation card.
- Gestation.
- Any abnormality in this pregnancy or in preceding ones.

Examination

- Abdominal examination
- Presenting part? engaged?
- State of the cervix — position — firmness/effaced — dilatation
- Is foetal heart present and normal?
- Palpate contractions

Entonox can always be used in casualty at any stage of labour.

It is important to clear the baby's airways and to keep him warm.

Bleeding in pregnancy

This can vary from spotting to catastrophic bleeding.

Causes

Placental: Placenta praevia; abruption — a bleed after 28 weeks.

Other: Vasa praevia; unknown.

Management in casualty

- Resuscitate: IV; cross-match.
- No vaginal examination.
- *Refer* immediately.

Pains in pregnancy

Obstetric:

> *Round ligaments*
> *Urinary tract infection (UTI)/Pyelonephritis*
> *Premature labour*
> *Abruption*
> *Fibroid:* red degeneration; torsion.
> *Ovary:* Torsion; rupture; haemorrhage.

Other:

> *General causes* of abdominal pain/acute abdomen.

Prescribing in pregnancy

If in any doubt — refer to BNF/drug information in pharmacy.

General

- Avoid if possible.
- Confirm which drugs are safe.
- Weigh up risk.

Avoid

1 Live vaccines (can give ATT).
2 Antibiotics: TTC; metronidazole; sulphonamides.
3 Analgesics: aspirins; NSAIDS.

Family planning

Combined pill

Notes for postcoital contraception (PCC). Ovran 50 (levonorgestrel 250 µg + ethlyloestradiol 50 µg).
ii stat and ii 12 hours later. Within 72 hours of unprotected intercourse. Needs for counselling, refer to local family planning clinic if possible.

IUCD

Remove any time during pregnancy if the threads are visible.

NOTES

11

Sick and injured children

Sick and Injured Children

A joint statement from the BPA, CSA, and BAPS reveals that between 20 and 25 per cent of the child population are seen annually in the A & E departments: that is approximately two to two and a half million children.

When children attend with trauma there may be associated medical problems; complicated social factors may also be involved in the aetiology of trauma and these need time for investigation by staff trained to work with parents and children.

A & E may be the first point of contact with hospital services for parents who have had difficulty in obtaining urgent primary care, particularly when infants and young children are unwell. At least 15 per cent of children who attend have medical conditions: of those children under two years estimates are as high as 40 per cent. Diagnosis and management can be difficult under these circumstances so full opportunities should be made for consultation with the paediatricians.

Particular care and attention must be paid to the special needs of the sick or injured child; diagnostic procedures and drug dosages particularly. Special facilities are required for waiting, examination, and treatment areas for the child and its parents, brothers, and sisters, apart from the usual hurly-burly of A & E. With increasing awareness of non-accidental injuries and of sexual abuse, privacy for talking to patients and families away from clinical areas is also required. These cases must be referred as soon as suspected.

Convulsions and coma

Emergency treatment of the convulsing child

- *Clear the airway*
- *Administer oxygen*
- *Rapid control of fits*

Diazepam: IV 0.25 mg/kg; rectally — up to 0.5 mg/kg. Repeat SOS.

If diazepam is unsuccessful, or maximum dose has already been given at home or by GP, *then try*:

Paraldehyde 0.1 ml/kg IM 1 ml/year of age up to 5 ml; or Phenytoin 5–8 mg/kg IV slowly with ECG monitor.
If convulsions not rapidly controlled: intubation and ventilation.

● *Exclude obvious causes*

Hypoglycaemia
Hypocalcaemia
Orbital cellulitis
Meningitis
Otitis media

● *Admit for observation*

(Watch carefully for respiratory depression where diazepam has been administered.)

1 Febrile convulsions

Most commonly in children 6 months–3 years. Should not be diagnosed in children over 5 years. Associated with febrile illness.

Treatment

Cool the child — antipyretics, paracetamol; adequate fluid replacement; and treatment of underlying infection. Always suspect meningitis if no cause for pyrexia can be found. Repeated convulsions with febrile episodes are common but always admit:

● 1st febrile convulsion
● children under 18 months
● prolonged fits more than 15 minutes
● fits not responding quickly to treatment
● any suggestion of other pathology, e.g. neurological signs
● and child where cause of pyrexia cannot be found

2 Epilepsy

This is a common cause for fits presenting between 5 and 15 years. It is important to exclude other causes, e.g. meningitis and to make a firm diagnosis so that long-term anticonvulsant therapy can be planned.

3 Meningitis

Fits, drowsiness, irritability, coma should always alert the clinician to the possibility of meningitis (see later). *When in doubt admit for LP.*

Remember — classical signs may be absent, especially in the infant, and illness can be very rapid in onset.

4 Birth injury

Serious causes of fits in the first month of life.

Hypoglycaemia
Neonatal tetany

5 Other causes

- Hypertension (nephritis)
- Poisoning (ingestion)
- Cerebral malformation/hydrocephalus
- Encephalopathy

Infections in childhood

Meningitis

This presents with an acute illness with headache, neck pain, and photophobia in the older child. However, in the younger child and infant, symptoms and signs are often misleading. Neck stiffness is difficult to elicit and may not always be present — get the child to 'kiss his knees'. A persistent, feverish headache may be the first sign. Feel the fontanelle in an infant — this may be tense and bulging. Drowsiness, vomiting and fits are common. A first convulsion in a child under 1 year should be assumed to be meningitis until proven otherwise. A purpuric purple, blotchy rash is typical of meningococcal meningitis but not always present. Lumbar puncture will help differentiate between viral and bacterial aetiology. Tuberculous meningitis — though rare — should never be forgotten. (See Table 11.1.)

TABLE 11.1

Cerebrospinal fluid

	Cells	Protein	Sugar content
Viral	Lymphocytes	Normal	−ve Normal
Tuberculous	Lymphocytes	Raised	+ve Lowered
Bacterial	Polymorphs	Raised	+ve Lowered

Treatment of meningitis is initially resuscitation of the sick child, control of fits, correction of dehydration and electrolyte disturbance. Antibiotic therapy is instituted after collection of blood and CSF for culture on the basis of the likely organism (commonly *H. influenzae* in a child younger than 5 years, pneumococcus or meningococcus at all ages, and *E. coli* in neonates). Meningitis with purpuric rash is treated with penicillin instantly.

Otitis media/earache

Otitis media is a common condition in childhood. Older children present with earache, with or without discharge, usually associated with upper respiratory tract infection (URTI) and fever. In the infant the diagnosis is less easily made so the ear drums should be inspected on all sick and pyrexial infants. Signs vary from loss of light reflex to a bulging red drum or perforation. Common organisms are streptococcus and haemophilus influenzae. Treatment is with antibiotics and analgesics.

Discharge from a child's ear

May be due to otitis media, otitis externa, or a foreign body lodged in the external auditory meatus. In the latter case do not try to remove the FB by probing. Occasionally gentle syringing is successul but it will be best removed, often under GA, by ENT surgeon.

TABLE 11.2

Infectious diseases

Disease	Incubation (range)	Isolation period	Symptoms/ management/ complications
Chickenpox (varicella)	2 weeks (1–3 weeks)	1 week from onset of rash	prodromal malaise macular rash on trunk first, progressing to vesicular pustules and crusting, seen at various stages. Symptomatic treatment. Can be fatal in immuno-compromised.
Measles (morbilli)	10–11 days to catarrhal stage (1–2 weeks)	1 week from onset of rash	URT symptoms fever, coryza, conjunctivitis and cough initially + Koplik's spots on mucous membranes; blotchy maculo papular rash on face and trunk. Otitis media, broncho-pneumonia may require treatment, otherwise symptomatic.

days of illness
0 1 2 3 4 5 6 7 8 9 10
T(°C) 40 39 38 37
– rash
– low grade fever

days of illness
0 1 2 3 4 5 6 7 8 9 10
T(°C) 40 39 38 37
– rash
– Koplik's spots
– conjunctivitis
– coryza
– cough
– general lymphanopathy

TABLE 11.2—*contd.*

Disease	Incubation (range)	Isolation period	Symptoms/ management/ complications
German measles (rubella)	17–18 days (2–3 weeks)	until rash fades	mild illness, flat pinkish maculopapular rash. Cervical lymphadenopathy. *NB* Congenital malformations in foetus — avoid contact with pregnant women.
Mumps	17–18 days (2–3 weeks)	1 week from subsidence of swelling and > 2 weeks from onset	parotid swelling and pain usually bilateral. Meningitis, orchitis (post-pubertal males), pancreatitis.
Whooping cough (pertussis)	1–2 weeks to catarrhal stage then further 1–2 weeks to whoop	at least 2 weeks from subsidence of whoop or > 4 weeks from onset	paroxysmal coughing is very serious in babies who often do not whoop but stop breathing with coughing. Bronchiectasis; encephalopathy.
Diphtheria	2–4 days (1–7 days)	>4 weeks until 2 negative swabs from nose & throat obtained	malaise, cervical lymphadenopathy, sore throat, croupy cough or stridor. Mild pyrexia + tachycardia. Grey-white *adherent* membrane on pharynx and soft palate.

For German measles, a chart shows days of illness 0 1 2 3 4 5 6 7 8 9 10, T(°C) 40 39 38 37, with bars for – rash, – ing. nodes, – malaise, – URTI, – general lymphanopathy (especially suboccipital nodes).

NB ANTITOXIN is required before swabs confirm diagnosis, urgent trache-ostomy may be needed. *Diagnosis easily missed because of rarity but is becoming more common with low inoculation states.*

Pyrexia of unknown origin (PUO)

Many children present with non-specific illness and pyrexia and are a problem for the Casualty Officer. Diagnosis is really one of exclusion of serious illness, and the majority turn out to be self limiting viral illnesses. The decision when to admit for further investigation rests upon the clinical condition of the child — but when in doubt refer for paediatric opinion. The history should include details of foreign travel and contact with infectious diseases as well as specific symptomatology. Do not forget typhoid and malaria can present with non-specific symptoms and misleading signs such as pneumonia, constipation, diarrhoea, fits and anaemia. (See Table 11.2.)

Investigations such as urine culture, microscopy, CXR, WCC, blood culture and lumbar puncture form the basis for diagnosis.

Respiratory problems

Stridor

Noise on breathing which is usually mainly inspiratory. It arises from the upper airway (above bronchi). Commonly laryngeal, as young child's· larynx is small and soft compared to an adult's.

Causes

Congenital: audible from birth in severe cases. Stops at 12–15 months, rarely problematic, but gets worse in respiratory infections, etc.

Acute laryngotracheitis

Common in 1–4 year-olds. Causes 'croup'. Pyrexial illness, cough, and malaise. Commonly viral but can be caused by *H. influenzae*. Generally responds to humidification and antibiotics but if severe, admission is indicated. Differential diagnosis is acute epiglottitis.

Acute epiglottitis

Inflammation of the epiglottis, often caused by *H. influenzae*, can produce very sudden onset of severe stridor, and difficulty in swallowing saliva, etc. Sudden laryngeal obstruction can be precipitated by rough instrumentation of the child's throat and fright may severely worsen an already alarming degree of stridor. The child should therefore be kept quiet (but not sedated), reassured, and admitted for treatment, usually tracheostomy.

Foreign body

A common cause of laryeal obstruction in children. Difficult to confirm if not radio-opaque. Laryngoscopy, cricothyrotomy, may be required.

Wheeze

Noisy breathing which is mainly expiratory.

Causes

Acute bronchiolitis — Common in infants. Often associated with URTI, snuffliness, and feeding difficulty. Onset is sudden; fever, dyspnoea and tachypnoea are features. On auscultation there is both wheeze and crepitations which are widespread. Up to 85% are viral (RSV) but bacterial causes necessitate treatment with antibiotics. The child should be admitted for oxygen therapy. Ventilation and careful fluid therapy in severe cases.

Asthma

The differentiation between asthma and wheezy bronchitis is difficult, and definitions vary. However, for the purpose of emergency treatment of the wheezy child the exact diagnosis is often academic. Asthma is characterised by recurrent bouts of wheezing, breathlessness, and cough. There may be a family history of allergy. Obstruction of peripheral airways is responsive to treatment and is reversible.

- In status asthmaticus give: oxygen plus nebulised salbutamol 0.5 mls of 0.5 per cent solution in 2 mls saline via a nebuliser, at high gas flow of 8 l/min of oxygen. This is inhaled over about 10 minutes.
- If the child remains breathless or cyanosed, or speech remains difficult, commence IV infusion and give aminophylline 6 mg/kg over 20 min (*provided no aminophylline/theophylline has been given in last 8 hours*) and a bolus of hydrocortisone 4 mg/kg.
- Continual infusion of aminophylline and hydrocortisone at 1 mg kg/hr.
- Monitor ECG, pulse, respiratory rate, and conscious level carefully and frequently. PEFR and blood gases should be estimated before, during, and after treatment.

Danger signs

- Rising pulse rate
- Rising $PaCO_2$
- Restlessness
- Fatigue
- Chest pain (beware of pneumothorax)
- Fall in level of consciousness
- Cyanosis
- Reduced amount of wheeze when associated with any of the above signs.

Ventilation should be considered early if not responding to therapy. *Asthma still kills* and this often occurs because the severity of attack has been underestimated.
Sedate with care.

DO NOT — use repeated doses of bronchodilator to which the child is not responding.
DO NOT — omit to ascertain which and how much bronchodilator has been used prior to admission.
DO NOT — discharge until a period of observation has confirmed lasting response.

Respiratory infection

Respiratory tract infections are very common in children: if not treated adequately they can result in severe disability. A child with respiratory tract infection and a respiratory rate over 40 per minute should be referred.

Bronchitis

Can occur at any age — the only signs may be cough and fever.

Bronchiolitis

Often occurs in winter epidemics and only in young children. It may develop suddenly and rapidly. Widespread crepitations and rhonchi are present.

Treatment
Humidified oxygen.
Antibiotics if superinfection is suspected.

Bronchopneumonia

This is usually viral but there may be bacterial superinfection. The onset is usually gradual. Crepitations and bronchi are heard and the x-ray may show patchy consolidation. *Refer.*

Lobar pneumonia

This is usually an older child. It starts rapidly and there may be some chest pain. There is usually an expiratory grunt.

Treatment
Penicillin.

Diarrhoea and vomiting

Infective causes

Vomiting and diarrhoea are commonly caused by gastroenteritis. The aetiology may be bacterial (salmonella or shigella or *E. coli* in small babies) but the majority are viral (commonly rotavirus). Antibiotics are rarely helpful and treatment is directed at prevention of dehydration and control of spread within the community. Treatment with oral fluids often suffices but where vomiting is severe or dehydration is present admission is indicated — see assessment and treatment of dehydration, page 147.

Giardia

This generally causes chronic diarrhoea with little constitutional upset. Diagnosis is by the identification of cysts in the stool. The condition responds to treatment with metronidazole.

Campylobacter

Campylobacter causes gastroenteritis, usually in older children, and is thought to be acquired from animals such as chickens, dogs, cats, sheep, cows. Abdominal pain may be a feature, and also blood in the stools.

Lactose intolerance

May be a temporary condition following gastroenteritis. Withdrawal of milk, followed by gradual re-introduction, will usually suffice. There is, however, also a genetic condition in which there is lactase deficiency causing intolerance of milk, but this is rare.

Food allergy

True food allergy is rare but when present can cause diarrhoea, vomiting, rashes and abdominal pain. Cow's milk, fish and fruit have been common culprits.

Feeding errors

Are an important cause of diarrhoea and vomiting in young babies. Particularly, feeding the wrong food can be responsible.

Pyloric stenosis

Projectile vomiting in the first few weeks of life. The child is hungry, miserable, and often dehydrated. On examination, a visible peristalsis or the palpation of a 'tumour' in the right hypochondrium. A test meal may aid diagnosis. Low sodium, chloride, and raised bicarbonate are often found. Diagnosis easily confirmed by ultra sound test.

Correction of dehydration

Oral rehydration

Oral rehydration with clear fluids or electrolyte solutions (e.g. Dioralyte/Rehidrat) is usually possible in mild dehydration. Small amounts frequently (e.g. hourly) are required up to 180 ml/kg for first 2 hours. After 24 hours, full strength milk is introduced. Persistent losses will necessitate hospital treatment after this time.

IV rehydration

If shock is present, commence with plasma 20 ml/kg over 25 minutes. If hypernatraemic, commence with plasma or 0.9 per cent saline, and replacement should be slower — rehydration taking 3–5 days.

Generally replacement is with 0.18 per cent saline in 4 per cent dextrose except in the above circumstances. (See Table 11.3.)

TABLE 11.3

Rehydration

Weight kg	5 per cent dehydration ml/hour	> 5 per cent dehydration ml/hour
2	12	17
3	19	25
4	25	33
5	31	42
6	40	50
7	44	58
8	50	67
9	56	75
10	63	83

TABLE 11.4

Maintenance IV fluid

Weight kg	Fluid mls/day	Na mmol/day	K⁺ mmol/day
<10	100–120/kg	2.5–3.5/kg	2.5–3.5/kg
10–20	90–120/kg	2–2.5/kg	2–2.5/kg
>20	50– 90/kg	1.5–2/kg	1.5–2/kg

Dehydration and fluid therapy

Any sick child may present with dehydration. Sick children require more fluid, and fluid requirement increases by 12 per cent for every degree centigrade rise in temperature.

Fluid replacement (litres) = percentage dehydration × body weight in kg. (See Tables 11.3, 11.4 and 11.5.)

Dehydration may be *Hypotonic* (sodium < 130 mmol/l; *Isotonic* (sodium 130–150 mmol/l); *Hypertonic* (sodium > 150 mmol/l).

The above signs may be absent in hypertonic dehydration so severity is underestimated. This can be very serious.

Abdominal pain in children

This can present many diagnostic difficulties. On the one hand, many childhood infections and illnesses present with 'tummy ache' — especially in younger children — though there is no abdominal pathology, and on the other hand acute appendicitis is notoriously difficult to diagnose in the infant and small child and is easily missed.

TABLE 11.5

Estimation of dehydration

<5% (mild)	Dry mucous membranes. Thirst. Skin turgidity.
5–10% (medium)	Worsening of above signs. Sunken eyes. Sunken fontanelle, tachycardia, oliguria, apathy.
>10–15% (severe)	Worsening of above signs. Drowsiness, hypotension. Peripheral shutdown.

Appendicitis

Though uncommon under age of 2 this should not deter you from making this diagnosis. In older children the diagnosis may be suggested by pain, tenderness over McBurney's point, vomiting, and fever, though classic signs are not always present. A small number of unnecessary laparotomies are preferable to a number of cases of peritonitis where the prognosis is much worse.

Intussusception

Characterised by colicky abdominal pain and rectal bleeding. Classically present are the 'red-currant jelly stools'. Attacks of pain are associated with vomiting. There may be a palpable mass, and bowel sounds are increased. Abdominal x-ray shows obstruction. The child is commonly less than 1 year old and often very ill. Diagnostic barium enema can sometimes reduce the intussusception — otherwise surgery is indicated urgently: resuscitation and correction of electrolyte status may be necessary first.

Inguinal hernia

Commonly congenital, can cause obstruction or damage to the testis if incarcerated.

Urinary tract infection (UTI)

Common in girls. Investigation for renal tract abnormality is indicated if recurrent.

Testicular torsion

Should not be forgotten, and may present as abdominal pain. If genitalia are not examined the diagnosis will be missed.

Examination of the abdomen

Liver

Normally palpable in infancy and in young children. 2 cm below costal margin is normal in babies.

Spleen

Tip often palpable in infants and small children.

Small bowel

Peristalsis often visible in thin or preterm babies.

Rectal

Examination is often unhelpful if the child is already distressed. Examination of the stool may be informative, however.

The skin

Skin diseases

1 Infantile seborrhoeic dermatitis

The child is usually less than 3 months old and presents with erythema and scaling which is usually flexural and in the axilla, behind the ears and on the face. There is a thick yellow scale on the scalp. It can often become secondarily infected with either bacteria or candida. The child is normally well.

Treatment

Topical steroid and antibiotic mix.

2 Atopic eczema (see adult)

Older than 3 months with a flexural erythematous eruption: there is usually a family history of eczema and also asthma or hayfever.

Treatment

Mild-topical steroid cream.

N.B. They are often susceptible to viral infections, e.g. herpes simplex, and molluscum contagiosum.

Nappy rash

The child develops erythema and there may be erosions, 85% are Monilia infections.

Treatment

Nystatin cream and frequent nappy changes.

4 Vascular naevi

  (a) Capillary — port wine stain

Treatment

Cosmetic cover.
Cryosurgery or laser treatment.

  (b) Cavernous/strawberry naevi.
       These increase in size over the first year and then over the succeeding years usually undergo spontaneous resolution.

No treatment

Reassure patient and parent.

5 Papular urticaria

Papular erythematous lesions which may vesiculate: they itch and scratching may lead to infection. They occur in crops often on the lower limbs: causes are insect bites or allergic reactions, for example to food dyes.

6 Juvenile plantar dermatitis

Fore-foot eczema with inter-digital cleft sparing. Occurs between the ages of 3 and 15 years.

Treatment

Regular cleaning of feet, cotton socks, mild steroid creams.

7 Allergic contact dermatitis (see adult)

8 Lip-licking dermatitis

Treatment

1 per cent hydrocortisone.

9 Epidermolysis bullosa

A group of genetic diseases, which vary in their severity and in-heritance, ranging from the commonest type (due to rare autosomal dominant gene), to the most severe lethal type (due to rare auto-somal recessive gene). All need dermatological referral for treatment and genetic counselling. Pre-natal treatment is now possible.

Burns

A child's head and trunk are proportionally larger than an adult's; therefore, the calculation of fluid replacement is slightly different. Calculate percentage area burned: complete chart (Fig. 11.1)

More than 10 per cent body surface area burned (BSB) will require fluid therapy IV.

$$\text{Give } \frac{\text{Percentage BSB} \times \text{weight in kg}}{2} \text{ mls in 1st 4 hours.}$$

Initially as colloid then crystalloid for metabolic requirements depending on severity and response. (Remember to calculate from time of burn, *not* time of arrival.) (See page 233.)

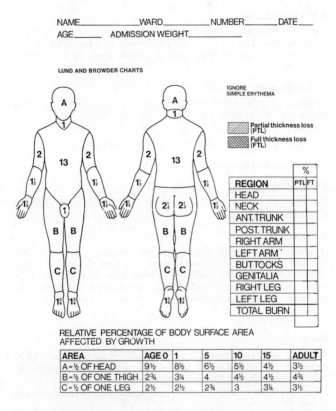

RELATIVE PERCENTAGE OF BODY SURFACE AREA
AFFECTED BY GROWTH

AREA	AGE 0	1	5	10	15	ADULT
A = ½ OF HEAD	9½	8½	6½	5½	4½	3½
B = ½ OF ONE THIGH	2¾	3¼	4	4½	4½	4¾
C = ½ OF ONE LEG	2½	2½	2¾	3	3¼	3½

Reproduced with the permission of Smith and Nephew Pharmaceuticals Ltd.

Figure 11.1 *Chart for estimating severity of burn wounds*

Analgesia

Small doses of IV opiate, e.g. papaveretum 0.2 mg/kg/8 hour.

Resuscitation

Resuscitation otherwise is as for adult burns and includes care of airway.

Treatment

- Monitoring of response to fluids by urine output and vital signs.
- Blood gas analysis and oxygen therapy.
- Replacement of blood where indicated depending upon severity.
- The threshold for admitting more minor burns should be lower than in the adult because of the difficulty of management of dressings in the child. Admit any child with burns to face, perineum, hands or burns more than 10 per cent.

  (See Tables 11.6 and 11.7.)

TABLE 11.6

| Resuscitation data | | | | | Size of bag |
Age	Heart rate	Systolic BP	Resp. rate	Tidal volume	for ventilation
Infant	<160	80	40	<20 mls	240–300 mls
Pre-school	<140	90	30		500 mls
				7–10 ml/kg	
School age	<120	100	20		500 mls
Post-puberty	<100	120	16	4–600 mls	Adult

Urine output in an infant should be at least 1–2 ml/kg/hr.

Failure to thrive

Normal heights and weights. (See Figures 11.2 and 11.3, page 156.)

Causes

1 *Poor feeding*

Neglect

Feeding problems: e.g. cleft palate; cerebral palsy. Vomiting — pyloric stenosis; vomiting — hiatus hernia.

2 *Failure of absorption*

Cystic fibrosis

Coeliac disease

Chronic infective diarrhoea

TABLE 11.7

Resuscitation data for children

Age	approx. wt kg	approx. maintenance fluid IV ml/hr	ET tube size mm	ET tube length (oral)	Defib paddle size	Defib charge J	Adrenaline dose of 1: 10,000	Atropine dose mcg
small neonate/prem	1.5	7.5	2.5	9.0		3–6	0.25	30
	1.75		3.0					
Larger neonate	3.5	17.5	3.5	10	4.5 cm	7–14	0.5	60
6 months	7.0	35	4.0	12		14–28	0.75	150
1 year	10	45	4.5	12		20–40	1.0	200
3 years	15	65	5.0	13		30–60	1.5	300
5 years	20	75	5.5	14	8 cm	40–80	2.0	400
7 years	22	80	6.0	16		45–90	2.5	450
10 years	30	85	6.5	17		60–120	3.0	600
15 years	50	110	7.0 + cuff	21		100–200	5.0	600

NB — Using paediatric giving set microdrops 60 drops = 1 ml: therefore No mls/hr = No drops 1 min eg 7.5 mls/hr = 7.5 drops/min.

    3 *Anorexia*
Chronic infection, e.g. urinary tract infection (UTI)
Heart failure
Metabolic disorders
    4 *Emotional deprivation*
Including NAI.

Sudden infant death syndrome

Sudden death in an infant between ages of 1 week and 2 years: this is very distressing for the parents. Typically the baby is apparently normal and healthy and then found dead in its cot. Peak incidence is between 2 and 5 months and is more common in boys. The infant may arrive dead but occasionally resuscitation has been attempted by parents or ambulance crew; this should be continued in the department until it is certain that the infant is beyond resuscitation.

Death should always be certified in the department and never in an ambulance.

A brief history should be obtained from parents of any recent infections, feeding, birth, health of the baby, etc.

It is necessary to consider the impact on parents and other members of the family who all need to be handled in an understanding manner in privacy where they can express grief and ask questions.
It will be necessary to involve:
- paediatrician
- social work department
- coroner's officer
- general practitioner and health visitor
- the hospital chaplain.

Foundation for the Study of Infant Deaths, Cot Death Research and Support — Information for Parents, 35 Belgrave Square, London SW1X 8QB. 071 235 1721.

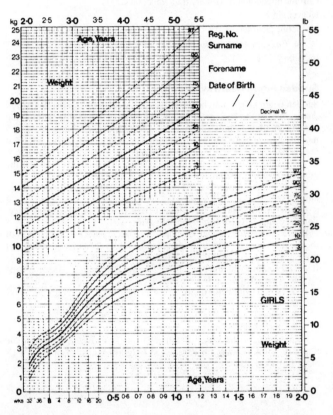

Figures 11.2 and 11.3 reproduced with the permission of Castlemead Publications.

Figure 11.2 *Weight standards chart for girls 0–5 years (J. M. Tanner and R. H. Whitehouse)*

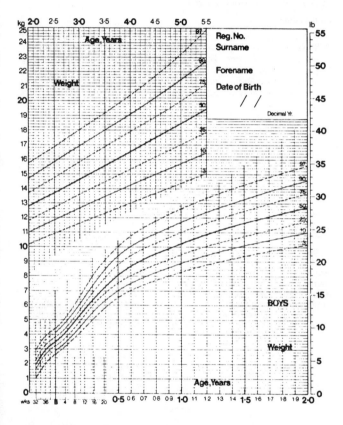

Figure 11.3 *Weight standards chart for boys 0–5 years (J. M. Tanner and R. H. Whitehouse)*

Fractures, sprains and dislocations

Treatment is generally along the lines as in the adult: however, certain areas are more commonly injured.

Pulled elbow

A very common condition in young children. There is often a history of walking hand in hand with an adult who pulls the child sharply onwards, or of swinging by the arms. The child refuses to use the arm and it hangs limply by the side. X-ray is normal. The condition is easily corrected by pronating and supinating the arm with a finger over the elbow. A click may be felt, and shortly afterwards the child is fully recovered and will resume the use of the arm.

   The condition is said to be caused by subluxation of the radial head from the annular ligament.

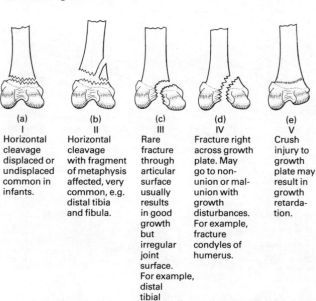

(a)	(b)	(c)	(d)	(e)
I	II	III	IV	V
Horizontal cleavage displaced or undisplaced common in infants.	Horizontal cleavage with fragment of metaphysis affected, very common, e.g. distal tibia and fibula.	Rare fracture through articular surface usually results in good growth but irregular joint surface. For example, distal tibial fracture.	Fracture right across growth plate. May go to non-union or mal-union with growth disturbances. For example, fracture condyles of humerus.	Crush injury to growth plate may result in growth retarda-tion.

Figure 11.4 *Classification of growth plate injuries (Salter)*

Sprains

Sprains do not generally occur in childhood, so post-traumatic pain and swelling arouse suspicion, e.g. a fracture or growth plate separation.

Disclocations

Rare in childhood, occasionally occur at elbow or hip. Dislocation of the patella may be traumatic or recurrent.

Fractures

Generally heal quicker than in adults. Common at distal radius, ulna, tibia. Often incomplete 'buckle fractures' or 'greenstick' fractures. One third of children's fractures involve a growth plate and can cause permanent damage to growth there. (Figure 11.4.)

Fracture tibia

Undisplaced spiral fracture tibia is common in toddlers.

Ankle

Sprains are rare. Injury is commonly to the distal growth plate tibia and fibula.

Associated arterial injury

The fracture associated with ischaemia is a fracture around the elbow joint, i.e. supracondylar fracture of humerus. If circulation is not rapidly restored, by reduction, and carefully watched, Volkman's ischaemic contracture is certain. Observe distal pulse, capillary return in finger nails and passive extension of fingers. If these are abnormal extend elbow. Always admit; elevate; observe.

Osgood Schlatter's disease

Painful swelling over tibial tubercle, usually in boys 10–15 years old. X-ray shows irregular ossification of the proximal tibial tubercle, often looking fragmented.

Spontaneous recovery is normal and most cases require no more than reassurance and rest from the provoking trauma. Very rarely symptoms necessitate a period of immobilisation.

Perthe's disease (avascular necrosis of femoral head)

Most common in boys, usually presenting with a painless limp — usually 5–10 years. There may be no x-ray changes but earliest sign is widening of joint space. There may also be 'uncovering' of femoral head out of the acetabulum, flattening, and irregularity. The child should be referred for orthopaedic assessment and follow-up. (Figure 11.5)

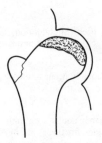

Figure 11.5 *Perthes' disease*

Irritable hip

This, unlike others, is a benign condition usually affecting children between 2 and 12 years. It presents with a limp and limitation of movement. There is often pain and tenderness. X-ray is normal. Important differential diagnosis is from Perthe's or septic arthritis, or slipped femoral epiphysis in the older child.

Slipped capital femoral epiphysis

Obese children; boys 12–16 years and girls 10–14 years. Pain in the hip or referred to the knee with a limp or cannot put the knee of the affected side over to the opposite shoulder. X-ray, AP and lateral, shows displacement of the epiphysis downwards and posteriorly. *Refer.*

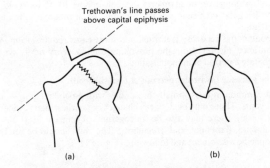

Figure 11.6 *Slipped capital femoral epiphysis*

Non-accidental injury and child abuse

This is a very specialist topic. The family implications of making this diagnosis are far reaching but the implications for the child of missing the diagnosis are even more serious, and in some cases fatal. If you suspect the diagnosis at all refer the child at once to a paediatrician for admission and/or involve a senior member of the Accident department. It is much safer to admit the child whilst the exact mode of injury and social circumstances are checked than to risk further injury. There is usually no need at this stage to confront the parents with your suspicions; a careful and detailed history should be taken, if possible from several different persons and the child. Undress the child fully and examine all parts, not just the injury. Make careful records with diagrams. Discussions with the general practitioner may be helpful in obtaining further background history. The family may already be known to social services. However, the absence of significant past history from these sources should not deter you from your diagnosis if the clinical signs are suspicious.

Features which should arouse suspicion

1 Delay — inexplicable delay — in seeking medical attention.
2 Discrepancy — between the appearance of the injury and the description of the mechanism of injury given by parents.
3 Disturbed behaviour or unusual reaction on the part of the parents in relation to the child's injury or reluctance to give information.
4 Injuries of different ages on the child, e.g. old bruises and cuts as well as the new injury.
5 History of attendance with previous injury either by child or a sibling (check 'at risk register').
6 Failure to thrive, obvious neglect, deprivation.
7 Unusually withdrawn child, or abnormal reactions to parents.

Particular injuries which should arouse suspicion

1 *Bruising*
    (a) especially on a baby less than 8 months old.
    (b) especially if on the cheek or head.
    (c) if bizarre — consider human bites.
        — 'grip' and 'pinch' marks.
        — printing from use of implements, e.g. belts, sticks, etc.
    (d) if multiple.
    (e) if of different stages of maturity.

2 *Black eyes*

Especially the type suggestive of fracture base of skull.

3 *Multiple sub-ungual haematomata.*

4 *Retinal and sub-hyaloid haemorrhage.*

5 *Fractures*

   (a) especially child less than 1 year of age.
   (b) rib fractures, especially multiple.
   (c) multiple fractures.
   (d) old multiple healed fractures. ⎱ May be revealed on skeletal
   ⎰ survey.

   (e) epiphyseal displacement.
   (f) double contour of periosteum on x-ray.
   (g) cortical thickening on x-ray.

6 *Burns and scalds*

   (a) circular burns or scalds — suspect cigarette burns.
   (b) old burn scars.
   (c) scalds in young children.
   (d) scald of legs or buttocks, but not hands or feet, from putting in
       boiling water.

7 *Bruising or laceration around the mouth*

Look for a torn frenulum — caused by ramming a fist or bottle into the
mouth.

Sexual abuse

Sexual abuse of children more usually comes to light after specific allega-
tions or after clues picked up from a child's behaviour or response.
Physical signs are frequently absent, and if present are often non-specific.
General signs may include failure to thrive, signs of neglect, recurrent
abdominal pain, recurrent UTI, faecal soiling or constipation, enuresis,
emotional problems.

   More specific signs may include vulval or anal soreness, tears or genital
bleeding, venereal disease, including pharyngeal gonorrhoea, absent
hymen, widened vaginal canal.

   The implications of diagnosing sexual abuse are far reaching. It is totally
inappropriate to carry out an extensive examination in the Accident
department, or to go into detailed questioning of the child or family. If the
question of sexual abuse arises in casualty as a presenting complaint, or in
the course of examination for other reasons, then the case is best referred
to the paediatric department initially as with cases of non-accidental
injury. The confirmation of the diagnosis is best handled by paediatricians, social workers, and police surgeons, experienced in dealing with
such cases. New protocols may be developed in the light of recent legal
enquiries.

TABLE 11.8

Dosages at a glance

Age	Wt kg	Percentages of adult dose
2 months	3.2	10%
4 months	6.5	15%
1 year	10	25%
5 years	18	33%
7 years	23	50%
12 years	37	75%

IPECACUANHA (paediatric syrup)	– up to 1 year 10 mls over 1 year 15 mls
SALBUTAMOL	– 2.5 mg i.e. 2.5 mls of 0.1% solution (Nebules) or 0.5 mls of 0.5% sol (nebuliser solution) diluted to 2 mls in saline.
PARACETAMOL (paediatric syrup)	– 60–120 mg (½–1 teaspoon) under 1 yr 120–250 mg (1–2 teaspoon) 1–5 yrs 250–500 mg over 5 yrs
PAPAVERETUM (omnopon) IM	– up to 1 yr 200 mcg/1 kg – over 1 yr 200–300 mcg/1kg } dilute 10 mg up to 10 mls with water for injection. This then contains 100 mcg 1 ml

¼ to ½ of above dose may be given IV.

ASPIRIN — *do not use in children under 12 years because of association between Reye's Syndrome and use of aspirin.*

NOTES

12

The elderly

Accident and Emergency departments in hospitals are now used more by the elderly. With the increased proportion of elderly people in the general population, and with a projected increase in the total number of elderly into the next century, attention must be paid to the needs of this age group. The attendance rate increases as the patient becomes older, and particularly in those who have social and physical isolation. The elderly single, widowed, and divorced will often use the A & E department in preference to other methods of obtaining primary medical care. In patients over 85 years especially, self-referral and the use of 999 ambulances will increase. The pain and loss of function of comparatively minor injuries will interfere with the patient's ability to live alone at home. The majority of patients will be able to return home after treatment, but special care needs to be taken in arranging support where needed to avoid early return to hospital.

The major causes for attendance are falls, faints, confusional states, hypothermia, wandering, and sometimes just inability to cope. Overdose is more significant in the elderly, and social and psychogeriatric factors are more of a problem. In trauma cases, because of the osteoporosis of age, a higher proportion of patients have fractures. They also die at a higher rate for the same amount of injury.

In addition to the normal medical history, more details of social circumstances need to be recorded and taken into account in deciding treatment and disposal. These factors will enable requests for social services to be made sooner.

- Where does the patient live?
- If alone, what help would he have from caring family, friends, neighbours, or GP?
- If living with family, is it spouse or children?
- What existing social services are used: home help, meals on wheels, or District Nurse?
- If sheltered accommodation, will the injury cause difficulties?
- If old people's home, will there be nursing supervision?

Communication

Many patients in this age group are hard of hearing and this can pose a problem. Communicators, with an amplifier between a microphone and earpiece, can give distortion-free amplification of speech. This can be very useful in a busy department.

Confusion

Whilst four out of five over the age of 80 are rational, the others will have grossly impaired cognitive functions. Other elderly patients who are not demented are easily confused following a fall, a fit, infection, or trauma. These confusional states are transient but it is important to establish whether they were present before the injury/illness.

Mild confusional states initially may cause slowness in thinking, but later disorientation in space and time may be present. Such confusion should be carefully noted for comparison with the later condition. It may also alter the patient's recollection of the occasion, examination, and treatment and this may have medico-legal significance for the department.

Gross confusion will be associated with paranoid ideas, with abnormal ideation, frank delusions, and hallucinations. Rarely it will be associated with anti-social behaviour such as abusive language and violence towards members of staff. Tranquillisers are best avoided before a psychogeriatric opinion is obtained, but it may be necessary to use neuroleptic agents before the diagnosis is established.

Additional information, on previous illnesses, what medications the patient is receiving, and any allergies he suffers from, should be obtained from relatives, friends, or even the home help. Unaccompanied patients present a particular problem and the help of a social worker can be invaluable. The patient's GP can also help with the above information.

Examination

Differences in the norm are seen in the examination of the older patient. The pulse rate in elderly patients is normally 70 beats per minute at rest. A slow pulse should alert you to the possibility that the patient is hypothermic, has raised intracranial pressure, or is jaundiced. Few old people have sufficient athletic training to cause bradycardia, but some may be taking beta blockers which cause a slow pulse. Heart block is an important possible cause and may contribute to syncope and a fall.

Mental state

A simple quick assessment of the patient's mental state can be useful when deciding whether a patient is confused, their normal state has changed, or they are demented. Simple questions are used:

1 Their own age.
2 Date of birth.
3 Today's date.
4 The present and past prime ministers.

The answers give a fair indication of state of short- and long-term memory. These can be recorded and repeated.

The eyes

The pupillary reaction is marginally slower and reduced in amplitude in elderly patients. Many drugs which they may be taking, such as opiates, can influence the size of the pupils. Arcus senilis, the concentric deposit of cholesterol around the iris, has no great diagnostic significance in the elderly.

Bruising

Many elderly people suffer from senile purpura and spontaneous bruising occurs readily. This results from an age-related reduction of elastic and collagen fibres in the subcutaneous tissue. Subconjunctival haemorrhages which also resolve spontaneously are not uncommon in the elderly.

Blood pressure

The blood pressure should be taken both sitting and standing as postural hypotension is a cause for the elderly patient to fall. It is usually caused by drugs like hypotensive agents and diuretics.

Auscultation

Heart

Some 50 per cent of elderly patients have a systolic murmur. These murmurs are important only if there are other signs of cardiac failure or pyrexia. If found as an isolated observation they may not have any significance.

Lungs

Some crackles may be heard over the lung bases. These are only significant if they do not clear on coughing. Otherwise pneumonia and heart failure can be misdiagnosed when not present.

Abdominal signs

A rectal examination will often demonstrate constipation, or occasionally a tumour which may account for confusion or general deterioration. Urinalysis may also be helpful.

Neurology

The ankle jerks are frequently absent in elderly patients. In many healthy old people the vibration sense might not be present over the antero-superior iliac spine.

Management

After a careful history and examination, it should be possible to reach a diagnosis. Do not forget that the elderly often suffer from multiple complaints and it is usual to make a number of diagnoses. A patient who suffers from heart failure associated with ischaemic heart disease, diabetes, or chronic bronchitis may now be suffering from hypothermia in addition.

Elderly patients have great difficulty in maintaining the *milieu interieur:* intravenous fluids, given with care, may be required to restore hydration. When rapid atrial fibrillation is present, digitalisation may be required. Remember that in the elderly with fractures moderate blood loss might be significant and oxygenation with restoration of circulation should be carried out at an early stage. Early treatment of fractures in the elderly, particularly those affecting mobility, is not only essential but life-saving.

These patients rapidly develop pressure areas, so should be placed on soft foam mattresses on trolleys; fractures should be splinted efficiently and then the patient should be moved quickly to an orthopaedic ward and a proper bed.

Problem list

In addition to the medical and surgical diagnoses, the casualty officer should draw up a problem list.

1 Can the patient walk unaided or not; does he fall frequently; does he live alone; can he look after himself?
2 Which problems have been adequately compensated, for example:

    (a) can walk safely with a frame, and has a frame;
    (b) room-bound but has a commode in the room;
    (c) cannot get in and out of bed unaided, but has a District Nurse who comes twice a day;
    (d) diabetes is adequately controlled by diet, but the patient has retinopathy and impairment of vision.

Drugs

Remember that in the elderly excretion of drugs is often impaired and the half-life is extended. Their reaction may also differ. When drug treatment is required, the existing regimen should be identified so that no interacting medications are given. Refer to *BNF*.

Among analgesics, paracetamol and aspirin have little effect on the mind, while stronger analgesics like codeine or dextropropoxyphene are more likely to cause confusion.

Among the tranquillisers, thioridazine in small doses seems to be well tolerated in the elderly.

In cases with left ventricular failure and pulmonary oedema, frusemide should be used to start diuresis.

Discharge of elderly patients

It is important to assess the patient's capability for returning home and to realise that the patient's independence may be lost. The cause of attendance at the hospital, accident or illness, may affect the independence of those elderly patients who were barely coping before. Although the patient may already be receiving some assistance at home there may be a need for further immediate help.

Patients attending the A & E department will fall into four groups:

A Discharged with no social help.
B Discharged but will need help.
C Discharged with immediate social help.
D Admitted (i) for social reasons; (ii) for specific medical cause.

There is a need to realise that A and B have a very narrow boundary and the early provision of social help may be needed in A to avoid later problems. Similarly group C and D (i) are closely related and with immediate help in the community, if possible from a community discharge team, admission to hospital may not be necessary. The use of overnight observation beds will often help in sorting out the patient's real needs and enabling the proper services to be obtained during the day. There is a need carefully to assess the patient and his home circumstances — e.g. to make sure that a patient with a broken arm in plaster, who is unable to use a key, is not discharged to an empty house in the early hours of the morning. Liaison with the district nurses from your nursing staff, about dressings and review of bandaging, may obviate troublesome journeys with long hours of waiting and travelling by ambulance. The patient's GP should always be notified of the patient's treatment, diagnosis, and return to home, with a request for an early visit.

A community liaison officer, Age Concern, or the social services, should also be notified when the patient is over 70 and has any disability.

NOTES

NOTES

13

The central nervous system

Head injuries

Acceleration or deceleration trauma from road traffic accidents (RTA), fighting, or sport, causes most of the head injuries seen in A & E. At the moment of impact, shearing stress and contusion cause displacement or distortion of brain tissue, particularly on sudden deceleration. The subsequent neuronal damage is related to the degree of stretch. See Figure 13.1. Patients in coma need their airway clearing urgently; intubation; and in traumatic shock restoration of the circulating blood volume. The effects of hypoxia, hypoxaemia and hypotension soon cause further injury to the damaged neurones. High-velocity accidents usually cause other severe injuries which will require specific treatment urgently in A & E.

The scalp

Lacerations bleed profusely, but haemorrhage can be stopped by direct pressure on wound edges after putting a gauze swab on the wound. Occasionally with torrential haemorrhage it is necessary to put 3 strong sutures through all layers to gain time.

Infection is not common because of the abundant blood supply, but it is still essential to clean the wounds and excise dead or contaminated tissue. Shave the wound edges first to ensure good apposition of the skin. *All scalp wounds must be probed to exclude an unsuspected fracture.* This fracture is compound with all the dangers of osteomyelitis, meningitis, and abscess formation.

Concussion

There has been a paralysis of function: the brief loss of consciousness is associated with neuronal stretch and may be followed by a post-concussional syndrome of varying severity.

Contusion

With sliding of the grey matter in relation to white rupture of fibres at various levels occurs: the clinical picture is more severe. Unconsciousness is more prolonged and recovery takes longer. Confusion, cerebral irritability, and shallow respiration are seen initially. On recovery the patient curls up and resents attention.

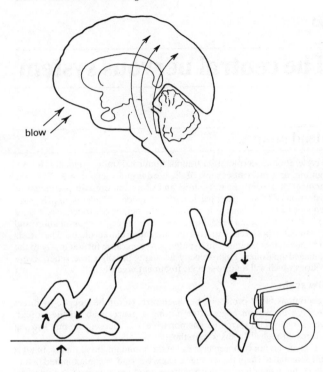

Figure 13.1 *Shearing force acting on the brain*

Laceration

Brain laceration and brain stem damage are indicated by signs of severe damage: deep coma, dilated pupils, Cheyne-Stokes' respiration and irregular pulse.

Cerebral compression

Accumulating blood — extradural, subdural, or intracerebral plus oedema — leads to raised intracranial pressure. If there has been a lucid interval, the headache becomes more severe, vomiting occurs, and the level of consciousness falls. If already semiconscious, the patient becomes more restless and fails to react to stimuli. The pupil dilates on the side of

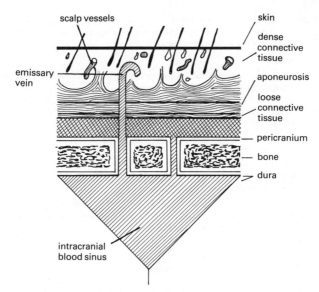

Figure 13.2 *Scalp and cranium. The scalp consists of five layers:*
S   *Skin*
C   *Connective tissue (superficial fascia)*
A   *Aponeurosis (galea aponeurotica or epicranial aponeurosis)*
L   *Loose connective tissue*
P   *Pericranium or periosteum*

the compression and does not react to light. Respiration becomes noisy and the pulse rate drops; these changes may happen very quickly as a critical pressure is reached.

Muscle power weakens and reflexes disappear, initially on the same side, but later — sadly too late — on both sides. With close observation and anticipation the serious head injury should avoid these catastrophic complications.

Clinical examination

Clinical examination should be thorough, timed, recorded, and repeated if there are any problems or doubts.

History

This should be taken from the ambulance crew or police. You need to know a brief description of the accident and the best level of consciousness between accident and arrival in A & E. Was he alert, speaking, rousable, reacting to pain from other injuries, or not showing any response? Is there retrograde or post-traumatic amnesia?

Examination

Carefully examine the cervical spine for tenderness or deformity: if there is any suspicion of injury apply a firm cervical collar or traction: x-ray through the collar. Be aware of the dangers of missing a lesion, look at C7, particularly if the patient is drunk or unconscious. If you are worried, go with him to the x-ray department yourself; do not leave the patient with a young nurse — the responsibility is still yours!

The Glasgow coma scale

The patient is assessed and his responses are measured to give a score which is suitable for comparison later. It is recorded, with pupils, pulse, and blood pressure, on a proper chart.

Pupils

Record size and reaction or whether the eye is closed by swelling. Inspect the fundi for haemorrhage or papilloedema.

Cranial nerves

    1 Olfactory: loss of smell, blood from nose.
    2 Normal vision, any loss or hemianopia.
    3⎫
    4⎬Nystagmus, double vision, or isolated lesion.
    6⎭
    5 Anaesthesia to touch or brush.
    7 Weakness.
    8 Blood from ear, whisper at 3 feet.

Reflexes

Record as manikin, note whether depressed or brisk.

Power

Record voluntary contractions of shoulder, elbow, hand, hip, knee, and foot.

Record involuntary movements

Localisation, flexion or extension, or no reaction to painful stimulus.

Sensation

Draw area of loss.

Draw any injuries to head and face

This is often of great value later when writing medico-legal reports.

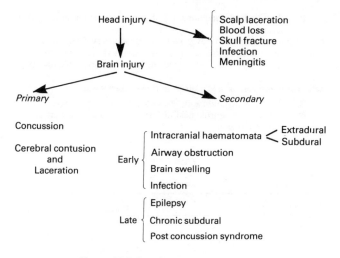

Figure 13.3 *Complications of a head injury*

X-rays

One of many problems associated with head injuries is whether to x-ray the skull or not. Radiologists say that we x-ray too many: the neuro-surgeon says that if a fracture is not shown then the risk of extradural haemorrhage is minimal. A policy should be clearly stated.

X-ray patients with one or more of the following:

- loss of consciousness/amnesia for 5 minutes
- neurological symptoms or signs
- CSF or blood from nose or ears
- suspected or obvious penetrating injury
- scalp bruising or swelling, often easier to feel when in the hair
- those difficult to assess, e.g. children, epileptics, drunks

It is important that the airway is cleared; with intubation in coma. With multiple injuries adequate treatment of shock must start immediately. Fractures must be adequately splinted.

Admit for observation those patients with

- confusion at time of examination: fracture
- abnormal neurological signs or vomiting or headaches
- difficult to assess/social reasons with no one to watch patient

● other medical conditions, e.g. haemophilia or on anticoagulant
  therapy.

This excludes those who have made a full recovery from brief post-
traumatic amnesia. All patients who are not admitted must be given a head
injury card, which they can understand and give to a responsible relation.

Refer to the surgeons or neurosurgeons those patients with

● fractures with confusion, fits, or focal neurological signs
● confusion or neurological disturbance lasting overnight in the
  observation ward

TABLE 13.1

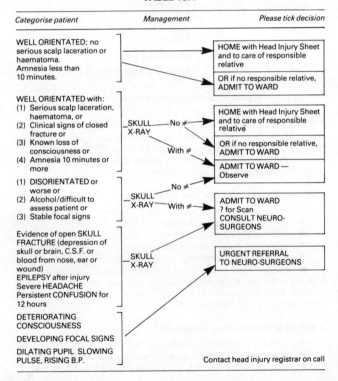

Categorise patient	Management	Please tick decision
WELL ORIENTATED; no serious scalp laceration or haematoma. Amnesia less than 10 minutes.		HOME with Head Injury Sheet and to care of responsible relative
		OR if no responsible relative, ADMIT TO WARD
WELL ORIENTATED with: (1) Serious scalp laceration, haematoma, or (2) Clinical signs of closed fracture or (3) Known loss of consciousness or (4) Amnesia 10 minutes or more	SKULL X-RAY — No #	HOME with Head Injury Sheet and to care of responsible relative
		OR if no responsible relative, ADMIT TO WARD
	With #	ADMIT TO WARD — Observe
(1) DISORIENTATED or worse or (2) Alcohol/difficult to assess patient or (3) Stable focal signs	SKULL X-RAY — No # / With #	ADMIT TO WARD ? for Scan CONSULT NEURO-SURGEONS
Evidence of open SKULL FRACTURE (depression of skull or brain, C.S.F. or blood from nose, ear or wound) EPILEPSY after injury Severe HEADACHE Persistent CONFUSION for 12 hours	SKULL X-RAY	URGENT REFERRAL TO NEURO-SURGEONS
DETERIORATING CONSCIOUSNESS DEVELOPING FOCAL SIGNS DILATING PUPIL SLOWING PULSE, RISING B.P.		Contact head injury registrar on call

- deteriorating level of consciousness following resuscitation
- suspected open or depressed fracture
- deterioration of any kind

All these would benefit from a CT scan.

Facial injuries

Seatbelts prevent the gross facial fractures but there are still many injuries from assaults, falls, and sport, etc. The face swells rapidly after a blow and depressed fractures of the zygoma and nose can easily be missed. Always examine the facial contours: palpate the cheek, orbit, nose, and check airway, teeth and bite for signs of fracture. In 'blowout' fractures of the orbit diplopia, restricted eye movements and anaesthesia of infraorbital nerve are found.

The facial bones unite very quickly so if delay in getting definitive treatment occurs extensive surgery will be required. If you have any doubts, consult the maxillo-facial surgeon early before the swelling has subsided.

X-rays of the face

The facial skeleton does not show well on the standard skull X-rays so always ask for occipito-mental (OM) views for maxilla or zygomatic fractures; mandible views for lower jaw; nose for nasal injury. Check for fluid levels in the maxillary, ethmoidal, and sphenoidal air sinuses.

Treatment

Abrasions are often impregnated with dirt; this must be removed immediately, or permanent ugly tattooing will occur. In bad cases a GA and a scrubbing brush are necessary, but use the brush gently.

Lacerations need minimal excision, but all dead tissue must be removed completely. Particular care is required at the mucocutaneous junction of the lip and at the eyebrow to get the alignment right. Wounds should be sutured in layers with deep fine 4 0 catgut and for skin 5 or 6 0 prolene on atraumatic needles. (See suturing, page 269.)

Incised wounds often involve damage to deep structures, nerve, muscle, or parotid gland and duct. If long, deep, or complicated refer to surgeons. Smaller ones do well with a combination of 6 0 sutures and steristrips. Remember to remove sutures from the face at 5 days; steristrips can then be applied for another 5 days on long wounds.

PLEASE RECORD WITH LINKED DOTS (*NOT* TICKS) TO MAKE A GRAPH AS WITH A
TEMPERATURE CHART

COMA SCALE:

1) <u>Eyes open</u>

— Spontaneously	All self evident,
— To speech	not a good indicator
— To pain	of conscious level
— None (no opening)	alone.

2) *Best* verbal response

Orientated — Knows, name, place, year, season and month.

Confused conversation — Attention held, conversational response, but disorientated and confused.

Inappropriate words — Intelligible articulation, non-conversational, abusive or swear words.

Incomprehensible sounds — Moans and groans, no recognisable words.

None — None.

3) *Best* motor response — Best arm response usually recorded, do not misinterpret reflex grasping.

Obeys commands — Best response. If negative use painful stimulus.

Localise pain — Causes the limb to move in an attempt to remove the stimulus.

Flexion to pain — Can vary in degree.

Extension to pain — U.L. : Arm adducted and extended at elbow, forearm pronated.

— L.L. : Extension at hip and knee, plantar flexion of foot.

None — None.

BLOOD PRESSURE, TEMPERATURE, PULSE AND RESPIRATION:
Record in the usual way.

LIMB MOVEMENT:

First three sections refer to voluntary movement, last three to painful stimuli.

Normal power — Self evident.

Mild weakness — Can move the limb against gravity.

Severe weakness — Flicker movement to power unable to overcome gravity.

Spastic flexion — Shoulder abduction, elbow flexion, hand closed, increased tone.

Extension — As for extension to pain above.

No response — No response.

FITS:
If fits occur put 'F' at bottom of chart and record details on a separate fit chart.

Figure 13.4 *Guy's Health District neurological observation chart*

GUY'S HOSPITAL

ACCIDENT AND EMERGENCY DEPARTMENT

HEAD INJURIES ONLY

SURNAME		A & E No.
FIRST NAMES		UNIT No.

Source	Classification	Disposal	ADDRESS

Source		Classification		Disposal	
G.P.	☐	RTA		ADMITTED	☐
SELF	☐	F/S PASSENGER	☐		
POLICE	☐	B/S PASSENGER	☐	TREATED TO CONCLUSION	☐
OTHER HOS.	☐	CYCLIST	☐		
		PEDESTRIAN	☐	DIED	☐
MODE OF ARRIVAL		HOME ACCIDENT	☐		
		WORKS ACCIDENT	☐	G.P.	☐
		SPORT	☐	O.P.D.	☐
AMBULANCE	☐	SELF INFLICTED	☐		
OTHER	☐	OTHER	☐	OTHER	☐

DATE OF BIRTH	MARITAL STATE	RELIGION
OCCUPATION/SCHOOL		DATE/TIME
OWN DOCTOR/ADDRESS		

BRIEF DESCRIPTION OF ACCIDENT: TIME

Ambulance Crew Treatment		
	IV Fluid	
	ET Tube	

TETANUS IMMUNIZATION	RELATIVE INFORMED	
If already immunized – Year of course	BY HOSPITAL	☐
New course commenced	BY POLICE	☐

BEST level of consciousness between Accident and Arrival in A/E: Definite period

ALERT		ROUSABLE		ANOXIA		
SPOKE		REACTED TO PAIN		HYPOTENSION		NO RESPONSE

INITIAL EXAMINATION   Time: Medical Officer examining:

COMA SCALE	EVM SCORE		POST TRAUMATIC AMNESIA	P.T.A. FOR MINOR INJURY		

EYES OPEN		BEST VERBAL RESPONSE		BEST MOTOR RESPONSE	
Spontaneously	E4	Orientated	V5	Obey commands	M5
To speech	3	Confused	4	Localize pain	4
To pain	2	Inappropriate Words	3	Flexion to pain	3
None	1	Incomprehensible Sounds	2	Extension to pain	2
		None	1	None	1

PUPILS:

		R	L					H	L
+ REACTS	REACTION				FUNDI:	NORMAL			
− NO REACTION	SIZE					HAEMORRHAGES			
c EYE CLOSED BY SWELLING									

PUPIL SCALE (mm):   • • ● ● ● ● ● ●
          1   2   3   4   5   6   7   8

CRANIAL NERVES	R	L	III, IV, VI	R	L		R	L
I. BLOOD FROM NOSE			NYSTAGMUS			V. ANALGESIA		
LOSS OF SMELL			DISCONJUGATION			VII. WEAKNESS		
II. NORMAL VISION			DEVIATION			VIII. BLOOD FROM EAR		
LOSS OF VISION						WHISPER AT 3ft		
HAEMIANOPIA			ISOLATED LESION III					
			VI					

REFLEXES:	B.J.	T.J.	S.J.	K.J.	A.J.	P	ABDOMINAL.
RIGHT							
LEFT							

POWER	Shoulder	Elbow	Hand	Hip	Knee	Foot	
VOLUNTARY: RIGHT							(GRADE 0-5)
LEFT							

SENSATION: Describe loss:

GUY'S HOSPITAL, S.E.1.
ACCIDENT & EMERGENCY DEPT.
Telephone: 01 407 7600 Ext. 2556

Name		
Date		Time

HEAD INJURIES

You should return immediately to the Accident Department of the Hospital if you experience any of the following symptoms:—

SEVERE HEADACHE

INCREASING DROWSINESS

VOMITING

FITS OR CONVULSIONS

**ANY OTHER UNUSUAL
                    SYMPTOM**

If you live some distance from Guy's you should contact your own doctor without delay.

GH 448

When you first attend the Accident and Emergency Department you may be examined by a medical student in addition to the casualty officer. In a teaching hospital we have to train doctors of the future, thus students may be present during your treatment. Although this may involve some waiting during your attendance this is not only in their interest but in yours and other patients.

We try to keep waiting time as short as possible but several hundred patients are seen each day and serious cases must take precedence over less urgent conditions.

If you have been treated for a head injury or an accident the following notes will apply to you and should be read carefully.

ACCIDENTS

You should return immediately to the Accident Department of the Hospital if the pain of your injury gets worse or if other symptoms develop.

If a plaster of paris or other splint has been applied, keep the injured limb elevated as far as possible—in a sling or resting on a chair. The limb and plaster should be kept dry, exposed to the air and away from direct heat. You should return without delay if the plaster or splint causes pain or if the fingers or toes of the limb in plaster go blue or white or become cold.

If you live some distance from Guy's you should contact your own doctor at once.

Please turn over

Figure 13.5 *Guy's Hospital head injury card*

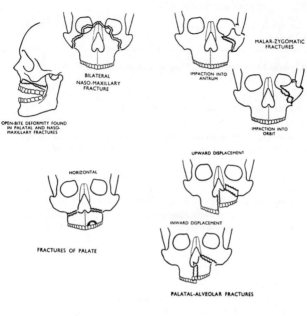

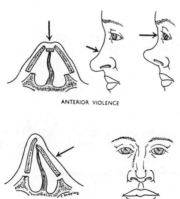

Figure 13.6 *Facio-maxillary fractures*

Coma

A system for management of the unconscious patient

Airway

Correct hypoxia: positioning of patient. Protection of airway with Guedel's airway or endotracheal tube, suction.

Breathing

Ventilation — ? respiratory stimulant — naloxone 0.8–2 mg initially.

O_2 therapy — 40–50 per cent concentration unless respiratory failure suspected.

Circulation

Assess and treat shock. Check pulse and BP. ECG monitor. Fluid therapy: obtain early IV access on all unconscious patients.

During the initial resuscitation check the history. Obvious findings on superficial examination may have already given clues to the diagnosis.

- signs of trauma
- neurological signs – papilloedema
- neck rigidity – pyrexia

Draw blood for

- FBC – Glucose — dextrostix/BM stix
- Electrolytes – Blood gases (arterial)
- Toxicology if drugs are suspected

X-rays

- Cervical spine on *all* unconscious head injuries
- Skull if *trauma* is suspected – Chest

Alcohol

Never assume depressed conscious level is due to alcohol alone — always positively exclude other pathology first. Check blood alcohol for a base line.

Overdose

If any overdose is suspected perform gastric lavage after protection of airway with cuffed endotracheal tube and send stomach washings for toxicology analysis.

Coma: causes of depression of level of consciousness

Trauma

1 Head injury
2 Multiple injury (secondary to hypotension, hypoxia, etc.)

Intracranial events

1 Epilepsy

2 'Stroke'
3 Subarachnoid haemorrhage
4 Tumour
5 Hypertensive crises
6 Subdural haematoma

Toxic

1 Poisoning by
    (a) drugs
        (i) self poisoning
        (ii) iatrogenic
    (b) chemicals
    (c) gases
2 Metabolic

(a) hyperglycaemia	(i) acidosis
(b) hypoglycaemia	(j) hypothyroidism
(c) hepatic coma	(k) hypopituitrism
(d) renal failure	(l) hypoadrenalism
(e) dehydration	(m) hypo and hypercalcaemia
(f) polydipsia	
(g) water intoxication	
(h) inappropriate ADH	

Infective

1 Meningitis
2 Encephalitis
3 Abscess
4 Secondary to infection/hyperpyrexia of other origin

Cerebral deprivation

1 Circulation
    (a) vasovagal
    (b) cardiac arrest/arrhythmia
    (c) hypovolaemia/hypotension
    (d) tamponade
2 Oxygen
    (a) airway obstruction
        (i) foreign body
        (ii) asthma
        (iii) chronic obstructive airway disease (COAD)
    (b) pneumothorax
    (c) consolidation/collapse
    (d) drowning
    (e) anaemia

Other

    (a) hypothermia
    (b) hyperpyrexia
    (c) hysteria

Syncope

- Epilepsy
- Transient ischaemic attacks
- Vertebrobasilar ischaemia
- Hypoglycaemia
- Cardiac arrhythmia/Stokes Adams attacks
- Pulmonary embolus
- Vasovagal
- Orthostatic as in intravascular volume depletion, antihypertensives, phenothiazines, diabetes
- Subclavian steal syndrome
- Cough, micturition syncope
- Hyperventilation

Convulsions

Fits

Can be secondary to treatable pathology, e.g. hypoglycaemia, arrhythmia, hypoxia, hypertension, drugs. Check for these.

Emergency treatment

- Protect the patient from harm by safe positioning and removal of harmful objects, but do not try to restrain forcibly.
- Airway — O_2 via face mask.
  An airway or soft gag may be inserted as soon as possible, but do not try to force this.
- Establish IV access — to enable anti-epileptic therapy to be given.
- Check glucose with a Dextrostix/BM stix. Give dextrose if low.
- Check calcium.

Drugs for use in a convulsion

(i) *Diazepam*: 10 mg IV slowly until fitting stops. Often up to 20 mg needed in adults. (0.2–0.3 mg/kg in children.) Works rapidly by IV. Does *not* work IM or subcutaneously. Can also be given rectally with good effect — very useful in children where IV access is difficult.

(ii) *Paraldehyde*: 5 ml into each buttock by deep IM injection. Useful if IV access impossible but can cause great irritation. (Must be given as soon as drawn up because it dissolves plastic syringes.)

(iii) *Thiopentone*: 25–100 mg slowly IV; watch for respiratory depression.

(iv) *Chlormethiazole*: 0.8 per cent solution for infusion — rapidly until fit stops, then slow down to minimal speed possible to control fitting. Useful because rapidly reversible on stopping infusion. Watch for hypotension.

Status epilepticus

Defined as two or more major fits without recovery of consciousness, or any fit lasting longer than 30 minutes (post-ictal unconsciousness lasting more than 30 minutes should be regarded with suspicion unless large amounts of sedative drugs have been given).

Treat as for convulsions. Large doses may be needed and you should be prepared to support respiration should respiratory depression occur.

Continuation of an infusion of anticonvulsant after control of the fit is usually required. This may be in the form of:

   (i) *Chlormethiazole:* 0.8 per cent infusion — easily reversed on stopping.

  (ii) *Diazepam:* 100 mg in 500 ml saline — tendency to accumulate.

 (iii) *Phenytoin* — 18 mg/kg in Normal saline infused at a rate no greater than 50 mg/min whilst cardiac rhythm is monitored. Contraindicated in 2nd or 3rd degree A–V block. IM route leads to tissue change.

      Drug of first choice in convulsions associated with head trauma as it does not depress level of consciousness.

 (iv) *Thiopentone:* 1 g in 500 ml saline — watch for respiratory depression.

Very occasionally if fitting is prolonged and cannot be aborted by large doses of anticonvulsants, severe hypoxia results. In such cases, intubation and ventilation are indicated, using muscle relaxant drugs to achieve this if necessary (e.g. Suxamethonium 50–100 mg IV).

Cerebro-vascular accident (CVA)

The classic 'stroke' may vary in presentation from mild unilateral weakness, speech defect, or visual field defect, to deep coma. It may be impossible to determine from the history and initial examination in A & E whether stroke is due to:

   (a) Cerebral haemorrhage
   (b) Thrombosis
   (c) Embolus.

Other causes of loss of consciousness must be excluded and treated. It is important to differentiate between primary CVA and an underlying treatable condition such as embolus or leaking cerebral aneurysm.

Conditions which may masquerade as CVA

  1 Post-ictal states — due to epilepsy — following a fit secondary to underlying disease e.g. hypoxia, hypoglycaemia, hypotension
  2 Subdural haematoma
  3 Tumour — primary or secondary

    4 Hemiplegic migraine
    5 Hypoglycaemia

Conditions which may present as CVA

    1 Polycythaemia/thrombocythaemia
    2 Leukaemia
    3 Vasculitis/temporal arteritis
    4 Sudden hypotensive episode e.g. gastro-intestinal bleeding (GIB), myocardial infarction (MI).
    5 Hypertensive crises

Therefore when examining and monitoring patients, always ask about previous medical conditions such as hypertension, MI, valvular disease, SBE, diabetes, and transient ischaemic attacks (TIA) in the history, and check BP and fundi for hypertensive changes and papilloedema. Listen over carotid arteries and orbits for bruits and check CVS for arrhythmias and cardiac murmurs. Investigations should include FBC, ESR clotting screen, blood glucose. A skull x-ray may be indicated if there is a history of trauma; if a subdural haematoma or cerebral tumour is suspected a CT scan will be invaluable.

Transient ischaemic attacks (TIA)

Transient neurological deficit completely resolving within 24 hours. These may be due to ischaemia in either carotid or vertebrobasilar territory.

Symptoms of TIAs

Carotid	Vertebro-basilar
Uniocular blindness	drop attacks
Hemianopia	vertigo
Transient hemiplegia	ataxia
monoplegia	dysarthria
unilateral paraesthesia	diplopia
Transient dysphasia	facial paraesthesia

Check for

- Bruits over carotid and subclavian arteries
- Anaemia
- Polycythaemia/thrombocythaemia
- Cervical spondylosis and symptoms on movement of neck
- Inequality of BP in arms (subclavian steal syndrome)
- Retinal emboli

Patients with neurological signs should be admitted. TIAs may herald a complete stroke; therefore treatable underlying conditions should be sought.

Malignant/accelerated hypertension

May present as fits, CVA, TIA, or simply decreased level of consciousness with or without cardiac failure: BP more than 140 mm Hg diastolic. Urgent treatment is required and patient should be admitted, but BP can usually be controlled with oral therapy within 24 hours using β blockers, nifedipine, and/or hydralazine. Very rapid falls in BP are to be avoided as cerebral infarction can ensue and renal perfusion deteriorates. Parenteral anti-hypertensives are therefore rarely indicated and should always be closely monitored on ITU. The emergency treatment of hypertensive encephalopathy with papilloedema consists of elevation of the head of the bed to 45 degrees, sedation with pethidine and chlorpromazine, supportive therapy such as oxygen, treatment of pulmonary oedema, etc. and rapid control of BP.

Subarachnoid haemorrhage

This may present in young and old alike and may be very dramatic. Though frequently preceded by hypertension it can tragically strike young, previously fit, adults.

Though the presentation may be with sudden loss of consciousness, accompanied by signs of meningeal irritation and brain stem compression, *less dramatic presentation with headache alone is not uncommon and should not be treated lightly.* The classic story of sudden headache like a blow to the back of the head should alert suspicions but any severe unremitting headache of fairly sudden onset must be regarded with suspicion.

Signs (often absent in a small bleed)

- Photophobia may be present or absent
- Neck stiffness — may be absent in mild or early cases
- Conscious level decreased
- Rising BP
- Falling pulse
- Papilloedema
- Subhyaloid haemorrhages

There may be proteinuria, glycosuria.

Lumbar puncture shows uniform staining but is contraindicated in the presence of raised intracranial pressure. (With modern techniques of CT scanning, the need for diagnostic lumbar puncture is declining.)

Treatment

At the slightest suspicion of subarachnoid haemorrhage all patients should be admitted for investigation. Even if recovery from a first attack is full, recurrence is common within the first two weeks. Surgery to ligate a bleeding site can be life-saving in the acute phase or as a planned procedure to prevent further bleeding. *Refer.*

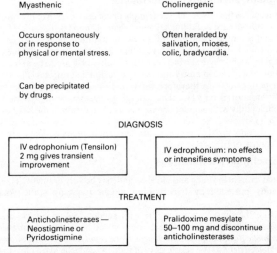

Figure 13.7 *Differentiation between myasthenic and cholinergenic crises*

Myasthenic crises

Myasthenia is a disease with muscle weakness due to failure of neuromuscular transmission. Weakness is usually most marked in the face and eyes. Treatment with anticholinesterases, neostigmine or pyridostigmine gives symptomatic relief. A crisis of muscular weakness can occur owing to an acute exacerbation of the disease process or to overdosage with anticholinesterase. Both can cause increased weakness, especially dangerous when respiratory and bulbar muscles are involved. In severe cases, intubation and ventilation may be required. (See Figure 13.7.)

Pain relief

Analgesic agents used in the A & E department

An important function of the A & E department is to reduce pain and suffering in the acutely ill or injured.

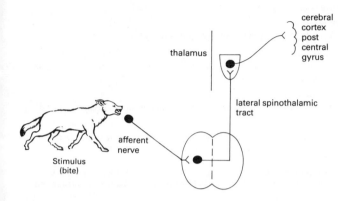

Figure 13.8 *Pain pathway*

Various studies have indicated that the majority of patients in severe pain in an A & E department get suboptimal pain relief.

Problems

    1 Inappropriate drug

    2 Wrong route

    3 Excessive wait before repeating the dose if pain not resolved

Sensory pathway (Figure 13.8)

    1 Chemical changes — PNS. A rise in bradykinin and prostaglandins sensitises and stimulates nerve endings to pain.

      The concentration of bradykinin is increased in damaged tissues.

      NSAIDs and aspirin: decrease the release of mediators by mechanisms including inhibition of prostaglandin synthesis.

    2 Within the CNS, opiate receptors are localised in the substantia gelatinosa and limbic areas of the brain.

      Endogenous opiates — enkephalins, released as neuro transmitters from specific opiate containing neurones — act at these sites to modify pain sensation.

      Leucine and methionine enkephalin are pentapeptides which are equipotent with morphine.

      Beta-endorphins, a pituitary hormone, has 48 times the analgesic activity of morphine.

Which drugs to use?

In acute trauma

Morphine is best and N_2O is safe and non-toxic.

Visceral pain

Pain is dull and poorly localised, relieved only by potent or narcotic analgesics.

Somatic pain

Sharply defined; will usually respond to milder, non-narcotic analgesics.

Dose

Adequate doses must be used in severe pain, small frequent doses of morphine give best pain relief; *titrated* to give complete pain relief.

It is effective and safe.

Respiratory depression is not a problem even if there are severe chest wounds as were seen in the Falklands War. (Except in chronic chest disease.)

Route

In severe pain, opiates should be given IV, not IM. This leads to: more rapid effect, predictable absorption; avoids accumulation of drug in poorly perfused muscle.

There is *no* place for use of the oral route in acute major trauma as there is often GI ileus and vomiting and so absorption is decreased and unpredictable.

Drugs available

Narcotics

Morphine

Morphine produces a range of depressant effects by central activity on specific opiate receptors in the CNS and peripheral tissues.

Products of metabolism are excreted in the urine. It should be given IV. Orally — high 1st pass metabolism. IM — peaks 30–45 mins: absorption erratic.

Side effects: Respiratory depression, nausea/vomiting, hypotension, constipation, tremor urticaria/rash/tolerance/addiction.

Use in A & E: Visceral and traumatic pain; anxiety and pain post MI/haematemesis, to decrease pre-load in LVF; before and during anaesthesia as part of anaesthetic technique.

Dose: 10–15 mg.

Papaveretum

Solution of opiate alkaloids. Use as morphine.

Dose: 20 mg.

TABLE 13.2

Analgesics

Injury	Drug	Dose	Route	Notes
Severe trauma crush injuries severe burns	MORPHINE	10 mgs	IV	small repeated doses
Visceral pain perforation	MORPHINE	10 mgs	IV	
Myocardial infarction	DIAMORPHINE	5 mgs	IV	less hypotensive
Biliary/renal colic pancreatitis labour	PETHIDINE DICLOFENAC	50–100 mg 75 mg	IM IM	is as effective as pethidine in Renal/Biliary colic
Gout ankylosing spondylitis	AZAPROPAZONE	1.8–2.4 g daily	0	is uricosuric
Soft tissue injuries, sprained joint, M/S chest pain, fracture ribs, dysmenorrhoea	NSAID IBUPROFEN/ Fenbufen Piroxicam	400 mg tds 300 mg bd 20 mg daily	0	side-effects see: Table 13.3 try NSAI from another group if there is a reaction
Earache, sore throat	ASPIRIN/ PARACETAMOL	600–900 mg 500 mg	0 0	Anti-pyretic
Migraine	+Ergotamine	up to 6–8 mgms	0	not to be exceeded
Herpes zoster Dental	NSAID Ibuprofen	600 mgm tds	0	⎫ can be very
Trigeminal neuralgia	Carbamazepine	100 mg bd	Oral: early in attack	⎬ severe

Diamorphine (heroin)

More potent (×2) and less emetic than morphine: used in myocardial infarction as has less hypotensive action.

Dose: 5 mg.

Codeine

Action similar to morphine but much less potent, used with aspirin or paracetamol as a mild analgesic agent.

Pethidine

Synthetic narcotic. Less potent than morphine. Used in renal and biliary colic, and labour. More nausea, less respiratory depression, more hypotensive than morphine. Rapid onset. Smooth muscle contracting is less prominent, can accumulate.

Dose: 75–150 mg.

Buprenorphine

Partial agonist.
Long lasting.
Potent.
Respiratory depressant, may cause drowsiness.
Not reversed by naloxone except in very high dose (15 mg or more). Not recommended in pregnancy.
IM, SC, sublingual.
Clinically *can* be used with agonists.

Dose: Sublingual initially 200 mcg every 8 hours, increasing if necessary 200–400 mcg 6/8 hourly.
IM, slow IV, every 6/8 hours.
300–600 mcg.

Naloxone

Opiate antagonist — no agonist activity, can precipitate withdrawal if given to addict.
Short action.
IV or IM.

Dose: 0.4–1.2 mg.

Non-narcotic analgesics

Simple analgesics

Paracetamol

Aniline derivative.
Negligible anti-inflammatory action.
For mild pain 500 mg–1 gm QDS. Toxic in overdose.

Non-steroidal anti-inflammatory drugs (NSAID)

All inhibit prostaglandin synthesis.
For moderate pain/inflammation, e.g. ibuprofen, fenbufen, naproxen, piroxicam.
Some evidence that the above are clinically superior in treatment of minor injuries.
NSAIDS have marked anti-inflammatory effects.
Note: drug interactions with Warfarin, lithium, diuretics, anti-hypertensive agents, and sulphonylureas.

Aspirin

Antipyretic.

Dose: 300 mg–900 mg.

Side effects: Dyspepsia, gastric irritation, bronchospasm, prolonged bleeding time, tinnitus.

Contraindicated in children and gout.

Indomethacin

As aspirin: more potent dose 25–50 mg QDS – 7 days.

Phenylbutazone

Due to side-effects for use only in gout and ankylosing spondylitis.

Local anaesthesia

Local anaesthesia produces a localised reversible block of nerve conduction by decreasing permeability of the nerve cell membrane to sodium.
When infiltrated they act locally:

- around wounds on nerve endings
- ring blocks on the nerve trunk

Adrenalin can be added to prolong the action of the drug. *Never* to be used on fingers/toes/penis as leads to ischaemic necrosis.

IV (after applying a cuff to the arm) — for anaesthesia of a limb, e.g. Biers Block. If absorbed systemically, will cause cardiac arrest.

Lignocaine

Membrane stabiliser.

An overdose can cause anxiety, excitement, confusion, fits.
1 per cent — 2 per cent solution.

Maximum dose/extradural dose: 200 mg (20 ml 1 per cent) (400 mg if with adrenalin). Takes 5 minutes to work.

Marcain (bupivacaine)

Prolonged local anaesthesia: good for nerve block — up to 8 hours' duration. Should not be used in Biers Block: risk of adverse CVS effects if bolus escapes into circulation by cuff release.

Other methods of reducing pain

Reduction — of dislocated/fractured limbs into an anatomical position.

Splinting — to reduce painful movement.

Elevation — to reduce swelling/pressure.

Special problems: avoid narcotics

(a) *Head injury patients with other injuries.* If in severe pain — entonox.
(b) *Addicts.*
(c) *Pregnancy.*
(d) Narcotics, e.g. pethidine — can be reversed with Narcan.

TABLE 13.3

Side-effects of anti-inflammatory/analgesic drugs: epidemiology and gastrointestinal tract

Kim Rainsford

Department of Pharmacology, University of Cambridge, Cambridge, UK

Side-effects of some anti-inflammatory/analgesic drugs

Drug	GI ulceration and haemorrhage	Other GI	Skin	CNS	Haematological	Liver	Kidney	Other (specified)
Alclofenac	+	+				?		
Acetylsalicylic acid	+++	++++	++	+	+	+ (SLE)	+ (SLE)	
Azapropazone	±	±	++	+	O	O	O	
Benorylate	+	++		++	O	O	O +	
Benoxaprofen	++	++	+++	O	O	+	+	
Carprofen	++	++						
Diclofenac	++	++	+	++	± ?	± O	O O	
Diflunisal	+	+	++	+		+ O		
Fenbufen	–	+						
Fenclofenac	+++	+++	++	O	O	+ O	O +	
Fenoprofen		+++	+	++ +++	O	O		
Feprazone	++	+++				O		
Flufenamic acid	++	+++	O O	++	O +	O	O O O	
Flurbiprofen	+++	+++		+	?	O	+	
Ibuprofen	+	++	++	+	+	O		+ (Pruritis)
Indomethacin		++++	++	++		O		+ (Respiratory)
Indoprofen		+++						

Drug						
Ketoprofen	++	+++	+++	O	O	++ (Flu-like syndrome)
Levamisole	++	+++	+++	++	+	±
Meclofenamic acid	+	++	++	O		O
Mefenamic acid	+	++	++	++	O	
Naproxen	+	++	++	+		O
Oxymethacin	+	++	++	+++		
Oxaprozin	+	+	+	+	+	+ (Cardiovascular)
Paracetamol	±			O		?
Penicillamine	+	++	++	O	+	++ (Taste loss)
						+ (Lupus syndrome)
						+ ('Goodpasture' syndrome)
Phenylbutazone and oxyphenylbutazone	+	++++	+++	+++	+	
Piroxicam	+++	++++	O	O	O	+ (Cardiovascular)
Pirprofen	+++	+++	+	O	+	O
Sulindac	+	+++	++	+	±	+
Tolmetin	+	+++	+	+		+ (Urticarial, water retention)

The incidence of the individual side-effects is graded on a scale according to approximate percentage namely, 0.1–5.0% = +, 5.0–10.0% = ++, 10–15% = +++, >20% = ++++. A zero rating denotes that the best clinical evidence indicates that no appreciable numbers of cases have been recorded which would give a reliable statistical percentage. A ? denotes that the drug may cause the side-effect. The absence of any rating means that no adequate data exist to enable a rating to be assessed.

It should be emphasised that these are at best only approximate ratings based on clinical trial data from groups of various sizes and studies of varying length of time and methodologies. For further details, see Refs 1–3.

TABLE 13.4

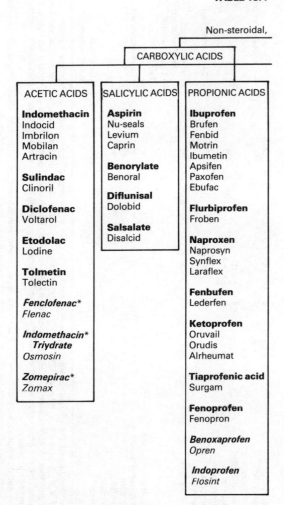

Non-steroidal,

CARBOXYLIC ACIDS

ACETIC ACIDS	SALICYLIC ACIDS	PROPIONIC ACIDS
Indomethacin Indocid Imbrilon Mobilan Artracin	**Aspirin** Nu-seals Levium Caprin	**Ibuprofen** Brufen Fenbid Motrin Ibumetin Apsifen Paxofen Ebufac
Sulindac Clinoril	**Benorylate** Benoral	**Flurbiprofen** Froben
Diclofenac Voltarol	**Diflunisal** Dolobid	**Naproxen** Naprosyn Synflex Laraflex
Etodolac Lodine	**Salsalate** Disalcid	**Fenbufen** Lederfen
Tolmetin Tolectin		**Ketoprofen** Oruvail Orudis Alrheumat
*Fenclofenac** Flenac		**Tiaprofenic acid** Surgam
*Indomethacin** *Triydrate* *Osmosin*		**Fenoprofen** Fenopron
*Zomepirac** *Zomax*		*Benoxaprofen* *Opren*
		Indoprofen *Flosint*

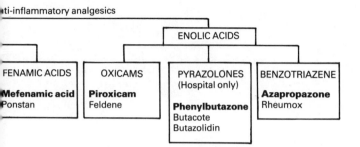

ti-inflammatory analgesics

ENOLIC ACIDS

FENAMIC ACIDS	OXICAMS	PYRAZOLONES (Hospital only)	BENZOTRIAZENE
Mefenamic acid Ponstan	**Piroxicam** Feldene	**Phenylbutazone** Butacote Butazolidin	**Azapropazone** Rheumox

*Drugs removed due to adverse reaction in italic type.
Generic names in bold type
Acknowledgements to A.H. Robins Co. Ltd.

NOTES

14

Spinal injuries

Spinal injuries

Injuries of the spine are common, and range from simple musculo-ligamentous strains to gross fracture-dislocations with spinal cord lesions. The injuries occur most commonly at the junction of relatively mobile and fixed areas, namely thoraco-lumbar and cervico-thoracic. They cause acute and chronic pain in the low back or the neck and this may be difficult to cure.

Anatomy of the spine (Figure 14.1)

The bodies of adjacent vertebrae are bound together by the strong inter-vertebral disc. The annulus fibrosus consists of many layers, with fibres at right-angles, and surrounds the nucleus pulposus which lies in the posterior part of the disc. The anterior longitudinal ligament connects the vertebral bodies whilst the posterior longitudinal ligament is attached to the discs. The synovial zygapophyseal joints are between the articular processes of the vertebrae. Interspinous ligaments are attached to dorsal and transverse spinous processes as are complex arrangements of muscles which move the spine. The anterior primary rami of the nerve roots pass through the intervertebral foramina, in close proximity to the disc, and give a nerve supply to the adjacent zygapophyseal joints.

Injuries of the spine

Listen

The commonest presentations are complaints of pain, stiffness (muscle spasm), tingling sensations, and weakness or paralysis. Patients presenting to A & E usually have a history of injury. This may be only minor and the underlying pathology may be more serious such as secondary, or rarely primary, tumours.

It is important to find out exactly how much force caused the injury; was it the result of a trivial fall or over 5 feet, a high-speed car crash with considerable damage to the vehicles, or the collapse of a rugby scrum with the patient underneath a heavy pack? The presence of nerve root signs at any stage makes the injury more severe.

Localise the site of the pain, preferably on a diagram, noting time of onset, intensity, frequency, radiation, and aggravation factors. Ask

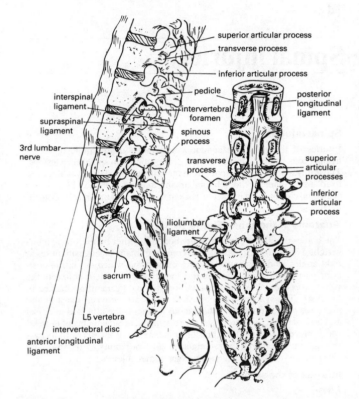

Figure 14.1 *Anatomy of the spine*

carefully about paraesthesia. Check which dermatome is affected and record this: it may change later or be bizarre in cases of compensationitis or hysteria. See Figure 14.2.

Look

Examination must involve a clear inspection of the normal curves of the spine, so that any abnormal angulation is easily seen. With severe bruising of neck, suspect brachial plexus injury.

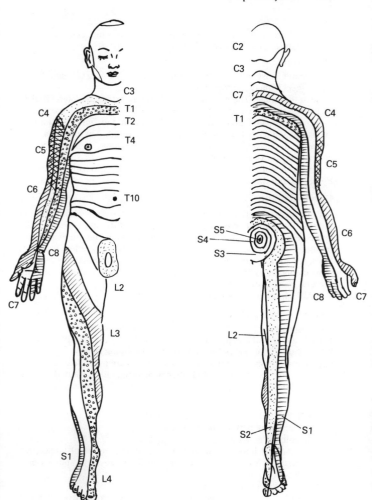

Figure 14.2 *The body's dermatomes*

Feel

Feel along the spine and press gently on the spinous processes. An angle may be felt with tenderness at its apex — then x-ray.

Movements

Movements must be tested, unless there is any possibility of instability. If you suspect from the history that there is a fracture, it is better to x-ray the spine at that stage. The normal range of flexion, extension, lateral flexion, and rotation is measured. It is best recorded as showing the loss of movement in any direction. Muscle power in the limbs is similarly measured and recorded. The reflexes are then tested. Any abnormality of sensation is charted: be careful, as hyperaesthesia is present in the dermatome above a spinal lesion.

X-rays are initially required in two planes, antero-posterior and lateral. If doubtful, or the junctional zones are not shown, ask for extra views.

Cervical spine

All unconscious patients must be presumed to have a neck injury until proven otherwise. If you suspect a cervical fracture, apply a stiff collar immediately. Whiplash injury is more common since the use of seatbelts became compulsory: gross facial and cerebral injuries are less frequent. Look for a retropharyngeal haematoma in high injuries. Assess range of movements gently: do not force patient to move neck if pain and spasm are present. See Figure 14.3.

A full neurological examination is obligatory.

X-rays

Antero-posterior and lateral views of the cervical vertebrae are required. If C7 is not seen then apply a downwards pull on the arms with the head held steady. If not successful then take the swimming view (crawl); finally ask for tomograms or a CT scan. Oblique views are useful in cases where there is doubt about the vertebral alignment as the tube is rotated, not the patient. The odontoid peg is shown by a coned view through the open mouth.

Looking at X-rays of the spine (Figure 14.4)

1 Identify all parts of the vertebrae.
2 Note the general alignment of the vertebrae:
   3 parallel lines: (a) anterior surface of the vertebral bodies; (b) posterior surface of vertebral bodies; (c) bases of spinous processes.
3 Note loss of normal curves.
4 Note the general height of the bodies; they increase from upper to lower end of the spine.
5 Depths of the disc spaces also increase downwards.
6 Note width of soft tissue shadow in the pharynx.

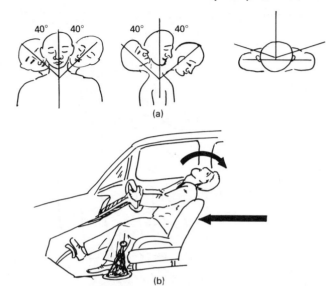

Figure 14.3 *The neck*
(a) Range of neck movement
(b) Whiplash injury to neck

Cervical spine injuries

Soft-tissue injuries are most frequently of the whiplash type, forward flexion is limited by chin on chest, extension by spinous process impingements. Hence 'whip lash' is hyperextension injury. Extensor-flexion musculo-ligamentous sprains of the intervertebral joints occur when a stationary or slow-moving vehicle is hit from behind; conversely flexion-extension injury results from sudden deceleration. Note position of head at time of activity or, if in car, whether hit from behind or front. The patient is usually held in the seat by the belt and the weight of the unrestrained head causes the injury. Pain may not be felt for several hours and then is noticed when the neck becomes stiff. Nerve root pain is frequently caused by these musculo-ligamentous sprains. Not uncommonly posterior headache results from a C2 lesion. With high-speed accidents moderate degrees of concussion can also occur from the whiplash effect.

Feel

There is often loss of the normal curve, muscle spasm, and tenderness over the interspinous ligaments.

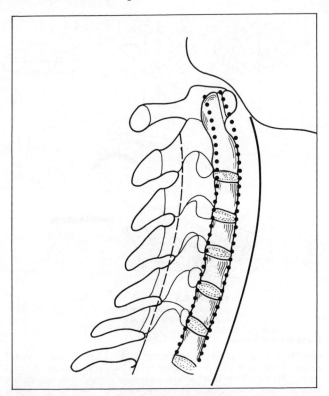

Figure 14.4 *Looking at cervical spine X-rays. Soft tissue in front of spine is widened in injury or infection*

Move

All movements are restricted, particularly rotation.

X-rays seldom show any signs other than loss of the normal curve. With persistent symptoms, lateral views in flexion and extension will often show a minor degree of subluxation at the relevant intervertebral space; this is of value later for medico-legal purposes. In extension injuries, the anterior border of a vertebral body may show a small flake avulsion — tear drop fracture.

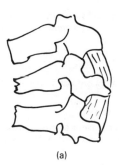
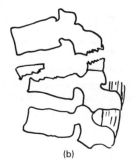

(a)   (b)

Figure 14.5 *Fractures of vertebrae*
(a) Wedge fracture — stable
(b) Fracture dislocation — unstable

Treatment

Treatment is initially by a cervical collar, NSAI tablets and start on exercises. Patients should be reviewed after a week and if not improving should be referred for physiotherapy. These injuries are often more severe than we suspect, and symptoms and signs frequently last up to 18 months, or in a few cases longer. Restriction of rotation, presenting as difficulty when reversing a car, is a common complaint. Even when litigation has been completed residual pain and stiffness are commonplace, particularly when the patient is tired or under stress.

Spinal cord injury

The main cause of concern in fractures of the spine is damage to the spinal cord (Figure 14.5). If the fracture is stable the cord is safe; if unstable the possibility of transection of the cord is ever-present. Suspected fractures must be treated as being potentially unstable until x-rays confirm the nature of the injury.

Transection of the spinal cord

- The patient feels cut in two at the moment of injury with referred pain along the spinal nerve.
- Voluntary movement below the level of the lesion is lost immediately and the muscles are flaccid.
- Sensation below the transection is lost but hyperaesthesia may be present at the level of injury.
- Bladder and rectum are paralysed. The bladder sphincter subsequently recovers to cause acute retention.

- Hypotension is severe and is not explained by any other injuries. The higher the lesion the more loss of sympathetic vasomotor control and the more profound the shock.
- There is loss of temperature control.

Cauda equina injury

Unstable fractures below the first lumbar vertebra produce lower motor neurone lesions because the cord ends at L1.

Examination in suspected spinal fractures

Do not move the patient unnecessarily, and endeavour to avoid further damage while he is being transferred from ambulance to A & E trolley. Only one move should be made: onto a trolley with a carrying-canvas on its top. In neck injuries apply traction or a collar. Move the patient as a whole, see Figure 14.6.

Carefully palpate the spine and note any deformity, bruising, tenderness, or hyperaesthesia.

Neurological examination must test reflexes (Figure 14.7), motor power and sensation. Record with time of examination.

Retroperitoneal bleeding may cause a paralytic ileus.

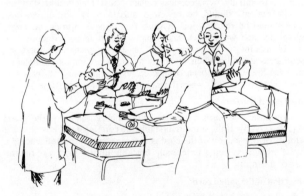

Figure 14.6 *Lifting the patient as a whole. Three nurses on one side lift the patient simultaneously, taking care not to bend or twist the spine. The casualty officer applies traction to the head and maintains proper alignment with the body*

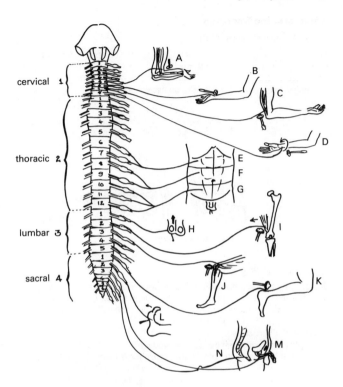

Figure 14.7 *Spinal reflexes*

A	Biceps	C5
B	Supinator	C6
C	Triceps	C7
D	Pronator	C8

E, F G Upper T67, middle T89, and lower T10, 11, 12, abdominal

H	Cremasteric	L1
I	Adductor jerk	L2
J	Knee jerk	L3
K	Ankle jerk	S1
L	Plantar	S2
M	Bulbo-cavernous	S3
N	Anal	S4

Cervical spine fractures

Wedge fractures (Figure 14.8)

Following a compression force acting on the flexed spine, the cancellous bone of the body is crushed anteriorly. As the posterior arch and ligaments are intact the fracture is stable. Common in elderly osteoporotic bone.

Apply a firm cervical collar, give analgesics, and *refer*.

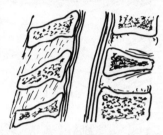

Figure 14.8 *Wedge fracture*

Burst fractures (Figure 14.9)

Result when a compression force is applied to a straight spine. The vertebral endplate is ruptured and the disc is forced into the body. The fracture is stable but the spinal cord may be damaged by bony fragments driven posteriorly. CT often shows injury to be more severe than plain x-rays so not all are stable.

Apply a firm collar, give analgesics and *refer*.

If partial lesions of the spinal cord occur then traction should be applied.

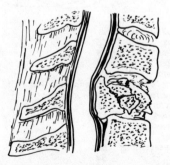

Figure 14.9 *Compression injury — burst fracture*

Flexion subluxation fractures (Figure 14.10)

Result from flexion and rotation, forward displacement of the body occurs but if the posterior arch is intact the injury is stable. The lateral x-ray shows loss of the cervical curve; flexion and extension views will demonstrate subluxation. (Figure 14.10a)

Apply a firm collar, give analgesics and *refer*.

Slight angulation at site of injury. Body of vertebra has subluxed forwards. May be disc space narrowing

Small wedge avulsion fracture. May be loss of disc space. Potentially unstable

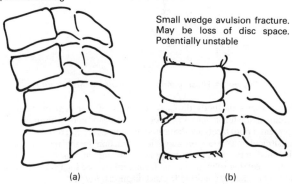

(a)   (b)

Figure 14.10 *Flexion and extension injury*
(a) Flexion subluxation injury — lateral X-ray in flexion
(b) Extension subluxation fracture

Extension subluxation fractures

Small avulsion fractures (tear-drops) off the anterior margin of a vertebral body follow an extension injury. They are essentially stable but the spinal cord may have been damaged by stretching. (Figure 14.10b)

If the anterior longitudinal ligament is torn, the disc and the cord are often damaged. In such cases x-rays will demonstrate a decreased intervertebral distance anteriorly.

Apply a firm collar, give analgesics and *refer*.

Fracture dislocations

Posterior ligaments or the vertebral arch are disrupted and the posterior facet joints displaced. This is a very unstable injury and is often accompanied by severe cord damage. (Figure 14.10c)

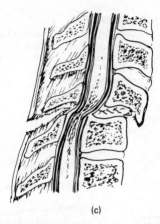

(c)

Figure 14.10(c) *Anterior dislocation of spinal column*

X-ray shows the body displaced less than 50 per cent of its antero-posterior diameter if only one facet joint is dislocated, with greater displacement if both facets are dislocated or pedicles are fractured.

Treatment must start on admission. Traction to the neck should be maintained until a firm collar is applied. The patient must be moved only as 'one piece' (log-rolling) to avoid further injury, see Figure 14.11. X-rays can then be taken to confirm the exact diagnosis. *Refer*.

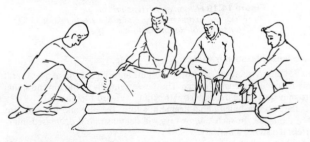

Figure 14.11 *'Log-rolling'*

Fracture of atlas

Usually follows a vertical compression force pushing the occipital condyles through the ring of the atlas. Often the ring splits in four places, the posterior fracture being the most easily seen. It is relatively stable and the cord often escapes injury initially. Particular care in handling is therefore essential to avoid the danger of a late quadriplegia and death. Treatment for fracture dislocation. *Refer*.

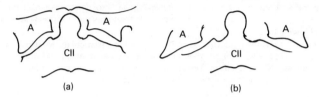

Figure 14.12 *Fracture of atlas (open mouth view atlas — odontoid process)*
(a) Note normal relation of body of atlas A to CII
(b) Note movement of body A

Fractured odontoid, fracture-dislocation of atlanto-axial joint

These fractures are usually seen easily on the 'open mouth' view x-rays, especially if there is displacement (Figure 14.13). Odontoid fractures commonly occur at the base of the process. Treatment as for fracture dislocation. *Refer*.

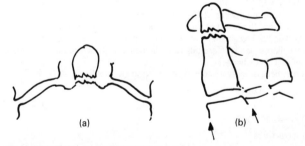

Figure 14.13 *Fracture of odontoid process*
(a) Open mouth view. If odontoid peg is not clearly seen because of teeth, repeat
(b) Lateral view. Follow the line of posterior and anterior longitudinal ligaments

Fractured spinous process

This is an avulsion injury due to strong muscular action. It is known as the 'shovellor's fracture' which usually damages the C7 or T1 spines. Treatment is conservative as for a whiplash injury.

Thoracic and lumbar spines

Musculo-ligamentous strains

These are frequently seen in the A & E department. If they are acute there is marked spasm of the erector spinae group and movement is painful and limited. X-rays should be taken to exclude the many more serious causes of back pain.

Treatment: If the tenderness is easily localised to a particular spot, this can be injected with a long-acting anaesthetic such as marcaine with depo-medrone. NSAI agents are started and the patient should be referred to an interested physiotherapist for further active treatment.

Low back pain (Table 14.1)

These frequent attenders are usually suffering from an acute exacerbation of a chronic condition, and are not suitable for A & E investigation and treatment. They should be examined to exclude acute nerve root involvement, particularly of bladder and S1, given NSAIs and referred to their GP.

Fractured transverse process

Usually due to an acute muscular rotational strain or a direct blow over the site. It is most important to exclude reneal or visceral damage (see Chapter 2). Treatment is rest and exercise.

Wedge fractures

These commonly occur at the junction of fixed and mobile parts of the spine and are the result of forced flexion. Thus they often involve T10.11, 12, or L1, L5. Occasionally the fracture is not seen on early x-rays but the body collapses later. (Carefully note the height from which the patient has fallen and check heels.)

Treatment is bedrest and early exercise so give analgesia and *refer*.

Extension fractures

These are less frequently seen and, as in the cervical spine, are stable. Give analgesia and *refer*.

Burst fractures

Results from compression applied to a straight spine, thus forcing the intervertebral disc into the body. Fragments may be driven into the cord, causing damage. CT shows these are not all stable fractures: look for ↑ width of vertebral body. Give analgesia and *refer*.

Fracture dislocations

These are unstable fractures with damage to the pedicles or facet joints, tearing of the posterior ligaments, and anterior displacement of the upper vertebra. Several vertebrae may be fractured. If the injury is above the

TABLE 14.1

Causes of low back pain

	Child	Young adult	Middle age	Elderly
Scoliosis	+			
Osteochondritis	+			
Posture		+		
Ankylosing spondylitis		+		
Spondylolisthesis		+	+	
Osteoporosis				+
Paget's disease				+
Rheumatoid arthritis		+	+	
Prolapsed disc		+	+	
Osteoarthritis			+	+
Tumours primary	+	+	+	
secondary			+	+
Fractures	+	+	+	+
Infections	+	+	+	+

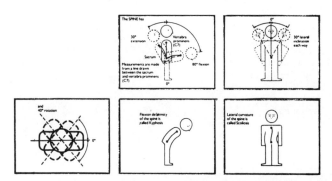

level of L2 the cord is at risk if below — the cauda equina. Treatment is exactly the same as for cervical spine fractures. The risk of further damage to the cord should be avoided by immobilisation after careful lifting in one piece onto a stretcher canvas on a non-yielding trolley. An adequate mattress must be placed on the firm trolley and full precautions taken from the time of admission to avoid the risk of pressure sores — all too frequently the result of lack of thought in the A & E department. Refer immediately, before the need for suprapubic catheterisation arises.

Fracture of the sacrum

Is uncommon and is usually associated with the much more serious fractures of the pelvis.

Fractured coccyx

A painful fracture of the tail which follows a fall or kick directly onto the bones. Diagnosis is made by a finger inserted into the rectum. X-ray does not help and is not advised. Treatment is to give analgesics, NSAIs, high-residue diet, rest for a few days, then gently progressive activity. The patient should be warned that, as with rib fractures, symptoms take some weeks to resolve.

NOTES

15

Poisoning

Poisoning

Acute poisoning is a common problem which accounts for ten per cent of medical admissions and 3 to 5 per cent of accident and emergency attendances. The most important thing to remember is that the great majority of poisoned patients make a full recovery with supportive care alone: only a small number require specialised investigations and treatments. The section on poisoning in the *British National Formulary* is very helpful and is useful for reference. This chapter provides general principles on diagnosis and management, together with notes on some common problems.

The unconscious patient

When a patient presents in coma with little or no history, and poisoning is a possibility, a rapid working diagnosis must be made and treatment given urgently — see Figure 15.1.

Resuscitation must be given for a cardio-respiratory arrest or severe shock, and the cardiac arrest team should be called if necessary. An intravenous line should be established and endotracheal intubation may be needed. The nursing staff should ensure that any relatives or friends of the patient do not leave, as you may wish to question them once the initial examination has been made. Once it is established that the patient's life is not in immediate danger, a fuller examination can be made, starting with an assessment of the patient's respiratory, cardiovascular, and central nervous system function.

Respiratory assessment

Ensure that the airway is patent. The next consideration is whether the patient needs mechanical ventilation. The colour of the patient, the pattern and depth of respiration and respiratory rate are useful clinical pointers. If there is any doubt, measure the minute volume, with the help of an anaesthetist if necessary, and take an arterial blood sample for estimation of gases. A minute volume of less than 4 litres/min is usually an indication for intubation and ventilation. The lungs should be examined. Localised crackles may indicate that aspiration of vomit has occurred.

Cardiovascular assessment

Attention should be paid to the state of hydration, pulse rate, and blood pressure; the central venous pressure should be measured if the patient is hypotensive. Table 15.1 gives some of the poisons which may be involved.

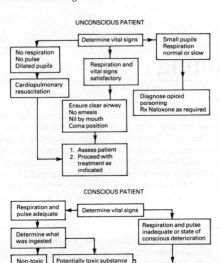

UNCONSCIOUS PATIENT

CONSCIOUS PATIENT

Figure 15.1 *Action in cases of suspected poisoning (John Henry)*

Neurological assessment

The conscious level should be observed and recorded. A simple coma grading can be used:

Grade 1 Patient drowsy, responds to verbal commands.

Grade 2 Response to painful stimulation.

Grade 3 Response to maximum painful stimulation.

Grade 4 No response to painful stimulation.

The usual painful stimulus is rubbing the sternum with the knuckles. Patients in Grade 4 coma are at much greater risk of complications and require special care to prevent respiratory complications.

The size and reaction of the pupils should be noted. Causes of changes in pupil size are shown in Table 15.1. Convulsions may be due to hypoxia or a metabolic disturbance, or may be directly due to the effect of the poison on the central nervous system.

History

A careful history should be taken from the patient (if conscious), and from relatives, bystanders, or ambulance personnel, who should be asked for bottles, tablets, syringes, suicide note, or any other evidence. Some patients who have taken a poisonous substance may give a misleading history, but the majority provide an accurate record. In childhood poisoning it is often difficult to know whether the child has actually taken anything. In all cases the following points should be noted:

1 Poison(s) involved or suspected, and the amount or concentration.
2 Mode of exposure: oral, intravenous, inhaled. Has there been any contact with skin or eyes?

TABLE 15.1
Symptoms and clinical and metabolic changes occurring in poisoning

HAEMATEMESIS	Corrosives Iron Theophylline
COMA, HYPOTENSION	Tranquillisers, opioids, antidepressants, anticonvulsants, alcohols, solvent abuse, carbon monoxide (Fig. 15.3, page 232)
CONVULSIONS	Tricyclic antidepressants, phenothiazines, antihistamines, theophylline, isoniazid, mefenamic acid
OCULOGYRIC SPASMS	Phenothiazines
INVOLUNTARY MOVEMENTS	Metoclopramide
HALLUCINATIONS, AGITATION	Atropine, hyoscine, tricyclic antidepressants, antihistamines, LSD, amphetamines (including MDMA, 'ecstasy'), psilocybe mushrooms (magic mushrooms), drug withdrawal
AGITATION, HYPERREFLEXIA, PYREXIA	Monoamine oxidase inhibitors, strychnine, phencyclidine, anticholinergic agents
PUPILS: DILATED	Hypoxia, hypothermia, atropine, tricyclic antidepressants, glutethimide, antihistamines, sympathomimetics, amphetamines, cocaine
PUPILS: CONSTRICTED	Opioids (including Lomotil), Organophosphorous compounds (insecticides)

TABLE 15.1 — contd.

TACHYCARDIA	Anticholinergic agents theophylline sympathomimetics
BRADYCARDIA	Digoxin beta blocking drugs organophosphorus compounds
METABOLIC ACIDOSIS	salicylates ethanol Iron tricyclic antidepressants methanol ethylene glycol
HYPOGLYCAEMIA	Insulin oral hypoglycaemic agents salicylates ethanol
RENAL FAILURE	Paracetamol salicylates paraquat inorganic mercurial essential oils organic acids
HEPATIC FAILURE	Paracetamol Amanita phalloides some chlorinated hydrocarbons

3 Time since exposure and duration of exposure.
4 Symptoms the patient has had.
5 Past medical history and current drug treatment.

Further examination and investigations

1 The physical examination of the patient should be completed.
2 The body temperature should be measured accurately. In all unconscious patients, the rectal temperature should be taken with a
   low-reading thermometer.
3 The mouth and skin should be inspected for corrosive burns or
   coloured stains in the mouth, blisters, injection marks, or other
   evidence of poisoning or drug abuse.
4 The smell of the breath may be characteristic of solvents, ketosis,
   and other substances. A smell of alcohol gives no guidance to the
   concentration in the blood.

5 Any vomit produced should be inspected for tablet residues or other evidence of ingestion.

6 Laboratory analyses: a blood sample should be taken for haematological examination, measurement of urea, electrolytes and glucose, and also for toxicological analyses. A chest x-ray and an electrocardiogram should be obtained. In unconscious patients, paracetamol and salicylate should be measured. Further toxicological analyses may be necessary. Some of these may be obtained from the local laboratory, while others may have to be obtained through a specialised poisons laboratory. Table 15.1 groups the main analyses which may be required. It is customary to save 10 ml heparinised blood, stomach contents, and 20 ml of the first sample of urine passed. Whole blood should be taken into an EDTA tube for carboxyhaemoglobin (carbon monoxide) methaemoglobin, and metals such as lead and mercury.

Resuscitation

If the patient is profoundly hypotensive, the response to a fluid challenge (250 ml saline given rapidly intravenously) may indicate that hypovolaemia is the major problem, and further volume replacement should be given as required. In other cases the problem may be a negative inotropic effect depressing the heart, and inotropic agents will be indicated (dopamine, dobutamine). If the blood pressure is very low or unrecordable, it may be necessary to support cardiac output with external chest compression until the cardiac output can be restored by other means.

Respiratory depression due to sedative and hypnotic agents produces shallow respiration; that due to opioids produces slow or irregular respiration; in either case, assisted ventilation may be required urgently to prevent cerebral hypoxia. Intravenous naloxone can be used to reverse opioid poisoning. Severe respiratory depression is rare in benzodiazepine poisoning, and flumezenil should not be used routinely.

Gastric lavage and emesis

If there is evidence that the patient has ingested a potentially toxic amount of a drug or poison, the stomach should be emptied. The general approach to management has been given in Figure 15.1 (page 216). Gastric lavage should be performed on adults presenting within four hours of ingestion (12 hours for aspirin, carbamazepine or tricyclic antidepressants) provided the patient is rousable and has a gag reflex. If the patient is comatose, or if the patient has swallowed a petroleum distillate, or the gag reflex is absent, gastric lavage can only be carried out after endotracheal intubation. Consent to the procedure can be assumed in the unconscious patient.

Syrup of ipecacuanha is used as an emetic in conscious patients and is the preferred means of emptying the stomach in children. The dose is 10 ml for children under 18 months, 15 ml for older children. When used in

TABLE 15.2
Antidotes which may be required urgently in severe poisoning

Poison	Antidote	Dosing regime
Beta-blockers	Glucagon	5 mg IV over 1 minute followed by an infusion of 1–5 mg/hour.
	Isoprenaline	5–50 μg/minute by IV infusion.
Carbon monoxide	Oxygen	Administer as high an inspired oxygen as possible until carboxyhaemoglobin concentration falls below 5%. Consider hyperbaric oxygen in severe cases.
Cyanide	Oxygen	Administer a high inspired oxygen until clinical recovery occurs.
	Dicobalt edetate	600 mg IV over 1 minute, followed by sodium thiosulphate (see below).
	Sodium nitrite	10 ml of 30% solution IV over 2–4 minutes, followed by sodium thiosulphate (see below).
	Sodium thiosulphate	50 ml of 25% solution IV over 10 minutes
Cholinesterase inhibitors	Atropine	2 mg IV (IM or SC in less severely poisoned patients) followed by further 2 mg doses at 5–10-minute intervals until clinical features of full atropinisation become apparent (dry mouth is the most reliable sign).
Organophosphates	Pralidoxime	30 mg/kg IV (at rate not exceeding 500 mg/minute) or IM every 4 hours for 24 hours.

adults the dose is 30 ml. It should be given with water or fruit juice, and the dose can be repeated once only if emesis has not occurred within 30 minutes.

Emesis is contraindicated if there is evidence of:

- Ingestion of corrosive substances, acids or alkalis
- Ingestion of petroleum distillates
- Increasing drowsiness, coma, or convulsions

Activated charcoal

This is finely powdered charcoal, available as 'Carbomix' (50 g plastic bottles; add water to produce suspension). Given orally shortly after ingestion, activated charcoal adsorbs many poisons, reducing the amount absorbed by the body. In repeated doses it can also remove some

TABLE 15.2—*contd.*

Poison	Antidote	Dosing regime
Digoxin	Fab antibody fragments	Dose should match the estimated dose of ingested digoxin.
Opioids	Naloxone	0.8–2.0 mg IV (children) 0.2 mg. This dose should be repeated if respiratory depression (assessed by respiratory rate and minute volume) is not reversed within 1–2 minutes. Continue with half the amount required to produce a response as an infusion over 30 minutes.
Anticholinergic agents (but not tricyclic antidepressants)	Physostigmine	2 mg IV over 5 minutes; continue with an infusion of 4–6 mg over an hour if there is a satisfactory response (adult dose).
Methaemoglobinaemia (nitrites, etc.)	Methylene blue	0.1 ml/kg of 1% solution (i.e. 1–2 mg/kg) slowly IV over 5 minutes, repeated as necessary to a maximum of 15 g.
Paracetamol	Methionine	2.5 g orally stat followed by 3 further doses at 4-hourly intervals (10 g over 12 hours). Children: 1.0 g in 4 doses 4 hourly.
	Acetylcysteine	IV infusion of 150 mg/kg in 200 ml over 15 minutes, then 50 mg/kg in 500 ml over 4 hours, then 100 mg/kg in 1 litre over 16 hours.

substances (notably phenobarbitone and theophylline) after absorption, reducing the severity of the poisoning.

It can be given after gastric lavage or after emesis, but should not be given with orally administered drugs (it can bind ipecacuanha and methionine). The dose required is at least 10 times the weight of the ingested poison; if this is unknown, give 5–10 g for a child and 50 g for an adult. Warn parents that the child's stools will be black.

Diuresis, haemodialysis and haemoperfusion

These procedures are occasionally indicated in severe cases of poisoning. Consult a poisons centre before using them.

Antidotes

Only a small number of antidotes are likely to be of immediate use in the Accident and Emergency department. These are given in Table 15.2. Note that dicobalt edetate is toxic in its own right and should only be given if poisoning is certain.

Consulting poisons centres

Advice on the toxicity, symptoms and management of poisoning can be obtained from a poisons centre. There are several centres in the United Kingdom which provide a 24-hour service (see list of phone numbers, page 232). Enquiries may be answered in the first instance by trained information staff with physicians available when a medical opinion is needed. Some centres also provide a laboratory analytical service.

To admit or not

In most cases of accidental childhood poisoning the parents can be re-assured and hospital admission is not required. Admission may be required for observation or active treatment in the case of some poisons, and is always indicated if non-accidental poisoning is suspected, for example when repeated unexplained episodes have occurred.

In adult poisoning which is deliberately self-inflicted, admission may be indicated for the medical complications of the poisoning episode. Once the patient is physically fit, the policy of the department should be followed concerning the patient's social and psychiatric welfare.

Sedative and hypnotic agents

Benzodiazepines are the most common group of drugs taken in overdose. They rarely develop severe complications, but can be fatal in massive overdose, particularly flurazepam. Many other drugs (including barbiturates, chloral hydrate, opioids, tricyclic antidepressants, and ethanol) may produce deep coma.

Clinical features

1 Sedative and hypnotic drugs may cause excitability and occasionally hallucinations, but more often drowsiness, with larger doses causing central nervous depression, flaccidity, and coma.
2 Aspiration of vomit is a major complication and respiratory depression may occur.

Management

1 Drowsy or comatose patients should be placed semi-prone, to protect the airway.
2 If the patient is comatose, gastric lavage should be performed after first passing an endotracheal tube.
3 Blood gas estimation should be made and assisted ventilation performed if respiratory depression is suspected or present.
4 It is usual to measure plasma paracetamol and salicylate in case these have also been ingested so that treatment can be given if blood levels indicate toxicity.

Salicylates

Salicylates can cause severe poisoning with relatively few symptoms. They are considerably more toxic in children than in adults, and salicylate-containing preparations should never be given to children under 12 months because of the danger of iatrogenic poisoning due to accumulation. Salicylates are found in aspirin (acetylsalicylic acid), benorylate, oil of wintergreen, liniments, and some teething preparations, though the latter rarely cause poisoning as the amount of salicylate is small.

Clinical features

1 Salicylates cause irritability, tinnitus, deafness, tremor, nausea, vomiting, hyperventilation, sweating and pyrexia.
2 Respiratory alkalosis, metabolic acidosis, ketosis, hypoglycaemia, and hyperglycaemia may all occur.

Management

- Every patient suspected of salicylate toxicity should be detained until the severity has been assessed biochemically.
- The plasma salicylate level should be measured on presentation, and again after 6 hours in case it is rising. At the same time, arterial blood gases and plasma biochemistry should be checked.
- Gastric lavage or emesis should be performed up to 12 hours after overdose. Activated charcoal should be left in the stomach.
- The patient should be rehydrated with intravenous fluids and any metabolic acidosis or hypoglycaemia corrected.
- If there are severe metabolic changes, accompanied by a salicylate level of over 800 mg/l, haemodialysis is indicated, and the patient should be referred for treatment urgently. If the level is over 600 mg/l, urinary alkalinisation (IV sodium bicarbonate 8.4%) and diuresis should be commenced. In children, salicylate levels of over 300 mg/l should be regarded as potentially toxic, and a poisons centre should be consulted.

Theophylline

Most preparations are sustained release. The patient may be asymptomatic on presentation, but treatment is urgent.

Clinical features

1 Symptoms may develop over several hours and include vomiting, abdominal pain, haematemesis, irritability, and hyperventilation.
2 A sinus tachycardia is usual, and there may be hypotension, cardiac arrhythmias (usually supraventricular tachycardia), convulsions, hypokalaemia and hyperglycaemia.
3 Coma is not common.

Management

- Give activated charcoal (10 g for a child and 50 g for an adult), plus a purgative (magnesium hydroxide or sulphate) if a delayed-release preparation has been taken. Severe vomiting should be suppressed by metoclopramide 10–40 mg IV as required. Activated charcoal should be repeated after 4 hours.
- Obtain a plasma theophylline level. Over 40 mg/l is a toxic plasma level after acute overdose. Measure plasma potassium and blood glucose.
- Hypokalaemia should be treated with a potassium chloride infusion in asthmatic patients, but propranolol can reverse both the haemodynamic and metabolic changes in non-asthmatic patients. An infusion of 5–10 mg can be given intravenously over one hour, and may be repeated if necessary.
- Convulsions should be treated with intravenous diazepam.
- If there are serious symptoms (such as convulsions or cardiac arrhythmias), charcoal haemoperfusion should be considered.

Methanol (methyl alcohol) and ethyl glycol

Both methanol and ethylene glycol are constituents of automobile anti-freezes. Model aircraft fuel also contains methanol, as do some screen-washes, varnishes and thinners, 10 ml of pure methanol can be fatal in a child, and 50 ml in an adult, causing profound metabolic acidosis, coma, convulsions and blindness. Ethylene glycol tends initially to cause signs of alcoholic intoxication followed later by convulsions, tachycardia, pulmonary oedema, and acute renal failure. The main principles of treatment are to correct acidosis, delay the metabolism of methanol or ethylene glycol to toxic metabolites by administering ethyl alcohol, and to hasten elimination by increasing the fluid output by the kidneys or using haemodialysis in severe cases.

Management

- Use gastric lavage or emesis to empty the stomach.
- Measure arterial blood gases, plasma electrolytes, urea, and osmolality. Correct acidosis with intravenous sodium bicarbonate. If plasma osmolality is normal, treatment will not be required.
- Consult a poisons centre for measurement of levels and for the regime of ethyl alcohol administration. Haemodialysis is indicated if plasma methanol is over 200 mg/l or ethylene glycol is over 500 mg/l.

Hydrocarbons, petroleum distillates and essential oils

These are found in the home as white spirit, petroleum jelly, polishes, waxes, window cleaners, turpentine substitute, paraffin, petrol, and solvents for garden pesticides. Ingestion of petroleum distillates and hydrocarbon oils and waxes causes two main problems: if aspirated during ingestion or subsequent vomiting, they can cause pneumonitis, and if absorbed via the lungs or the gut they can cause central nervous system depression.

Clinical features

1 Hydrocarbon ingestion can cause irritation of mucous membranes, with nausea, vomiting and diarrhoea.

2 Hydrocarbons destroy pulmonary surfactant properties. Aspiration of even very small amounts of paraffin or petrol can cause acute pulmonary damage similar to shock lung, developing 12–24 hours after exposure. Mineral oils and waxes cause low grade chronic inflammation. Clinical signs include cough, a rapid respiratory rate, cyanosis, and crackles. Radiological signs consist of dense patchy shadowing, usually in the lower lobes.

3 If sufficient is absorbed, central nervous system involvement can lead to restlessness, drowsiness, confusion, and coma.

4 Essential oils (such as oil of turpentine — not turpentine substitute — camphorated oil and oil of eucalyptus) are highly toxic and can also cause convulsions and renal failure.

Treatment

● The patient should be admitted for at least 24 hours after ingestion.

● A chest x-ray should be performed on admission.

● *Emesis is contraindicated because of the risk of aspiration.*

● If a large amount (over 10 ml/kg) has been recently ingested or the patient is losing consciousness, the patient should be intubated in order to prevent aspiration of gastric contents, and gastric lavage should be performed. In the case of essential oils gastric lavage is indicated if over 10 ml have been swallowed by a child or 25 ml by an adult. Activated charcoal should be given.

● Oxygen, humidity, or bronchodilators should be used as required if aspiration is suspected or if lung damage has occurred. Recovery will take place within 1–2 weeks but may take longer with waxes and polishes. There is no specific treatment: high-dose steroids will not help.

● If other organs are involved, management is symptomatic and supportive.

Dry-cleaning solvents

Dry-cleaning agents are usually chlorinated solvents such as trichloro-ethylene or trichloroethane. Carbon tetrachloride is now rarely used.

Chlorinated solvents are in general highly toxic, causing marked gastro-intestinal irritation, central nervous depression, and potentially serious hepatic damage.

Management

- Chlorinated solvents are radio-opaque, and significant amounts recently ingested should appear on an abdominal x-ray.
- This type of solvent is not an aspiration risk, and so emesis can be induced safely, after first ascertaining the ingredients, since some formulations also contain petroleum distillates.
- Acetylcysteine should be used as an antidote, as in paracetamol poisoning, since the mechanism of hepatic toxicity appears to be similar. Consult a poisons centre regarding toxicity.

Corrosive ingestion

Many household preparations contain acids and alkalis. The main symptom is pain, but shock and coma can develop rapidly. Three or four cups of water or milk should be given by mouth, and the face and hands, if contaminated, should be washed with copious amounts of water. There is no point in neutralising acids or alkalis.

Management in hospital

- Ensure the airway is clear; exclude glottal or laryngeal oedema.
- Liquid (as above) should be given at once, unless perforation is suspected.
- Emesis and gastric lavage are contraindicated, as they may produce further damage. However, if the substance taken is poisonous as well as corrosive (e.g. paraquat), emesis is indicated.
- Opioid analgesics should be used as required for pain, and plasma and saline should be given for shock.
- Where there is an experienced endoscopist, endoscopy should be performed early to assess the extent of damage.
- if perforation has occurred, urgent surgical intervention is essential. Time should not be wasted in attempting to improve metabolic or cardiovasular state.

Accidental ingestion of plants, mushrooms and berries

Young children often ingest plants and berries, but this seldom gives rise to serious problems. Generally a mild gastrointestinal disturbance is the most that will occur, and symptomatic and supportive treatment is all that is required. It is important to identify the plant material in case it is one capable of causing significant or serious toxicity. Table 15.3 gives the more commonly found toxic plants in the British Isles, together with indications for emesis; the toxic amounts are much larger. If there is doubt about the ingestion, identification, or the toxicity of plant material, emesis is a

TABLE 15.3
Plant ingestion for which emesis is indicated (this is not an exhaustive list of poisonous plants in the British Isles, but includes the more common ones)

Plant	Amount ingested
1 Deadly nightshade: all parts	Any amount
2 Other species containing atropine-like compounds e.g. Datura stramonium (thorn-apple)	Any amount
3 Woody nightshade: all parts	Any amount
4 Christmas/Jerusalem cherry: leaves or unripe berries	Any amount
5 Yew-leaves and seeds (the red fleshy part is not toxic)	Any amount
6 Snowberry	More than 3 berries
7 Holly berries	More than 5 berries
8 Foxglove: all parts	Any amount
9 Privet: leaves and berries	More than 1 berry
10 Bryony	Any amount
11 Daffodil bulbs	Any amount
12 Amanita phalloides	Any amount
13 Gyromitra esculenta (poisonous if eaten raw)	Any amount
14 Laburnum: all parts	Any amount
15 Cuckoo pint or lords and ladies (Arum maculatum)	More than 1 berry
16 Cherry laurel	Any amount
17 Daphne (laureola and mezereum): all parts	Any amount
18 Mistletoe	More than 10 berries

sensible precaution, as the vomitus can be inspected and kept for identification if necessary. Subsequent treatment will be generally supportive. The management of suicidal or accidental ingestion by an adult depends on the case and the amount taken.

Paracetamol

Since this is an easily available, over-the-counter drug, it is commonly taken in overdose and in accidental ingestions by children. Serious toxicity is rare in children, possibly because they are more resistant to the effects of the drug.

Clinical features

1 The patient may have nausea, vomiting, dizziness, or sweating, but may be symptomless for up to 36 hours after ingestion.
2 By 24–48 hours there may be hepatic tenderness and jaundice may become apparent. Prolongation of the prothrombin time by 15–18 hours is an early sign of hepatic damage; if it is over 20 seconds at 24 hours, or 44 seconds at 48 hours, the prognosis is poor. Serum transaminases start to rise by 18–24 hours and peak about three or

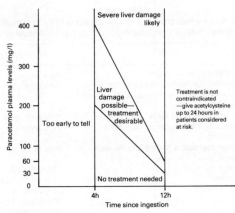

Figure 15.2 *Treatment nomogram for cases of paracetamol poisoning (applies to both adults and children).*

four days after ingestion, returning to normal within 7–10 days in those who recover.

3 Monitor for hypoglycaemia, coagulation disturbances, and renal impairment. Renal tubular necrosis can occur, sometimes with minimal evidence of liver damage.

Management

- Blood should be taken for plasma paracetamol measurement.
- Gastric lavage or emesis should be used if the patient presents within 4 hours.
- If a large amount has been ingested and the patient presents within 8 hours, start treatment with antidotes at once, without waiting for blood paracetamol results. Treatment is much less likely to be effective after 10 hours.
- Oral methionine should be given if the patient presents within 10 hours and is able to swallow. Acetylcysteine should be given intravenously, if the patient is comatose or vomiting, or presents 10–24 hours after ingestion.
- The blood paracetamol level will tell you whether treatment needs to be continued or not (see nomogram, Figure 15.2).

Opioids

As well as heroin, morphine, and pethidine, the narcotic analgesics di-hydrocodeine, pentazocine, dextromoramide, and dextropropoxyphene are potentially fatal in overdose. Proprietary cough mixtures and pain relievers contain amounts of opioids which are potentially toxic in children and the antidiarrhoeal preparation Lomotil (diphenoxylate combined with atropine), can produce respiratory depression.

Clinical features

1 The typical signs of opioid overdose are:
- drowsiness or coma
- pinpoint pupils
- slow or irregular respiration

2 Hypotension, convulsions, vomiting, and pulmonary oedema may also occur.

3 The pupils may dilate due to cerebral hypoxia or hypothermia, or other drugs taken in combination with the opioid, e.g. the atropine in Lomotil.

Management

- If the patient is cyanosed or convulsing, or if naloxone is not available, assisted ventilation should be started immediately.
- Naloxone is the antidote of choice and should be given intravenously in doses of 0.8–2.0 mg as required. A response should occur within 30–60 seconds, with reversal of the signs of toxicity. A partial response may be due to the presence of another sedative or hypnotic agent, and further doses of naloxone should be given.

Tricyclic antidepressants

These are likely to be taken in overdose by patients who being treated for depression. These drugs are particularly dangerous in children, who may take their parents' drugs or the syrups prescribed for enuresis.

Clinical features

1 The patient may deteriorate over several hours following ingestion, with deepening coma.

2 Convulsions are common, and muscle tone is often increased.

3 Dilated pupils and tachycardia are due to the anticholinergic effects of the drug.

4 The most dangerous problem is cardiac toxicity which causes widened QRS complexes, ventricular arrhythmias, severe hypotension, metabolic acidosis, heart block and asystole.

5 Respiratory depression is also common in severe cases.

Management

- Emesis for a conscious child, and gastric lavage for an adult or an unconscious child, should be performed up to twelve hours after ingestion, after which activated charcoal should be left in the stomach.

- Plasma electrolytes and arterial blood gases should be measured and the electrocardiogram monitored.
- Sodium bicarbonate should be given intravenously to correct any metabolic acidosis, and to raise the arterial pH to 7.5 in severe cases. This often produces a marked improvement.
- Practolol should be given for arrhythmias (2–5 mg IV repeated as necessary). Lignocaine is contraindicated. Phenytoin can also be used (18 mg/kg intravenously over 20 minutes).
- Intravenous diazepam can be given for convulsions.
- If there is severe unresponsive hypotension or if a cardiac arrest occurs, the circulation should be supported by external cardiac massage for as long as necessary, as recovery can occur after long periods, even hours.
- If respiratory depression is causing hypoxaemia, assisted ventilation should be commenced.

Iron

This is a very common cause of childhood poisoning. It is not difficult for a child to ingest a toxic amount, except in the case of multivitamins with iron which contain only a small amount of iron. Deaths have occurred from iron poisoning, and all overdoses should be regarded as potentially serious. The fatal dose of ferrous sulphate is 0.9 g/kg.

Clinical features

1 Vomiting is an early symptom.
2 Haematemesis and severe, possibly bloody, diarrhoea may occur.
3 Shock may develop within 6 hours of ingestion.
4 Metabolic acidosis, fever and convulsions may occur.
5 There may be an apparent recovery between 12 and 24 hours, but hepatic and renal failure are late sequelae appearing 24–48 hours after ingestion, accompanied by metabolic acidosis, hypoglycaemia and hypotension.
6 Perforation of the bowel is a possibility, and intestinal stricture may occur after 2–6 weeks.

Management

- Admit all symptomatic patients. If the patient is severely shocked, resuscitate.
- Iron is radio-opaque. An early abdominal x-ray may confirm ingestion and show the position of iron tablets in the gut. Absence of opaque material does not exclude iron ingestion.
- Emesis can be used if the patient has few symptoms; gastric lavage with 5 per cent sodium bicarbonate should be performed if

the patient is shocked or comatose. Oral administration of desferrioxamine is not recommended.

● Serum iron levels and iron binding capacity should be measured if possible. A serum iron above 0.5 mg per cent (90 μmol/l) is usually seriously toxic, and a serum iron considerably greater than serum iron binding capacity indicates serious toxicity.

● If there are only minimal symptoms by 6 hours after ingestion, the patient can be sent home and late sequelae should not be anticipated.

● If the plasma iron is in the toxic range or the patient is symptomatic, 1 g desferrioxamine in 5 ml water should be injected IM and an IV drip set up so that 15 mg/kg/hour desferrioxamine is given by continuous infusion.

● Adequate urine flow should be ensured, otherwise the ferrioxamine chelate is not excreted and may cause toxicity. Haemodialysis or peritoneal dialysis are therefore required if the patient is developing renal failure.

● Ferrioxamine chelate gives the urine a red or *vin rosé* colour, which may be used to confirm the presence of toxic amounts of drug and the need for continued treatment.

National Poisons Information Service — telephone numbers

For information and advice in cases of poisoning contact the following centres and ask for 'poisons' information.

National Poisons Information Service — telephone calls

1 The caller should be ready to give the name of the suspected agent(s) involved as accurately as possible. Since the manufacturer's name or other details may also be needed, container(s) should, if possible, be at hand. In addition, the following information is usually required.
   (a) the patient's name and age
   (b) time of exposure
   (c) any apparent signs or symptoms
   (d) treatment already given

2 Patients or relatives should not be given the telephone number of the information service (except Leeds) since inquiries from the general public cannot be answered. The emergency information service answers inquiries only from hospitals, general practitioners, and other emergency services.

3 The caller may subsequently receive a follow-up questionnaire requesting information regarding the outcome of the poisoning. This should be filled in and returned to the information service as it is essential to compile records of acute poisoning in man, especially where new or uncommon compounds are involved.

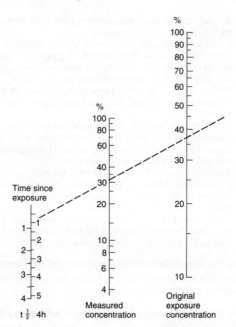

Figure 15.3 *Nomogram for calculating carboxyhaemoglobin concentration at time of exposure*

National Poisons Information Service

Guy's Hospital	Ordinary enquiries	071-955 5095
(London)	Emergency enquiries	071-635 9191
Belfast	Royal Victoria Hospital	0232-240503
Cardiff	Llandough Hospital	0222-709901
Dublin	Beaumont Hospital	Dublin 379966
Edinburgh	Edinburgh Royal Infirmary	031-229 2477

Poisons information also available from other centres:

Birmingham	Dudley Road Hospital	021-554 3801
Leeds	Leeds General Infirmary	0532 432799
Newcastle	Royal Victoria Infirmary	091-232 1525 (day)
		091-232 5131 (night)

16

Management of burns

Cause

Burn injury commonly results from wet or dry heat: with either the effect on the patient and his skin is the same so treatment is the same. The depth of the damage depends on the combination of temperature and duration of application of the source: e.g. hot-water bottle, low and long; petrol fire, high and short. See Figure 16.1.

Acid and alkali chemical burns are common, but radiation, except as a result of arc-lamps, sun, or sun-lamps, is fortunately rare.

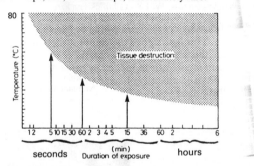

Figure 16.1 *Depth of tissue damage depends on combination of temperature and duration of the heat*

Pathophysiology

Burn wound

The burn creates a large wound in the skin — a vital organ — which is slow to heal, particularly if infected. Red blood cell (RBC) destruction results from increased fragility. Marrow depression and loss of RBCs from the burn cause anaemia.

Burn shock

Loss of circulating blood volume occurs rapidly as serum exudes from damaged capillaries, from surface or into deep tissues. Roughly one third is lost in each period of 8, 16, and 24 hours, calculated from time of burning. Transudation of electrolytes also occurs as the vapour barrier of skin has been lost; haemoconcentration is soon present. RBCs are destroyed; hyponatraemia and acidosis occur.

Aims of treatment

Clear and maintain patient's airway: give 50 per cent oxygen.
Prevent: shock by early transfusion; sepsis by early wound cover; excess scarring by early grafting.

Depth of burn

Use a functional classification (see Figure 16.2)

    (a) Erythema — redness as in mild sunburn
    (b) Partial skin loss (PSL)
        (i) Superficial, epidermal, heals in 7–10 days.
        (ii) Deep, dermal: heals 21 days from sweat glands, hair follicles.
    (c) Whole skin loss (WSL) is full thickness loss.

Estimation of depth

	PSL	WSL
(i)	Pink, blisters.	White, leathery.
(ii)	Pain to needle.	No pain.
(iii)	Blanching to needle.	No blanching.

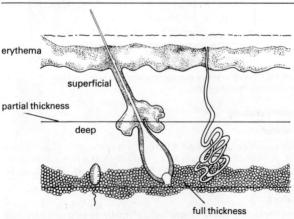

Figure 16.2 *Cross section of skin*

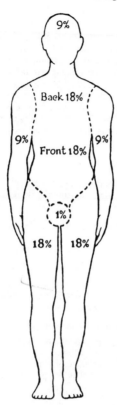

Figure 16.3 *Rule of nines*

Percentage body surface burnt (per cent BSB)

Plasma and RBC loss are related to per cent BSB. This is quickly estimated using the rule of nines. (See Figure 16.3.) The patient's hand is one per cent.

Major burns — are those on face or neck or perineum. Thermal/smoke injuries to respiratory tract; over 15 per cent BSB in adult; over 10 per cent BSB in child.

First actions

- Check airway: if consciousness level is depressed or airway is involved consider early endotracheal intubation. Administer humidified oxygen; WSL circumferential burns of chest need escharotomy soon if restricting respiration.
- Take blood for arterial blood gases, carboxyhaemoglobin, haematocrit and grouping.
- Wet and cool burn with saline; remove clothing; place patient on sterile polyurethane foam and cover with sterile sheet.
- Evidence of trauma/medical conditions.

Start records

- Time of burning
- Age, weight, sex
- Draw burn on chart to estimate per cent BSB — use rule of nines or, better still, Lund and Browder chart, see Figure 16.4.

Fluid replacement

This must start immediately. Insert large IV cannula, through unburnt skin if possible.

Intravenous fluid replacement is essential in major burns:

adults 15 per cent BSB: children 10 per cent BSB

Calculate per cent BSB from chart: start infusing with Hartmann's solution while doing your calculations. Use time from burning.

Catheterise: check urine for blood: measure.

Formula for transfusion in A & E department

$$\frac{\text{per cent BSB} \times \text{weight in kg}}{2} = \text{ml of fluid for first 4 hours after burning, as colloid}$$

Colloid: Haemaccel, dextran 70, gelofusine or PPF.

Plus metabolic requirement = 50 ml/kg/per day Hartmann's solution.

Use haematocrit control hourly. If this is satisfactory, and there is delay in moving patient to burns unit, repeat the same formula for the next four hours.

Serial observations

- Record fluid intake and output carefully:
    (i) Input: shock requirements and metabolic needs.
    (ii) Output: urine should measure between 35 and 50 ml/hour.
- Haemoconcentration should be avoided: increase rate of transfusion if this occurs.
- Measure pH, PCO_2: treat acidosis (if below 7.2) by intravenous bicarbonate.
- Measure PO_2: carefully check lungs and respiratory tract: if PO_2 falls IPPR may be lifesaving.

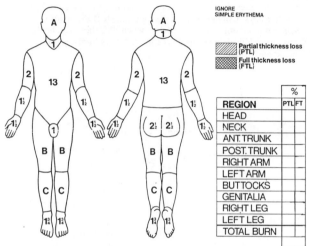

NAME_____WARD_____ NUMBER_____DATE____
AGE_____ ADMISSION WEIGHT_____

LUND AND BROWDER CHARTS

IGNORE
SIMPLE ERYTHEMA

Partial thickness loss (PTL)
Full thickness loss (FTL)

REGION	%	
	PTL	FT
HEAD		
NECK		
ANT. TRUNK		
POST. TRUNK		
RIGHT ARM		
LEFT ARM		
BUTTOCKS		
GENITALIA		
RIGHT LEG		
LEFT LEG		
TOTAL BURN		

RELATIVE PERCENTAGE OF BODY SURFACE AREA
AFFECTED BY GROWTH

AREA	AGE 0	1	5	10	15	ADULT
A = ½ OF HEAD	9½	8½	6½	5½	4½	3½
B = ½ OF ONE THIGH	2¾	3¼	4	4½	4½	4¾
C = ½ OF ONE LEG	2½	2½	2¾	3	3¼	3½

Reproduced with the permission of Smith and Nephew Pharmaceuticals Ltd.

Figure 16.4 *Lund and Browder charts*

- Bacteriological control should start after shock phase is under control. Check ATT status.
- Pain relief and sedation: titrated doses of morphine or pethidine and valium.

Local treatment

Small burns: treat early.
Major burns: after treating shock phase, clean burn wound gently.
Remove débris and aspirate blisters.

Closed dressings

Apply silver sulphadiazine (Flamazine) on non-adherent Melolin dressing, or a semi-occlusive dressing such as Synthaderm or Granuflex burnpak, and place on burn; 6 cm thickness of wool or Gamgee; crêpe bandage. See Figure 16.5.

Closed dressings, like all dressings, should be left as long as possible. Review at 5 days. Change when dressing is moist. If the cover is dry and the burn is not hurting, leave for 10 days when PSL should be healed.

Transparent film such as Opsite is good for small burns: aspirate excess exudate at early stage.

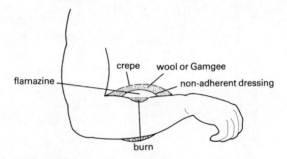

Figure 16.5 *The 'burn sandwich' — closed dressing*

Exposure treatment

Face, buttocks, perineum: apply Flamazine cream daily.

Escharotomy

Full thickness burns encircling chest, limbs, digits, need dividing with a scalpel down to fat. No anaesthetic is required in WSL burns.

General

Transfer major burns to burns unit as soon as shock is under control and they are fit to travel.

PSL burns, if not infected, will heal in 10 to 21 days.

WSL burns require excision and grafting as soon as depth is certain.

Eyelids need urgent grafting in 48 hours so *transfer*.

Hand burns

These heal quicker and remain mobile if they are treated in a moist atmosphere; this is the virtue of the Bunyan bag. (See Figure 16.6.)

Clean gently with Savlon and remove blisters and débris. Cover the

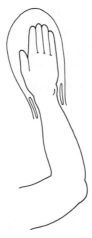

Figure 16.6 *The Bunyan bag — a polyethylene bag containing Flamazine, not too small or too large (but large enough to exercise fingers). Seal over gauze band at wrist*

TABLE 16.1

LARGE BURNS: URGENT ACTION
  1 Quickly assess % body surface burnt.
    15% + BSB in adults; 10% + BSB in child.
    Inhalation injury.
  2 Place on sterile sheet.
  3 Clear airway: ? Intubate.
    Administer humidified oxygen. ? nebulised Salbutamol
  4 Intravenous: large cannula.
    (a) Blood for PCV, Hb, group and save.
    (b) IV Hartmann's to start.
    (c) IV analgesic sos: titrate morphine.
  5 Blood gases and CO in inhalation injury.
  6 Catheterise; start fluid chart.
  7 Chart %BSB: calculate exact needs from formula.
  8 Cover with sterile sheet; silver sulphadiazine (Flamazine) to face.
  9 Escharotomy if required.
 10 Antibiotics; check ATT, reassess.
 11 Stabilise; admit or transfer.

TABLE 16.2

SMALL BURNS (2%): manage in A & E
1 Estimate area; depth: chart
2 Clean, Savlon; aspirate blisters
3 Silver sulphadiazine (Flamazine) cream
4 Closed dressings:
   (a) non-adherent dressing, granuflex; opsite
   (b) wool/Gamgee,
   (c) crêpe bandage.
   Review 3 days
5 Hands: Flamazine, Bunyan bag
   Review after 24 hours
6 Face: exposure treatment;
   inspect eyes carefully
   Review after 24 hours
7 Oral analgesics
8 Tetanus toxoid

burn with Flamazine then place the hand in a plastic bag which is fastened over a band of gauze at the wrist. Raise the hand and start exercise immediately.

Warn the patient and nurses that there will be a lot of exudate. Initially change the bag every 24 hours; the fingers will look sodden, but persevere. Review at 2/3 days to check depth of burn: if deep dermal or WSL better results follow grafting. Review every 2/3 days to change bag; they often require renewing. Ensure that the hand is raised and exercised: it will help the patient's morale to use the hand for simple jobs like using a fork.

Chemical burns

Immediate action

Irrigate profusely and continue irrigation. This will dilute and wash off offending liquids — acid or alkali.

- Phenols will require washing off with ethyl alcohol.
- White phosphorus: irrigate and keep moist. Irrigate with copper sulphate: particles become dark and can be picked out.
- Hydrofluoric acid: irrigate with water. Follow with topical calcium gluconate gel. Ice relieves pain.

Eyes

- *Irrigate profusely with water*: use a steady stream from an IV infusion bag.
- Look under the lids for irritant particles, such as lime, which are best irrigated and removed with sterile glucose solution.
- *Then* seek urgent ophthalmological advice as the cornea may have been damaged.

Electrical burns

These are always deeper than immediately apparent, particularly at the exit point. An electrocardiogram is important as arrhythmias may occur. Myoglobinuria can lead to renal failure, therefore check urine colour and output — maintain with IV fluids and diuretics if necessary.

Radiation burns

Skin damage depends on the energy of radiation. β particles are much more likely to burn subcutaneous and skin tissue than α particles or x-rays. The effects are often not evident for several hours and may take days to develop. A history of radiation exposure (e.g. in industry or hospital) should be sought in burn lesions with no obvious precipitating cause. Radiation burns heal slowly because of destruction of the blood supply and supporting tissues. Acute management includes decontamination procedures.

Morale

Burnt patients are often scared and need strong support during the difficult, and often painful, first few days. Adequate pain relief, elevation, and early movement are essential. Frequent changes of dressings are to be avoided: they are painful, damage growing epithelium and expose the burn to infection.

Healed burns are often dry and itch: apply a bland unguent:
lanoline 6 parts, liquid paraffin 1 part, arachis oil 1 part.

NOTES

NOTES

17

Hepatitis and AIDS

Virus B hepatitis

Hepatitis B is an acute viral hepatitis from which 90–95 per cent of patients make a full recovery. Sequelae in the remainder are acute and chronic liver failure, cirrhosis, hepatocellular carcinoma and, in 5–10 per cent, a carrier state.

Groups/activities at risk

- IV drug abusers sharing needles.
- Homosexuals and prostitutes.
- Health care workers (dentists particularly).
- Recent travel to high-incidence areas — tropics, Africa.
- Tattooing.
- Contaminated blood and products: now screened in UK.
- Sexual contact with above.
- Vertical transmission (mother to foetus).

Diagnosis

1 History of anorexia, nausea, diarrhoea, vomiting, followed by jaundice, dark urine and pale stools. Patient may complain of right hypochondral pain, arthralgia, and give a definite contact.

2 Examination reveals a low-grade fever, jaundice and tender, smooth hepatomegaly; 10 per cent have splenomegaly. A petechial, maculo-papular or urticarial rash may be seen.

3 Laboratory tests must be made but full precautions must be taken while the blood sample is obtained. Gloves must be worn while doing the venepuncture and the needle disposed of in the proper 'sharps' container. The blood must be transported in a secure container legibly marked 'danger of infection'; the request form to the pathologist must also be clearly marked with the provisional diagnosis.

    (a) Full blood count: shows an elevated white cell count (a non-specific reflection of viral infection).

    (b) Liver function tests: high aspartate aminotransferase, alanine aminotransferase and total and conjugated bilirubin.

(c) Clotting screen: a prolonged prothrombin time may occur.
(d) Viral hepatitis screen (hepatitis B antigen/antibody).
Hepatitis B surface antibody is the first to appear.

Differential diagnosis includes:

1 Other viral hepatitis: A, non-A–non-B, D, Epstein-Barr.
2 Biliary tract disease.
3 Toxic liver damage including drugs and alcohol.
4 Right ventricular failure.

Accidental exposure to infection

- Scratch/injection with needle from hepatitis B carrier.
- Hepatitis B positive blood splashed into eye.
- Hepatitis B positive blood splashed onto cut or a large quantity onto clothes (enough to make a change necessary).

Action

- Blood should be taken from both parties to confirm the correct Australia (Au) antigen status unless this is known for sure.
- Passive immunisation with immunoglobulin must be organised. Each A & E department should know where this can be carried out or where the immunoglobulin can be obtained. This should ideally be done within 48 hours, but can be of use up to 72 hours.

Acquired immunodeficiency syndrome (AIDS)

AIDS is the end-stage of infection with the human immunodeficiency virus (HIV). Other manifestations include, in diminishing severity:

- AIDS-related complex (ARC)
- persistent generalised lymphadenopathy (PGL)
- carrier state.

Acquired immunodeficiency syndrome (AIDS)

AIDS is at present an incurable and fatal disease. It is the result of a defective cell-mediated immunity due to a reduction in quality and quantity of T helper cells. This is associated with an increase in β cell activity leading to hypergammaglobulinaemia and autoimmune phenomena; with a decrease in β cell efficiency the response to new antigen is decreased.

The impaired immune response permits severe infections by various opportunistic agents and allows certain malignancies to progress. The terrible prognosis is due to overwhelming infections and/or tumours rather than the HIV itself.

Aids-related complex (ARC)

1 History is of non-specific symptoms for which no other cause is found: significant weight loss, persistent pyrexia of unknown origin (PUO), night sweats, lethargy, and diarrhoea.

2 Examination may reveal a generalised lymphadenopathy, hepato-splenomegaly, and minor infections such as impetigo, tinea pedis, herpes, or candida.

3 Laboratory investigations must be carried out with full precautions if the diagnosis is suspected and with the patient's consent. Full blood count may show a pancytopenia or a reduction in one or more cell lines; ESR is elevated; electrophoresis shows an increase in immunoglobulins; HIV antibodies, or the virus itself, are identified in the blood.

4 To make the diagnosis of ARC there should be at least two clinical and two laboratory abnormalities.

Persistent generalised lymphadenopathy (PGL)

PGL is characterised by painless lymphadenopathy, a non-specific hyperplasia, associated with HIV antibodies. It may persist for many years, change to ARC or AIDS, or revert to a carrier state. The patients are usually well, and development of systemic symptoms and deterioration of general health should alert to the possibility that the disease is progressing to a more sinister phase.

Carrier state

The patient looks, feels, and is completely well with a slightly increased incidence of infections including herpes, impetigo, TB, and pneumococcal pneumonia. Healthy carriers may progress to AIDS directly or via PGL and/or ARC.

Diagnosis

AIDS should be considered in 'at risk' groups — homosexuals, bisexuals, IV drug users sharing needles, travellers from high-risk areas (e.g. Haiti, central Africa), haemophiliacs and the sexual contacts of the above. Like hepatitis B it can spread by vertical transmission (mother to foetus).

For diagnosis the patient must have one or more of the opportunistic infections or malignant diseases listed by the USA Center for Disease Control. These include *Pneumocystis carinii* pneumonia, Kaposi's sarcoma, toxoplasmosis, mycobacteria, cryptococcus, β cell lymphoma, and high-grade non-Hodgkin's lymphoma.

Skin conditions may be the main presentation. Kaposi's sarcoma may be bruise-like, nodular, plaque-like or similar to pyogenic granuloma. Patients may have seborrhoeic eczema, folliculitis (often due to pityrosporos yeasts), candidiasis (oral, bronchial or oesophageal), cryptococcus, histoplasmosis, herpes simplex, molluscum contagiosum, severe tinea pedis, vasculitis and, finally in this depressing list, hairy cell leukaemia.

Central nervous system involvement may be due to an infective agent such as herpes encephalomeningitis or to direct infection by HIV, resulting in presenile dementia.

Gastrointestinal symptoms may occur because of tumour or infection and similarly diffuse pulmonary disease may be present.

AIDS and the A & E department

Precautions as outlined in the section on hepatitis B should be observed when handling blood or other body fluids. It should be remembered that HIV is not as robust or infective as the hepatitis B virus. Blood samples taken from patients known to have, or suspected of having, HIV should be labelled with 'DANGER OF INFECTION' stickers and put into robust bags for transit. 'Risk of AIDS' stickers abuse patients' confidentiality.

The HIV antibody test should be performed only with the patient's informed consent. There is no place for it in the A & E department as the patient cannot be satisfactorily followed up there.

It takes 2–3 months for the infected patient to sero-convert and 2 per cent do not show the antibody anyway. If surgery is required urgently the result will not be ready in time. Informed consent is not possible in the true emergency. Cases suspected of PGL, ARC or AIDS should be referred to the duty physician to ensure continuity of treatment.

Patients requesting screening should be referred to the genito-urinary medicine department or a centre where they can be properly counselled; they must be made aware of and understand the implications to their life of a positive result.

At-risk patients who require urgent invasive procedures should be treated as outlined for hepatitis B suspects. Medical and nursing staff should wear masks, gowns and gloves; sharp instruments and needles should be used with extra care and disposed of in the proper container. The theatre is cleaned after the case.

NOTES

18

Diabetes

The diagnosis of hypoglycaemia (blood glucose < 2.5 mmol/l) should be considered in any patient, especially a diabetic, who presents with confusion, aggressive or irrational behaviour, drowsiness or coma, a fit, or even focal cerebral dysfunction. Death is uncommon but irreversible brain damage can occur if the condition is not recognised and treated promptly.

Diabetic patient

Diagnose hypoglycaemia if a diabetic taking insulin or a sulphonylurea presents with sudden deterioration of consciousness (within minutes or during sleep). This contrasts with the gradual onset of hyperglycaemic coma over several hours. Dehydration and hyperventilation are not features of hypoglycaemia.

- Take blood for glucose measurement before initiating treatment but do not wait for laboratory result. Instead use one drop for a rapid bedside check with a glucose test strip, e.g. BM glycemie 1–44.
- Inject 50 ml of 50 per cent glucose (available in a prefilled syringe) IV or if the patient is too restless, inject 1 mg of glucagon IM. The patient recovers dramatically within minutes. If the patient is not totally unconscious and is able to drink, glucose or sucrose in solution can be given orally, e.g. a glass of lucozade or other sweet drink or 5 teaspoonfuls of sugar in water or fruit juice.
- When the patient has fully regained consciousness, give additional carbohydrates, e.g. milk and biscuits orally to prevent recurrence before the next meal. Enquire about a precipitating cause, e.g. missed or delayed meal, prolonged exercise or alcohol. Advise on the prevention, early recognition and self-treatment of hypoglycaemia. Arrange to see GP or diabetic clinic. Consider reducing the dose of insulin or sulphonylurea. Admission to hospital is not routinely necessary; if an overdose of insulin or sulphonylurea is suspected infuse 5 per cent dextrose and admit as a medical emergency.

Non-diabetic patient

Hypoglycaemia in the non-diabetic is often subacute and recurrent. In the absence of a history of diabetes to prompt the diagnosis, hypoglycaemia may not be suspected clinically. Missed meals and/or alcohol may be factors. Blood glucose should thus be checked routinely with a test strip in any confused or unconscious patient or any unusual symptoms, particularly if related to fainting, and a sample sent for laboratory measurement. Treatment is similar to that in the diabetic. Admission is necessary to investigate the cause, e.g. an insulinoma, an extrapancreatic tumour or self-administration of insulin or sulphonylurea.

Diabetic ketoacidosis

Diabetic ketoacidosis (DKA) is the consequence of severe insulin deficiency in a known or newly presenting diabetic. It is characterised by hyperglycaemia, ketonaemia and hence ketonuria, and metabolic acidosis. The clinical manifestations are polyuria, polydipsia, lethargy, anorexia, vomiting, sometimes abdominal pain, which may mimic a surgical emergency, dehydration, hyperventilation and gradual deterioration of consciousness (drowsiness, stupor and coma) over several hours. The breath smells of acetone. The condition occurs most frequently in insulin-treated diabetics who fail to increase (or omit) their normal insulin dose during an intercurrent illness. Some are overwhelmed by acute illness, a definite minority engineer it deliberately. It is a serious emergency with a considerable mortality in inexperienced hands. The outcome is related to the delay in onset of treatment so it is vital that treatment is started immediately without waiting for laboratory results.

Investigations

1 *Laboratory investigations*: Plasma glucose, sodium, potassium, bicarbonate, urea and arterial pH should be measured urgently. Blood count is less urgent; a raised white cell count is not diagnostic of infection.

2 *Bedside investigations*: While awaiting laboratory results, check blood glucose level rapidly with a test strip such as BM glycemie 1–44, and test urine and plasma for ketones. To test plasma for ketones, collect 5 ml of blood into a heparinised bottle; allow the red cells to sediment for a few minutes or spin the sample in a centrifuge; then dip a ketone test strip into the separated plasma. A high or moderate level of ketones in urine and plasma with blood glucose > 20 mmol/l establishes the diagnosis.

3 *Other investigations*: These are carried out at an appropriate stage to exclude a precipitating factor especially an infection or a myocardial infarct. The most important are chest x-ray, ECG, cardiac enzymes, and bacteriological culture of blood, urine, stools, throat swab, and any septic skin. ECG is also useful for detecting hypokalaemia and hyperkalaemia.

Initial treatment

● *IV fluids*: Infuse N-saline, rapidly initially to re-expand blood volume, and then more gradually. A useful guide is 1 litre/hr for the first 2 hours, followed by 1 litre over 2, 4, and 6 hours,

● adjusting the rate according to the clinical state and fluid balance. A CVP line is useful in the elderly, the patient with heart disease, or renal disease. Treatment and investigation should always commence before CVP insertion. This should be an aid to treatment not a cause of further delay. If patient is shocked consider use of colloid and bicarbonate.

Hypokalaemia
ST depression and T wave flattening or inversion
Prominent U waves, which may fuse with the succeeding P

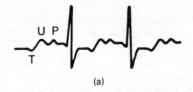

(a)

Hyperkalaemia
Small P waves with tall peaked T waves
QRS complex widens, and ventricular fibrillation may follow

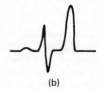

(b)

Figure 18.1 *ECG changes in (a) hypokalaemia and (b) hyperkalaemia*

● *Potassium*: K^+ replacement will always be needed because with the start of insulin therapy, K^+ ions are driven rapidly into the cells. To prevent hypokalaemia add 20 mmol of KCl to each litre of fluid once the serum K^+ is known to be less than 5 mmol/l; increase to 40 mmol/hr if plasma level is > 3.0 mmol/l. Withhold K^+ infusion if plasma level is > 6.0 mmol/l or if ECG shows peaked T wave changes of hyperkalaemia. Check plasma K^+ 2-hourly.
● *Soluble insulin*: Give 10 u IV stat followed by 6 u/hr by IV infusion. Use a syringe pump (e.g. Treonic IP3, Vickers Medical) or a paediatric burette and load with 50 u of soluble insulin diluted in 50 ml of N-saline (1 u/ml). Monitor blood glucose 1–2 hourly. The level usually falls by about 5 mmol/hr. If not, check the infusion set for malfunction before increasing the rate to 10 u/hr.

Alternatively inject 20 u IM stat followed by 6 u IM every hour. Blood glucose should fall at a similar rate.

● *Bicarbonate*: This is required only in the most severe acidosis. If arterial pH is < 7.0, infuse 50–100 mmol of sodium bicarbonate in dilute solution (1.2 per cent or 2.4 per cent or 8.4 per cent diluted in N-saline) over an hour with additional 20 mmol of potassium. Then repeat arterial pH and if > 7.0, no further bicarbonate is required. Its use is controversial and is declining. It is possible that intra cellular acidosis worsens with HCO_3 therapy.

● *Supportive treatment*: Nasogastric aspiration is indicated for nausea and vomiting and for the unconscious patient. It should be preceded by endotracheal intubation in the deeply comatose patient without a cough reflex. Catheterise the bladder if the patient is unconscious or anuric.

● *Precipitating cause*: If a bacterial infection is suspected; start IV antibiotics after taking the appropriate specimens for culture. Myocardial infarction or stroke are managed in the usual way but the prognosis is worse than in non-diabetics.

Management when blood glucose is 10–15 mmol/l

Continue the above treatment regimen until blood glucose has fallen to 10–15 mmol/l. Then modify as follows to prevent hypoglycaemia:

● Infuse 5 or 10 per cent dextrose at about 100 ml/hr.
● Reduce IV insulin infusion to 2–3 u/hr (or 10 u in every 2 hrs) and keep on giving 20 mmol/l.

Monitor blood glucose with test strips 2-hourly aiming to maintain a level of 4–10 mmol/l. If necessary, adjust the IV insulin infusion rate using a 'sliding' scale. Check plasma K^+ at least twice daily and if outside the normal range, adjust the potassium infusion rate. N-saline may also be infused if the patient is still dehydrated.

Discontinue IV therapy when the patient is able to eat and drink normally (usually after 12 hrs) and administer insulin subcutaneously when much improved and not vomiting. Continue with IV insulin until the ketones have cleared from the urine. The patient should receive appropriate education to prevent further episode of DKA.

Diabetic non-ketotic hyperosmolar coma

This condition resembles diabetic ketoacidosis but differs in several aspects as there is some residual insulin reaction:

1 Severe ketosis and acidosis are absent.
2 Blood glucose is very high, usually > 40 mmol/l.
3 Plasma osmolality, which is equal to $2(Na^+ + K^+)$ + urea + glucose concentrations in mmol/l, is very high, usually > 350 mOsm/l.

This is due to the very high plasma glucose and the raised plasma Na$^+$ and urea caused by severe water loss in the urine. The high plasma viscosity and dehydration predispose to arterial and venous thromboses.

4 The condition usually occurs in elderly non-insulin-dependent diabetics, and may be the presenting feature. It is often precipitated by an acute infection, a myocardial infarct, stroke or an increase in carbohydrate consumption such as glucose drinks to combat 'weakness' or thirst. Morbidity and mortality remain high.

Management

This is similar to that of DKA but with the following modifications:

- Rehydrate with 1/2 N-saline if plasma Na$^+$ > 150 mmol/l. Insert a CVP line to monitor fluid replacement.
- Lower blood glucose slowly (< 5 mmol/l per hr) with insulin to prevent rapid fall in plasma osmolality which can precipitate cerebral oedema.
- After the acute episode, insulin may not be required as hyperglycaemia can often be controlled with diet, supplemented if necessary with oral hypoglycaemic drugs. Careful diabetic education and regular follow-up are important to prevent recurrence.

N.B. Children and pregnant women present special problems which need expert help. Diabetic foot problems are either neuropathic, vascular or mixed. They are soon complicated by infection. Need expert opinion and chiropody. If cellulitis or gangrene — *refer* for admission.

NOTES

19

Medico-legal aspects of Accident and Emergency medicine

Medico-legal aspects of A & E medicine

Introduction

This section is intended to raise the issue of medico-legal aspects of A & E medicine. Medico-legal litigation is increasingly common as the general public's expectations are raised. Not only is the number of cases increasing each year, but also the value of damages, as judges become more realistic on the monetary consequences of injuries, psychological damage, loss of time and life style. The courts do not expect 'super doctors' but are advised as to the standard of care which can reasonably be expected.

The general principles of managing accidental injuries

1. *Do* be careful to act responsibly in history taking, examination of the patient and inspection of x-rays.
2. *Do* be diligent in writing comprehensive notes.
3. *Do* be thoughtful about possible present and future complications.
4. *Do* be watchful of the patient's progress.
5. *Do* be ready to seek help and advice.
6. *Do* try and convey a sympathetic and caring attitude.
7. *Don't* readily accept someone else's diagnosis without confirming it for yourself.
8. *Don't* rely on the spoken word and your own memory.
9. *Don't* believe that you are too experienced to make a mistake.
10. *Don't* go off duty without handing over properly to a colleague.
11. *Don't* exceed your own limitations and 'have a go'.

Due to their very nature, a great many accidents and emergencies have legal consequences, often emerging some time after the incident. The thinking doctor assumes that each case may have some future medico-legal complications.

A guideline for cases which frequently become 'medico-legal'

- Any case where compensation for injury may be obtained from a third party or the Criminal Injury Compensation Board.
- Any case involving the police.
- Any case where the patient feels that his treatment by the department or doctor was unsatisfactory.

More specific incidents which may involve litigation

- Road accidents — even if there is very little apparent injury — and especially 'whiplash' spinal injuries.
- Assault — no case is too trivial, even sports injuries have been subject to litigation.
- Injuries sustained on public transport or council-maintained property. Again no case is too trivial, and the police and security services are particularly susceptible.
- Rape and other sexual offences.
- Injuries to children — including accidental, non-accidental injuries, psychological, sexual abuse, neglect and cot deaths.
- Murder or other serious injury, from whatever cause.
- Unexpected death — especially accidental deaths.
- Late presentation of injuries — especially after consultation with a solicitor.

Recording of information

Every patient presenting at A & E should be considered as a possible medico-legal case. These cases sometimes take a number of years (up to seven) to come to court, and therefore it is essential that you write accurate, concise, and legible notes (you may not be the only one to read them) as this may be the only material available to you as a witness. Be very careful in your notes not to display a flippant, disrespectful or prejudiced attitude — this usually backfires in court. A routine format is the best way to ensure all relevant information is recorded, and should cover the following headings:

1 Date and time of examination.
2 Short accurate history, which must include the date, time, place, and mechanism of injury as stated by the patient, or if he is unconscious, by a witness. For example, 'tripped over broken paving stone at 2 pm today, injuring right ankle'. Also include the general state of the patient, e.g. 'distressed'.
3 The size, shape, site, type, and approximate age of each injury or absence of any signs of injury. Diagrams are a useful aid.
4 Other relevant findings of the examination, e.g. old median nerve injury.
5 Any treatment given, including reassurance, verbal or written advice.

6 Details of any resuscitation attempt, even if unsuccessful, and discussion with a senior doctor if this occurred.
7 Disposal of the patient — e.g. discharged home with a relative.
8 Note of any communication, e.g. letter to GP and if possible a copy.
9 Referral to other team and time.
10 Your legible signature and time.

Remember that every sheet of paper on which you make notes should bear a date and the patient's full name. Abbreviations should be avoided where possible.

Injuries

An injury should be recorded accurately according to its type — bruise, abrasion, laceration, incision, puncture, or stab wound (see section on wounds), and you should at least be able to say whether it is fresh or old.

Some injuries clearly reflect the implement used. However, it is unwise to jump to conclusions unless you have considerable expertise in this field. However, patterns of injuries should be noted and recorded — e.g. patterned bruising around the neck from fingers; patterns of clothing imprinted as bruising; linear multiple superficial incisions of self-inflicted injury, etc.

Record if patient left without being seen.

Cases of multiple injury

As soon as feasible after the victim has been fully resuscitated and is in a stable condition, make a comprehensive list of his injuries. To do this the patient must be completely undressed and examined systematically from crown to sole, front and back, and all injuries recorded. Be sure to remember to examine as part of your full examination:

- the eyes (petechial, haemorrhage, retinal haemorrhage);
- the ears (bleeding from middle ear, tears, or petechiae on tympanic membrane);
- the nose;
- the interior of the mouth;
- all of the skin surfaces, front and back;
- the genitalia and perineum.

Record all injuries in legible diagrammatic and written form. If there are lots of injuries or more than one victim it is expedient for one person to examine and dictate to another person (medical student). Use a ruler or tape measure to measure injuries and record their site as distance from a bony landmark.

Documentated examination should always be done before any exploration, extension, or suturing of wounds is carried out. Photographs (with consent) are an invaluable method of recording injuries. Blood samples for cross-matching and toxicology should be taken before any blood or dextran is infused. In cases of serious criminal injury — e.g. stabbing, hit-and-run accidents, the police may require a pre-transfusion cross-matching sample for their investigations and it is sensible to take this at the same time.

Minor injuries

Again it is important to record the details of the injury as above. The patient should be able to give you a better history; although you may have less reason to suspect that the case will become medico-legal it is still important to cultivate a habit of good note-taking. After examination of the actual injury, it is most important to examine and record the function of structures which might feasibly have been affected by the injury. In limb injuries the function of distal nerve, vessel, and tendons must always be recorded, however briefly, whether normal or not.

In note-taking, NAD ('nothing abnormal detected') is not sufficient and may be interpreted Not Actually Done.

In cases of injury to the eye, the visual acuity must be recorded, and in any case of trauma to the globe (even blunt trauma from a punch) an ophthalmic opinion should be sought. For specific injuries see relevant sections.

Consent

Consent is an important legal consideration, especially in A & E medicine. Consent may be implied or expressed, and the latter either verbal or written.

Implied consent covers most casualty attenders who imply their consent to examination by their very attendance. However, if anything is to be actually done to a patient then his express consent should be obtained — usually this is covered by the doctor obtaining the patient's verbal consent before actually carrying out any procedure such as an x-ray examination or suturing a wound. If you are worried concerning express verbal consent, a witness to the consent is good practice.

If the patient is to receive a general anaesthetic or have any more serious procedure done, then informed written consent should be obtained to protect the doctor from charges of assault and battery. Standard consent forms are available for general anaesthetic.

It is not unusual for casualty officers to have to examine and treat a patient who is in police custody, and it is wise to obtain written consent. If the patient refuses then the doctor *has no legal right to proceed*, except in rare cases where examination is likely to yield important criminal evidence — and these cases are best dealt with by the police surgeon.

Often adults are unable to give informed consent for emergency treatment due to unconsciousness, concussion, intoxication with drugs or alcohol, septicaemia, etc. and a doctor may then provide necessary treatment as *his* duty of care under common law. It is not unusual for concussed patients to be most unpleasant, often smelling of alcohol, but this duty of care must not be forgotten or omitted. It is generally agreed that if a patient presents at A & E there is a duty to treat if required.

When a patient refuses care and wishes to leave 'against medical advice' signing a self-discharge form does not exonerate the doctor from a duty to provide treatment, advice, and follow up, and communication. The patient may not be compos mentis (e.g. drugged, head inj. etc.) hypoglycaemia! It may be necessary to detain them against their will until the usual causes have been excluded and they can look after themselves.

- hypoglycaemia
- alcohol
- drugs
- H.I.
- sepsis
- meningitis/encephalitis
- Acute psychosis
- miscellaneous

More unusually, a victim of attempted suicide may be brought to hospital against his will, and refuses treatment. In a life-threatening emergency, care should be given and the legal niceties sorted out later; a psychiatric opinion on the patient's state of mind might permit treatment under the Mental Health Act, and in other cases of doubt, seek the opinion of your medical defence organisation, and the A & E consultant. The inability to treat the Jehovah's Witness who refuses a blood transfusion against advice would not be held against the casualty doctor.

In the case of children up to the age of 16 years the consent of a parent or guardian is needed for anything other than a cursory examination and children must not be x-rayed, investigated or treated without such consent — except in circumstances where there is risk to life or limb, where the duty of care to the individual overrides the need for consent, e.g. in reduction of a dislocated ankle or arresting haemorrhage. However, a *realistic attempt* should be made to locate a parent or guardian and verbal consent in the presence of a witness will suffice in an emergency. Children of 12–16 years can give informed consent for minor procedures if a parent cannot be contacted and delay would be detrimental. Should parents or carers refuse treatment for a child who urgently requires it (e.g. Jehovah's Witness refusing blood products for their child) despite every effort to persuade them, the child must be made a ward of court for treatment. Contact your A & E consultant, paediatrician, social work department and the police as necessary.

Confidentiality

This is another legal minefield for doctors. Generally speaking, doctors must keep confidential their professional findings, and act in the best interest of the patient. The best advice to follow is never to release *any* information on a patient to *any* other party without the patient's consent. This includes reports to employers, the police, solicitors, and insurance companies, and copies of all such reports should be retained with a copy of the patient's notes for future reference.

The doctor must preserve secrecy on all he/she knows. However, there are five exceptions to this general principle:

1 The patient gives consent.
2 When it is undesirable on medical grounds to seek a patient's consent.
3 The doctor's overriding duty to society.
4 For the purposes of medical research (which is governed by strict rules).
5 The information is required by the legal process (i.e. the court orders the doctor to disclose information).

Even if another doctor asks for a copy of your patient's case notes, you must ascertain (a) that he is acting with the consent of, or in the interest of, your patient (occasionally he is acting for the other party); (b) that there is no intention to take action against your hospital or HA. Information or medical reports on a deceased patient should be released only with the consent of the nearest surviving relative.

Should the police require your evidence without the patient's consent you may be subpoenaed to court and directed by a magistrate to give evidence as a 'privileged communication' or be in contempt of court. Your duty to society overrides your responsibility to an individual patient, and so if you have evidence that a serious crime has been committed (gunshot wounds, stabbing, etc.) the police must be informed. Likewise if a patient represents a danger to society — e.g. an epileptic train driver — and he will not voluntarily take sensible action, you have a duty to notify the appropriate body, preferably the doctor, again by way of sealed 'privileged communication'. However, every effort must be made to persuade the patient to disclose the information. If in doubt, consult your protection organisation and obtain the advice of seniors and/or colleagues. Other cases where confidentiality may be breached are in cases of notifiable disease and the treatment of unregistered drug addicts.

Rape and sexual assault of adults

Victims and alleged victims of rape and sexual assault attend A & E — some because they have been sexually assaulted, and others because they have sustained injuries, often serious, in addition to the sexual assault. The investigation of these crimes is a matter for the police and the police surgeon, who should be informed, and who will come and conduct the examination. Casualty officers, by and large, do not have the necessary experience or expertise in this respect, and should not undertake to perform the examination. However, any necessary medical treatment —

e.g. resuscitation, arrest of haemorrhage, etc. — should be carried out as usual, and any clothing removed carefully and kept in plastic bags. Where the victim has not otherwise been injured she should be sympathetically treated in a private place and asked not to wash or change clothes until the arrival of the police surgeon.

Occasionally a woman attends the A & E Department saying that she has been raped in the previous few days but does not wish the police to be involved. This view should be respected but it may be considered advisable to persuade her to make a statement to the police for the public good. The time of the alleged rape may concur with injuries to another person, and this should be identified to the consultant for him/her to decide on further action. It is important that the woman be protected against unwanted pregnancy and venereal disease, and during clinic hours referral to the genito-urinary clinic is the best option for treatment and follow-up; otherwise a gynaecologist should arrange examination, treatment, and appropriate follow-up. It is important to obtain the woman's written consent before any examination or treatment is carried out and to make detailed case notes.

Children: Non-accidental injury, sexual abuse and neglect

Non-accidental injury to children may come to light in the A & E department and a child protection register is kept. While there may be a 'typical case', no social classes or groups are exempt from suspicion. Generally the distribution and severity of the injury does not fit with the parent's story; there may be bruises and injuries of differing ages, the child may have a distant, unusual affect, or there may be obvious neglect. If there is any doubt about the cause of an injury the child should be admitted under the care of a paediatrician: preferably with the consent of the parents. Whatever your feelings, it is most important not to antagonise the parents and to gain their co-operation. If the parents do not consent to the child's admission to hospital, an emergency care order must be speedily obtained (with the help of a duty social worker) from a magistrate. The paediatricians and senior casualty staff and social worker must be involved from an early stage in these cases.

Children who have been allegedly sexually abused may be brought to casualty for one reason or another. These children should be dealt with by senior paediatricians, police surgeons, and social workers; it is not the place of a casualty officer to attempt to take a history from or examine them. To do so needs considerable experience and might actually prejudice the child's case or render any subsequent examination invalid, and be a further source of anxiety and distress to the victim.

Deaths

A casualty officer is rarely in a position to sign a death certificate. Death certificates must be issued by a doctor who has recently treated the patient for the same condition and this excludes most casualty officers. The coroner's officer must be informed of any death from unnatural causes (i.e. all accidental deaths) and he will arrange for a post-mortem examination and certification of death. If tissue transplantation from a dead (or brain-dead) accident victim is contemplated the consent of the coroner and the deceased's nearest relative should be obtained.

(The coroner does not actually give consent for tissue or organ removal, he just refrains from objecting to it.)

Where the death is that of a late spontaneous abortion or apparent stillbirth, the paediatrician should be called urgently and resuscitation started as these infants can apparently survive prolonged anoxia even if they initially appear quite dead. When death is confirmed in an A & E department the *time* should be noted as it occasionally has medicolegal significance (e.g. cases of inheritance).

Negligence

Negligence may be a criminal or a civil offence. The term 'medical negligence' usually refers to the civil offence, also called a 'tort'. The tort of negligence requires three ingredients:

1 A duty of care,
2 A breach of that duty, and
3 Harm as a result of that breach.

For example: A doctor may make a serious error but no *harm* results — perhaps because someone else (nurse, pharmacist, etc.) spots the mistake and arranges for its correction before harm is done. In addition, for a finding of medical negligence, it is necessary to show that the doctor fell below the expected standard of care. A doctor need not possess the highest expert skill; it is well-established law that it is sufficient if he/she exercises the ordinary skill of an ordinary competent doctor exercising that particular art.

A great many accusations of negligence are the result of poor communication, lack of courtesy, or an arrogant attitude by the doctor, compounded by defensiveness and worse communications. If you have not been negligent in your care of the patient you may have to rely on your notes of the examination and treatment to prove it. If you have been negligent, or think you have, then inform your consultant, and seek the advice of your medical protection organisation at the earliest opportunity and take steps to ensure that the patient receives appropriate treatment if there is still this option (e.g. recall the patient to treat a missed fracture). A full written report should be made and kept while the incident is still fresh in your mind, whether or not the case is pursued.

The results of tissue and blood specimens sent for investigation must be checked, and any abnormal reports acted upon. Failure to do so sometimes results in litigation, particularly if the patient has suffered as a result.

Medico-legal report

Doctors working in Accident & Emergency departments are frequently asked by solicitors to write reports on injuries sustained by patients attending the A & E department.

On occasions they just require a short account, taken from the casualty card, which they will use to start any subsequent actions. This report can be taken quite easily from the documents and x-rays in the department. Usually, however, they also want to know about progress, and in most cases a prognosis. In these cases it is better to review the patient and check exactly what changes have happened since. The solicitor is naturally interested in his client getting fair compensation for the injury and this must be borne in mind whilst you are writing this report. What is really needed is a fair report which will describe the injuries, the treatment required, the amount of pain and disability, and finally a prognosis — when is the patient ready to get back to work and how will the effects of the injury affect the plaintiff's life and future care? Is it going to effect long-term loss of earnings? Many of these cases, of course, include serious injuries when the patient will have been admitted, so it is better for the request for a report on these cases to be forwarded to the doctors who carried out the long-term treatment. However, many cases are dealt with in the Casualty department, finish their treatment, and need only a brief report.

Content of report

The first section of the report should give:

Patient's name:

Address:

Date of birth:

Occupation — should include details of what the job actually entails, the type and degree of work, and effort required.

Hobbies — quite frequently people are engaged in hobbies requiring dexterity or stamina, or take quite a lot of physical exercise. Quite trivial injuries of the hand can interfere seriously with these hobbies. It is useful to notice at this stage whether the patient is right-handed or left-handed and whether the injury affects his occupation or hobbies.

Date of accident:

Date of examination for medical report:

History of accident

Try to elucidate the details of how the accident occurred; obtain an indication of how much trauma was inflicted on the patient. If the patient was knocked out or dazed it is important to note this and also if travelling by ambulance the ambulance number or any PCs in attendance should be noted. Notes made in Casualty on examination should be described with copies of diagrams for multiple injuries and lacerations; include x-ray reports and treatment given. A note on disposal: follow this with notes on further attendances.

Progress

Include the times of attendance in the department and details of treatment, e.g. for removal of sutures when the wound has healed. Here it is important to register any time spent off work: when he returned to work did he return to full duties or only partial duties — i.e. was he protected from his normal duties for a further period?

Present condition

Ascertain exactly how he is, how the injuries have progressed, are there any permanent disabilities from the injury, does he complain of any persistent disability or deformity? Carefully list these present complaints.

On examination

A thorough examination must be made of the patient and it is important to examine the patient as a whole. Note any persistent scars, size, site, visibility, colour, and sensation. It is useful at this stage to note if there is any numbness distal to the site of the scar. During the course of the examination note the general agility of the patient — how easily he walks in, sits, stands, and moves during the course of the examination. It is also useful to note whether he manages to get dressed quite easily after the examination, and if there has been any change for the better in the degree of agility, etc.

X-rays

A review of all x-rays that are obtainable should be made at this stage.

Opinion

This must include the injury that has been sustained with a description of its cause and its effect on the patient, a brief résumé of the details of the patient and the effect that the injury has had on his work and hobbies. Notice the presence and duration of pain and the present type of treatment required to deal with the pain — whether there has been any change in its frequency, severity, or duration.

The effect of the accident on the patient's reactions in general: is he worried about driving or riding, and in the case of the elderly are they worried about going out by themselves?

Prognosis

This is quite important because the solicitor will need to know if the patient has reached a static position. Have the wounds healed satisfactorily, has the scar matured, are the effects of the strain of a ligament going to improve, or do you think this has reached its final degree? Will he return to all his sports and activities? Scars of the face: you should note whether there is a cosmetic deformity or not and whether this will need further treatment or needs make-up etc. to cover it.

Sign the report with your name, medical qualifications, and the position you hold, and if, as commonly happens, you are moving on to another appointment it is useful to put a permanent address through which you can be contacted. The address given in the Medical Register is recommended.

End of report: keep a copy in your file.

Appearing in court

Medical evidence remains a most important part of the administration of justice, both civil and criminal. The following guidance applies to all courts that you may be called to.

1 *The witness summons or subpoena*

A lawyer may subpoena you as a witness and there is no escaping this. However, much can be achieved by good communication with the lawyer to ensure minimum disruption to the A & E department and your personal life. Take all notes, reports and x-rays with you: revise them the day before and consult reference books if need be.

2 *Dress up*

You should attend court looking like a doctor — a smart and sober appearance will impress.

3 *Stand up*

It impresses the court if the practitioner stands up in an interested and attentive manner.

4 *Speak up*

You should speak in a firm voice, audible to all, using language which all can understand.

5 *Shut up*

You should listen carefully to the question, and should think carefully before replying. Give your reply as concisely as possible, consistent with your oath or affirmation. You should then shut up (i.e. remain totally silent).

6 *Visual aids*

Since you should avoid medical jargon, any diagram (copies if possible), chart, model, or surgical instrument can be a great help in expressing yourself.

7 *Fair play*

Do not be bullied: if a yes or no answer is impossible say so. The trial judge will usually be sympathetic and can be turned to for help if the going gets rough.

8 *Enjoy it*

With adequate care and preparation an appearance in court can be an interesting rather than a harrowing experience.

N.B. Keep in contact with the A & E department for the next couple of years as they may need to know where to contact you.

TABLE 19.1

Medico-legal reports Aide memoire

PATIENT'S	name,
	address,
	occupation,
	hobbies,
	right or left handed.
DATE	of birth,
	of accident,
	of examination.

HISTORY	of accident.
HOSPITAL PROGRESS	findings and treatment.
PRESENT	condition and complaints.
CLINICAL EXAMINATION: positive and relevant negative findings.	
X-RAYS	review.
OPINION PROGNOSIS	remember pain, disability, work, hobbies, scars, fears.
YOUR NAME,	qualifications, appointment.
PERMANENT ADDRESS.	

NOTES

20

Soft tissue injuries, bites and infections

Soft tissue injuries

These are injuries to the skin, muscles, tendons, and ligaments, where damage to bone, nerves, vessels, and viscera have been excluded.

Types of injuries sustained are: Bruises, abrasions, lacerations, incisions, and puncture wounds, and these may be complicated by haemorrhage, infection, or other complications, depending on the site of the injury. Bites are common and may be dangerous or disfiguring — they are discussed separately below.

Soft tissue injuries must be examined carefully to exclude damage to underlying structures such as tendon, bone, nerves, and blood vessels. The possible involvement of underlying joints, ligaments, organs, or viscera must also be considered. Measure and record the number, size, and site of the injuries, with diagrams where appropriate. These details and diagrams are particularly important in medico-legal cases which may go to trial years later.

Bruises

Tender swellings appear gradually after blunt trauma. The blood may track for some distance before appearing under the skin. Note the colour of the bruise and, in non-accidental injury, the presence of bruises of differing colours suggesting they were inflicted at various times, see Table 20.1. Check that the patient is not on anticoagulant therapy, and exclude bony injury. When fresh apply ice-pack, then compression with wool and a firm crêpe bandage. Elevate the limb if possible and ease the pain with an effective non-steroidal anti-inflammatory agent (NSAI). If the bruise does not resolve and a fluctuant haematoma forms, incise this under LA and expel the semi-solid clot. Apply wool and a firm crêpe bandage afterwards. (Antibiotics are usually required at this stage.)

Abdominal bruising with marks from a seat belt or boot points to the possibility of visceral injury.

Post-auricular bruising may indicate skull injury.

TABLE 20.1

Age of bruises

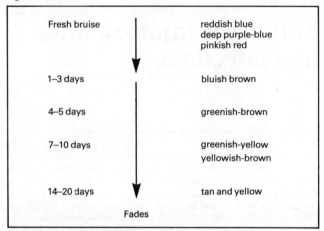

Fresh bruise	reddish blue
	deep purple-blue
	pinkish red
1–3 days	bluish brown
4–5 days	greenish-brown
7–10 days	greenish-yellow
	yellowish-brown
14–20 days	tan and yellow
Fades	

These changes show the general trend of changes, depending on amount of blood and depth: influenced by skin pigment. N.B. blood may appear at a distance from site of blow. These times are approximate only.

Open wounds

Abrasions

The skin damage may be full or partial thickness, similar to burns, and is frequently impregnated with grit or gravel and clothing.

- Clean thoroughly, usually under local anaesthetic, with a small brush and antiseptic.
- Apply an antiseptic cream such as povidone-iodine and a non-adherent dressing (NAD) which should be left for seven days if patient remains symptom free.
- Large or multiple areas require full cleaning under general anaesthetic.
- Deep friction abrasions over joints, frequently seen in motorcyclists thrown from their machines, may involve damage to the joint capsule.

Facial

1 After cleaning all impregnated grit, apply silver sulphadiazine (Flamazine) and leave exposed.
2 Review after a few days.

3 Any grit not removed will cause permanent tattooing, disfigurement, and possibly litigation, later.

Lacerations

Full thickness skin wound, with ragged edges, often with tissue damage to underlying structures.

Examination

1 Think of the underlying anatomy and examine carefully for tendon, nerve, or vessel damage, especially in the hand (see Chapter 23).
2 Even small (1 cm) wounds may sever tendons or nerves.
3 All wounds caused by glass must be x-rayed before treatment, though not all glass is radio-opaque. Soft tissue film with special x-ray. Tiny fragments which remain after debridement may be noted and left.
4 Clean and explore under local anaesthetic.

Laceration: irrigate copiously with normal saline, evacuate haematoma, excise carefully any dead tissue and remove any foreign material such as clothing, etc. Secure haemostasis. Lacerations should be closed with sutures — unless presentation was delayed.

● Pretibial area — steristrips are the method of choice.
● Ragged, extensive lacerations, particularly of children, of the face, or involving deep structures such as joints, tendons or nerves, require formal repair under GA so the patient should be admitted.
● In major injuries consider delayed primary suture after 3–4 days.

Flexor tendon or nerve injury

Obtain orthopaedic or plastic surgical opinion.

Muscle laceration

Expel any haematoma, carefully excise dead muscle (does not contract when pinched) then suture loosely with catgut. Obtain haemostasis. Leave a drain if muscle is oozing.

Facial lacerations

1 Examine the facial nerve, parotid duct and interior of mouth. If nerve or duct is damaged, *refer* to facio-maxillary surgeon immediately.
2 Clean thoroughly with an antiseptic and then saline.
3 Excise all foreign or dead material and irrigate dirty wounds well with normal saline.
4 Convert to a tidy wound with straight edges by excising untidy fragments. Suture carefully with 5.0 or 6.0 prolene or ethilon.

TABLE 20.2

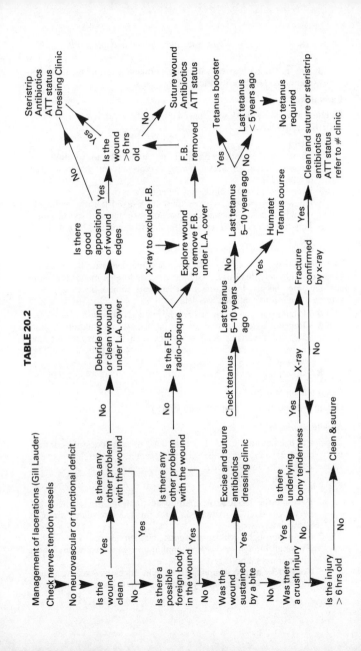

Management of lacerations (Gill Lauder)

Check nerves tendon vessels

No neurovascular or functional deficit

Is the wound clean — Yes → Is there any problem with the wound — No → Is there a possible foreign body in the wound — No → Was the wound sustained by a bite — No → Was there a crush injury — No → Is the injury >6 hrs old — No → Clean & suture

Is the wound clean — No → Debride wound or clean wound under L.A. cover → Is there good apposition of wound edges — Yes → Is the wound >6 hrs old — No → Yes → Steristrip Antibiotics ATT status Dressing Clinic

Is the wound >6 hrs old — No → Suture wound Antibiotics ATT status

Is there any problem with the wound — Yes → Is there a possible foreign body in the wound — Yes → X-ray to exclude F.B. → Is the F.B. radio-opaque — No → Explore wound to remove F.B. under L.A. cover

Is the F.B. radio-opaque — Yes → Explore wound to remove F.B. under L.A. cover → F.B. removed — Yes → Suture wound Antibiotics ATT status

Check tetanus — Last tetanus 5–10 years ago → Tetanus booster

Last tetanus 5–10 years ago — Yes → Tetanus booster
Last tetanus <5 years ago — No → No tetanus required

Was the wound sustained by a bite — Yes → Excise and suture antibiotics dressing clinic

Check tetanus — Last tetanus 5–10 years — No → Humatet Tetanus course
Last tetanus 5–10 years — Yes → Tetanus booster

Was there a crush injury — Yes → Is there underlying bony tenderness — Yes → X-ray — Yes → Fracture confirmed by x-ray — Yes → Clean and suture or steristrip antibiotics ATT status refer to # clinic

Is there underlying bony tenderness — No → X-ray — No

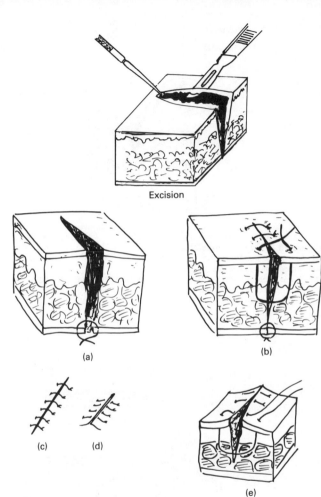

Figure 20.1 Wound excision and suture
(a) Fascial suture
(b) Suture needle introduced vertically through skin and subcutaneous tissue
(c) Ordinary
(d) Eversion
(e) Eversion suture

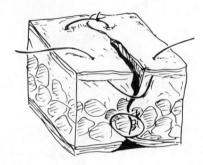

Figure 20.2 *Common errors of suturing*
- *Fascia not closed*
- *Subcutaneous sutures too tight*
- *Angle of needle entry and exit wrong, causing skin edge inversion*
- *Sutures too far from wound edge*
- *Skin suture too tight*

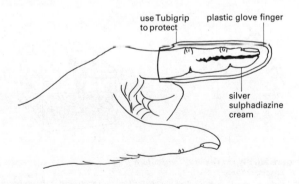

Figure 20.3 *Burst injury of finger*

Acknowledgements to Smith & Nephew Pharmaceuticals Ltd.

Steristrips will provide extra support and act as a dressing. With lips and eyebrows do not excise tissue, and make sure that the alignment of the mucocutaneous junction or hair line is exact. Mark these points before injecting the LA; it is impossible to define them after. Preferably a 'field block' or nerve block rather than infiltration with LA.

Eyelids

Damage to the tarsal plate or lacrimal duct or tissue loss requires opthalmological opinion — *refer*.

Scalp

Examine the underlying bone for fracture with a probe. Expel haematoma and close in one haemostatic layer with 3.0 silk sutures. Single accessible bleeding vessels should be ligated with cutgut.

Wound excision and suture

Full thickness skin loss

Obtain surgical opinion, especially if a facial wound. If in doubt, or to temporise for up to eight hours, cleanse and apply moist saline dressing and bandage. Cover exposed tendons with split skin graft or synthetic wound dressing such as Granuflex or Opsite.

Points to note

- Systemic antibiotics are not required for the above injuries: unless tendon or bone exposed or bite wound to the hand.
- Thorough cleaning and meticulous excision of dead tissue prevents infection.
- Tetanus prophylaxis — see Table 20.3.

Puncture wounds

1 Exclude internal damage in all stabwounds to chest and abdomen (page 25): x-ray the chest; *refer* for a surgical opinion — exploration may be necessary.
2 Other puncture wounds should be cleaned and thoroughly irrigated. If there is a possibility of a retained foreign body, x-ray and then explore. Remember to check tetanus status in all lacerated and puncture wounds.

Crush injuries

These will swell amazingly. If a limb has had a significant crush injury, admit patient for elevation of the limb, analgesia and observation of the distal circulation. Monitoring of the internal pressure in the osteo-fascial compartment may be necessary.

Urgent fasciotomy may be required to avoid the compartment ischaemia syndrome. *Pain*, made worse by movement of the digits — particularly extension, is an early warning sign. The limb is tense. If the

TABLE 20.3

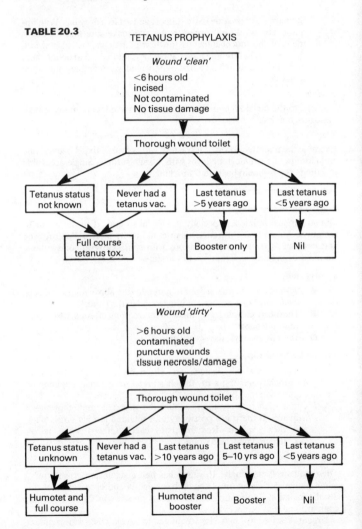

TETANUS PROPHYLAXIS

Wound 'clean'

<6 hours old
incised
Not contaminated
No tissue damage

Thorough wound toilet

Tetanus status not known | Never had a tetanus vac. | Last tetanus >5 years ago | Last tetanus <5 years ago

Full course tetanus tox. | Booster only | Nil

Wound 'dirty'

>6 hours old
contaminated
puncture wounds
tissue necrosis/damage

Thorough wound toilet

Tetanus status unknown | Never had a tetanus vac. | Last tetanus >10 years ago | Last tetanus 5–10 yrs ago | Last tetanus <5 years ago

Humotet and full course | Humotet and booster | Booster | Nil

Anne McGuiness

patient's limb has been trapped with compression for one to two hours, then crush syndrome may occur with myoglobinuria and renal failure. *Refer*.

Minor

1 Cleanse wounds, steristrip.
2 If no abnormality, apply wool and tubigrip, then rest with elevation.
3 Review within 48 hours.
4 Do not suture crushed fingers.
5 Use occlusive silver sulphadiazine dressing (Figure 20.3).

Delayed primary treatment of wounds presenting late

A different method of treatment is required for wounds presenting after 24 hours or if dirty or infected.

1 Take a bacteriological swab for culture and sensitivity before cleaning.
2 Cleanse thoroughly and drain any pus.
3 Enlarge the skin wound if necessary, carefully excise any dead tissue and subcutaneous fat and split the deep fascia to inspect the muscle.
4 Excise any muscle which does not contract on pressure with forceps or bleed on cutting.
5 Approximate skin loosely with steristrips.
6 Dress with povidone iodine and a non-adherent dressing. If cellulitis or lymphangitis is already present, give antibiotics, leave open and elevate. Remember tetanus toxoid.
7 Inspect wound in three days, when it may be suitable for delayed primary suture.

Wounds over a tendon or ligament

Examine the movements of the joint but remember that other muscles may produce the same movement. Wounds should be examined in the position in which the injury occurred so that injured structures are 'in line' for inspection. Examine the joint for instability to exclude ligamentous damage. Explore the wound under local anaesthetic. If a skin wound only, suture with 4.0 prolene.

Extensor tendon

Division, or partial division, is repaired with 4.0 prolene if you are surgically competent; a splint is applied in extension. If one end only of a tendon is found or if the flexor tendon is involved — *refer*.

Wound over joint

A superficial injury to a joint ligament can be repaired with catgut and the joint splinted. Wounds exposing the interior of joint require orthopaedic

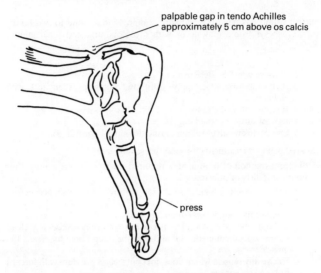

palpable gap in tendo Achilles
approximately 5 cm above os calcis

press

Figure 20.4 *Rupture of tendo Achilles*

referral urgently. Note that the knee joint is superficial adjacent to the patella: the interphalangeal joints are easily opened by teeth in a fight.

Closed injuries

Closed tendon and ligament injuries

Sprain

An overstretching, with partial tearing, of the ligaments around a joint. The joint is moderately swollen and bruising appears slowly. Tenderness is localised to the area of the ligament and should be carefully defined to differentiate from bony tenderness, the sign of a fracture.

Strain

Overstretching of the muscle or muscle-tendon unit. Patients complain of pain on movement: on examination there is tenderness on palpation of the structure and muscle spasm may be present around the bruise. A complete tear of a muscle belly, commonly in the biceps, quadriceps, or gastrocnemius, presents with pain, swelling, bruising, and the contracted belly can be felt proximally. A tear of the long head of the biceps is often associated with a rotator cuff tear which should be looked for as operative repair is indicated.

Treatment: apply an icepack if a recent injury (within 8 hours). An elastic cotton bandage such as tubigrip will give support and possibly reduce oedema. Analgesia is obtained with an NSAID, which will reduce swelling and allow early movement and use of the limb. The patient is encouraged to start non-weight-bearing muscle exercises and movement immediately. This is particularly important in the knee and ankle.

This regime of rest and exercise, if properly supervised by a physiotherapist, will restore the patient to full fitness more quickly. Unfortunately this supervision is not always possible, so the patient must be encouraged to carry out the regime himself.

Muscle/tendon rupture

Often there is a visible or palpable gap in the tendon but this may fill with bloodclot quite quickly. The Achilles tendon is commonly torn, usually when playing tennis or golf when sudden force is applied. The patient complains of a sudden blow on the tendon with loss of power in the ankle. He walks with a limp and is in severe discomfort. On examination, with the patient kneeling and pushing against your hand with his foot, there is a palpable tender gap at an early stage, later the gap fills with clot. (Figure 20.4.) Plantar flexion against resistance is lost, so he is unable to rise on his toes. *Refer* for opinion on operative repair. If this is not possible a POP splint, with the ankle plantar flexed and the knee flexed, is required.

Ligament rupture

Ligament rupture is accompanied by severe pain, sudden swelling, and bruising. The joint is unstable, and if there is any doubt a stress x-ray is done; a general anaesthetic allows the test to be done more reliably.

The swollen leg

A patient complaining of swelling of a leg commonly attends A & E.

History

Acute or gradual onset? Painful or painless? Note previous episodes which may be a factor in the present complaint: varicose veins, deep vein thrombosis (DVT), white leg of pregnancy, clots in leg requiring heparin or warfarin. Ask specifically about oral contraceptives and check them in the BNF. Prolonged immobility, such as long-distance flights, or the excessive activity of jogging or marathons may also cause swollen legs. Old injuries, operations or IV drug injections may also interfere with venous or lymphatic drainage. Remember that fractures immobilised in POP cause an oedematous swelling which elevation would have prevented; DVT may also occur in a leg in POP.

Clinical diagnosis

Deep vein thrombosis: classically oedematous leg with venous engorgement; the colour may be either red or white. There is tenderness in the deep calf muscles, and forced dorsiflexion of the ankle causes calf pain (Homan's sign). An urgent venogram is required to establish the diagnosis: the patient is admitted for anticoagulant therapy.

Lymphatic obstruction: pitting oedema is present; lymphadenopathy in the groin or a pelvic mass may be found. Service in the tropics may have resulted in Bancroft's filariasis.

Superficial thrombophlebitis: varicose veins are present, usually in both legs. The superficial veins are tender and the area along the vein shows inflammation. There may be tenderness extending along the long saphenous vein.

Infection — cellulitis: the skin is red, hot, and swollen with a throbbing pain. An ascending lymphangitis may extend to the groin with lymphadenopathy; usually with pyrexia. Look for small wounds, including between the toes.

Management

If no other causes can be found for a swollen leg, assume that there is a DVT present. An urgent venogram or Doppler ultrasonography is required. Admit for treatment as a DVT with heparin drip until proven otherwise.

A rectal examination is mandatory for a unilateral swollen leg.

Infection: Start flucloxacillin and ampicillin; attempt to find source and obtain swab for culture and sensitivity. Apply tubigrip and rest patient with leg elevated. If the infection is spreading rapidly, or the patient is septicaemic, then admit for further investigation and treatment.

Superficial thrombophlebitis: Apply a supporting tubigrip shaped bandage, advise rest, elevation, and gentle muscle exercise. An NSAID will give relief from pain. Review in three days or *refer* to GP for further follow-up

Lymphatic obstruction or pelvic mass: Apply tubigrip support bandage, rest with elevation, analgesia. *Refer* for urgent surgical opinion.

Bites

Bites should be considered as crushing and tearing wounds rather than incised. The majority of bites seen in the UK are minor dog bites, usually of the hand or leg. The dirtiest wounds often follow human or cat bites. Complications are skin necrosis, infection, tetanus, rabies.

History

● Carefully record where the bite was sustained and in which

country. If this was outside the UK suspect rabies. (See 'Travellers' Diseases' page 381.)
- Whether animal or human, and if an animal whether it was diseased, enraged, or provoked. What happened to the animal — was it observed, captured, killed, or examined?
- Time elapsed since bite?
- Look: bruising, abrasion, puncture marks, or laceration? Is wound inflamed or infected?
- Examination should exclude damage to underlying nerve, tendons or joints. In human fights the metacarpo-phalangeal joints in the hand are commonly injured.

Management

Early primary care of the wound is most important.

Simple abrasions: after cleaning apply povidone iodine and a non-adherent dressing.

In deeper wounds: thorough cleansing then excision of damaged sub-cutaneous tissues are essential to prevent wound infection. If the deep fascia has been penetrated it should be split and any underlying dead muscle excised to prevent clostridial infection.

Human bites

These are particularly prone to infection, especially to the hand and ear. They need excision under local anaesthetic and a broad-spectrum antibiotic (Augmentin), with review in 24 hours. If there are any signs of spreading infection, admit for intravenous antibiotics. Consider the risk of hepatitis or HIV infection if anything is known of the biter. A punch wound from teeth is the same as a human bite.

Monkey bites

These are also prone to infection and may be infected with herpes simplex virus. In addition to antibiotics, start oral acyclovir therapy, 400 mg 5 times daily and review.

Snake bites

- Poisonous bites are infrequent in the UK, the only poisonous snake being the adder (viper) — see Figure 20.5. Most bites are peripheral.
- Contact the nearest Poisons Unit with details of the snake and clinical details of the patient's condition since the bite.

(a) *If there has been no local reaction or swelling* at the bite, evenomation has not occurred.

(b) *Mild evenomation* — there is slight swelling at the bite with or without nausea.

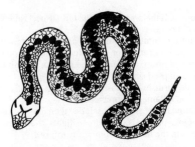

Figure 20.5 *European viper*

(c) *Moderate evenomation* — there is local swelling at the bite. Patient has vomiting, diarrhoea, transient hypotension, and collapse resolving within 30 minutes. Swelling of the limb as far as elbow or knee may progress slowly in the next 48 hours.

(d) *Severe poisoning* — there is severe hypotension and collapse which persists. A bleeding diathesis lasting 30 minutes and swelling of the limb occurs more rapidly. There may be ECG changes. Blood examination usually show a leucocytosis, rarely an elevated CPK, and SGOT. There is, occasionally, renal damage.

Treatment

1. No evenomation — treat as any bite.
2. Signs of evenomation — admit to ITU for monitoring.
3. Zagreb anti-venom must be used only for severe evenomation. Be careful with known allergies.
4. The more central the bite and the more poisonous the snake, the greater the urgency for supportive treatment.
5. Local treatment
   Clean: Pressure — immobilisation. A firm bandage and splints; elevate.

Soft tissue infections

Abscesses

Pus must always be drained as soon as diagnosed and never deferred to a minor operating session days later. Fluctuant infected sebaceous cysts generally have staphylococcal infections.

Incisions

1 Clean skin, incise adequately, and drain under LA. If the abscess is already leaking, the opening is enlarged with forceps and the cavity is curetted.
2 Send swab culture and sensitivity.
3 Irrigate cavity and pack with fusidic acid (Fucidin).
4 Re-dress in 24 hours.

Larger abscesses

These include axillary, breast and all perianal abscesses and require a GA. Remember that a red, hot, tender area over a child's bone may be an early osteomyelitis. X-ray will show nothing other than soft tissue swelling at the early stage. The child rapidly becomes toxic and may show signs of bronchopneumonia. *Refer* urgently.

Recurrent skin infections

These may result from diabetes so urine and blood sugar levels should be taken. Reinfection from a chronic staphylococcal nasal infection may occur. Nasal swab and culture should be done. In a patient showing general cachexia and weight loss, consider drug abuse or immune deficiency disease.

These infections, however, frequently occur as troublesome problems associated with stress, overwork, or inadequate diet. General health counselling is required with follow-up arrangements so refer to the General Practitioner.

Streptococcal infections

Cellulitis

Red, hot, swollen, oedematous, and tender area appearing after a short history. Usually there is a portal of entry for the infection such as a distal blister or laceration, although this may not be obviously infected.

Lymphangitis

A red line tracking proximally from a wound or area of infection leading to lymphadenopathy with systemic toxicity. Check patient's temperature and drain any pus. Give oral flucloxacillin and ampicillin every six hours (or erythromycin) and review in 24 hours. If the patient is toxic and his temperature rises quickly, associated with other signs of toxaemia, malaise and vomiting beware of septicaemia. Take blood for culture, then admit and treat with intravenous antibiotics.

N.B. Cellulitis of the upper lip, nose, and maxillary area still carries a risk of cavernous sinus thrombosis so requires special care and observation. Periorbital cellulitis carries a high risk of mortality (~10%) and should be admitted.

Acute bursitis

The bursae that frequently develop an acute bursitis are the olecranon, pre-patella, infra-patella and that over the metatarso-phalangeal joint of the great toe. There is usually a history of recurrent intermittent pressure on the area. On examination the area is painful, red, and swollen, and the bursa is tense or fluctuant.

Treatment

1 Clean the skin and aspirate through a large bore needle under LA. Usually a thick serous fluid is obtained.
2 Dress the wound with providone iodine cream, apply non-adherent dressing, wool and tubigrip.
3 Rest the joint by a sling or elevation of leg.
4 Send the aspirate for culture and sensitivity: uric acid crystals.
5 Start an oral broad-spectrum antibiotic and analgesics.
6 Review the patient and culture results within 48 hours.

Orf

A chronic viral infection usually associated with butchers or farm workers dealing with sheep. Clinical appearance is a red, friable, granulomatous, chronic condition usually on a finger. The condition usually resolves spontaneously, but the finger needs protecting from the risk of further infection. Treat with povidone iodine and NAD. The patient should not handle animals or meat until the condition is cured.

Pyogenic granuloma

A rapidly growing granuloma, usually on hand or foot, associated with a small, often trivial, skin wound. The granulation tissue is abundant and bleeds on contact. Treatment is to clean and curette excess granulation tissue, apply povidone iodine. If this does not cure then complete excision under LA might be necessary.

Leg ulcers

There may be loss only of epithelium, but frequently the skin loss is full thickness and infected, and healing proceeds slowly from its edge. The ulcer occurs commonly on the medial aspect of the lower leg, and usually follows minor trauma or pressure associated with various predisposing conditions:

(a) Chronic venous insufficiency from varicose veins or DVT is the principal cause, but in many cases this is aggravated by (b).
(b) Arterial insufficiency, arteritis with ischaemia such as Buerger's Disease in the young person, or atherosclerosis in the elderly.
(c) Diabetes or sensory loss, together with connective tissue disease, has an effect on the healing process.
(d) Pyoderma gangrenosum should be considered especially in younger patients. Always examine the limb carefully to establish the correct diagnosis.

A profuse exudate does not always mean infection, so look at the skin edges carefully to see if infected. The wounds heal best in warm moist conditions; in the absence of pathogens; under moderate pressure to relieve venous back pressure and adequate nutritional state. Many of the limbs are oedematous and this requires elevation and rest treatment otherwise healing is delayed.

Treatment

1 If ulcer is clinically infected take a bacteriological swab and treat with appropriate systemic antibiotic for 5 days.
2 Clean ulcers with saline, apply antiseptic such as povidone iodine for 5 days if infected. Apply an occlusive wound dressing such as granuflex. Modern foam dressings work on the principle of keeping the wound microenvironment moist, so encouraging epithelium to grow rapidly from the margins of the ulcer. Cover with adequate layer of wool or Gamgee dressing and support the leg with firm compression by a Dickson Wright blue line bandage.
3 Do not dress too frequently. Every 5 to 10 days is sufficient.
4 To prevent recurrence after these ulcers have healed compression supporting stockings must always be worn by the patient when venous insufficiency is present. With obvious varicose veins the patient is referred for a surgical opinion.

Vertical leg drainage

When the leg is oedematous it is important to reduce the amount of fibrin-rich oedema fluid in the leg, and this can be done at weekends without loss of work. The legs are elevated as long as possible for Saturday and Sunday (see Figure 20.6). The patient has a viscopaste bandage or the granuflex/Gamgee/blue line bandage applied weekly at first, then monthly until the ulcer is healed. See Figure 26.26, page 423.

Infected ulcers

Excise any obvious slough. The base is usually insensitive. Cleanse with saline or hydrogen peroxide solution. Dress with antiseptic cream, every 48–72 hours until infection has settled.

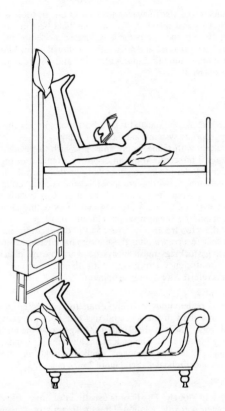

Figure 20.6 *Vertical leg drainage*
Leg ulcers will heal only in the absence of oedema. Vertical leg drainage is the best method of reducing oedema. This can be done for 48 hours over the weekend. Elevate the legs and keep them at an angle of at least 60°, the patient getting up for bodily functions only. There should not be any pain or change of colour of the foot. When the oedema has disappeared, bandage the leg with viscopaste. The bandage needs changing only every 2–3 weeks.
Use vertical leg drainage every day whenever you can, even if only for a short period

NOTES

21

Joints

Joints allow movement between the ends of bones. Articular cartilage and synovial fluid make movement easier by lubrication and reduction in friction. They are stabilised by the bone ends and ligaments. Surrounding joints there are muscles and tendons which facilitate movement. Sensory branches of the motor nerves to these muscles give a rich nerve supply to the joint on which they act, hence the marked perception of pain and reflex loss of movement. The tendons are covered by sheaths to allow easier movement where they cross other structures; these allow tendons to slip between bone and skin, over joints.

Painful joint

A joint will become painful when the structures either within or around it are damaged through injury, inflammation, or infection. Inflammation may result from either joint disease or abnormal use. The following conditions cause pain in joints.

Osteoarthritis (OA)

Chronic pain which gets worse over years with acute exacerbations; worse on moving, 'like a door creaking'; caused by wear. Best *referred* to GP.

Rheumatoid arthritis (RA)

Painful joints: worse in morning, better in evening. Many other long-term manifestations of the rheumatoid state are present. Best taken care of by GP or rheumatologist. Will probably be on tablets — do not change.

Gout

Gout usually occurs in the MTP joint of the great toe but should be suspected in acute excruciating monoarticular pain in any joint. Patient hates any contact, or jarring of joint. Serum uric acid is raised.

The drug of choice in acute gout is Azapropazone, as it increases uric acid excretion and is also an anti-inflammatory analgesic. Aspirin is contraindicated.

Long-term treatment is best supervised by the GP.

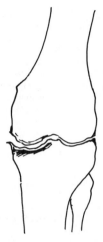

Figure 21.1 *Osteoarthritis of knee. Varus deformity, narrowing of medial joint space, subarticular bone sclerosis, osteophytes*

Septic arthritis

There may be a history of minor trauma. The patient is pyrexial, toxic and feels ill. The joint is tense, very painful and movement is impossible because of muscle spasm. Differential diagnosis: rheumatoid arthritis, acute bursitis and gout.

If suspected, immediate orthopaedic *referral* is essential. Admission and lavage of the joint is mandatory.

Effusion

A rapidly developing effusion indicates the presence of a serious injury. An effusion that comes up overnight is usually due to a sympathetic synovitis.

Bloody effusion is usually the result of trauma and necessitates orthopaedic *referral*.

A fat–fluid interface on an x-ray of joint indicates a fracture. Effusions should only be tapped for good clinical reasons, e.g. sepsis for C & S.

Locking joint

A joint will lock when a loose fragment impinges between the articular surfaces. This may be a loose body or a displaced piece of joint tissue, e.g. knee menisci or synovial frond.

Gentle manipulation may unlock the joint, but they should in any case be *referred* to an Orthopaedic Clinic.

Joint gives way

Usually affects the knee. This is caused by a reflex inhibition of the quadriceps muscles when the knee is about to lock. The quads relax to avoid damage to the joint. This should be taken seriously as it denotes a mechanical derangement and may occur at an inappropriate moment, e.g. when crossing the road. *Refer* — further investigation and arthroscopy are required.

Clicking joint

Clicks occur in many normal joints and as a sole symptom should not be pursued.

TABLE 21.1

Treatment of acute joint injuries

ACUTE MUSCULO-LIGAMENTOUS STRAINS TREATMENT
R = REST
I = ICE
C = COMPRESSION
E = EXERCISE

Tendonitis

Tendonitis occurs where tendons either cross structures, pass through osteo-fascial tunnels, or the insertion into bone.

Mobile tendons are covered by sheaths which lubricate them. Overuse or unusual use causes inflammation of these sheaths. Pain on movement of the tendons then occurs. If the tendon passes through an osteo-fascial tunnel then a painful arc will occur while the inflamed part of the tendon is in the tunnel.

On examination

There may be palpable crepitus over the tendon. The point of maximum tenderness moves with movement of the joint.

Treatment

Rest, NSAID, physiotherapy. Steroids should not be injected in the acute stage (wait at least six weeks from initial symptoms).

Overuse can cause pain at the insertions of tendons. Local point tenderness is present.

Bursitis

Inflamed bursae are hot and tender. They are not usually infected.

Treatment

Rest, NSAID and tubigrip support. If they persist aspirate through wide-bore needle.

X-ray of joints

Always have two views. Look at the alignment of bones. Note if there is abnormal rotation of one bone with regard to another. Look at the bony outlines: even a 1 mm depression of a joint surface is important. Look for fractures around and into the joint. Look at the peri-articular soft tissue for swelling. Look for a fluid level (blood–fat interface) in the joint. This is pathognomonic of a fracture (especially useful in elbow and knee).

Temporo-mandibular joint

This is just in front of the ear. It can be felt opening and closing just anterior to the external auditory meatus. Often gives problems after whiplash injuries.

Movements

Opening and closing of mouth; side-to-side glide.

Examination

Look at occlusion of the teeth. Look at how widely the mouth can be opened. Can the mouth be slid from side to side while shut?

Dislocation

This joint can be dislocated by a yawn or by a blow. In traumatic dislocation a fracture is also usually present. All fractures should be referred to a Facio-maxillary department.

Reduction

Adequate relaxation. Press downwards on the lower molars with thumbs. While doing this, rotate the jaw upwards and it should click back into place.

Shoulder

The shoulder is a highly mobile joint. It has a relatively lax capsule and is held in place by muscle tone.

Injuries can be caused by traction or falls onto the arm.

Movements

See Figure 21.2.

Examination

Look at the outline of the joint. Has the rounded outline disappeared? Are there any tender points? Is there a hollow where the head of humerus should be? Check movements. If dislocated, the patient cannot put hand onto opposite shoulder.

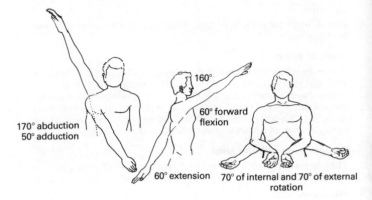

Figure 21.2 *The shoulder movements*

Check

    (a) axillary nerve (triangle of sensory loss in upper arm over the deltoid and paralysis of deltoid).

    (b) brachial pulse.

X-ray

Two views. Look for alignment of humeral head on the glenoid. Note the acromio-clavicular distance. Look for fractures. True lateral is essential to exclude posterior dislocation. (See Figure 21.3.)

Dislocation — anterior (Subcoracoid)

The humeral head lies below and in front of the glenoid. This is usually easy to spot. However, if the x-ray is taken with a sling on, the humerus can be lifted up and the x-ray is hard to interpret.

Dislocation — posterior

Usually occurs after a fit or ECT. The arm is medially rotated and external rotation is not possible. The dislocated head is best seen and felt looking from above. These can easily be missed on x-ray if two views are not taken.

Reduction — anterior

Adequate relaxation and analgesia are essential. Diazepam and pethidine IV are usually sufficient unless patient is very muscular, when a GA is essential.

Kocher's method: With an assistant stabilising the trunk, apply firm traction for 3–4 minutes. Slowly externally rotate and abduct the arm while

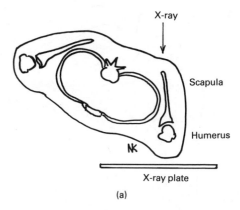

X-ray

Scapula

Humerus

X-ray plate

(a)

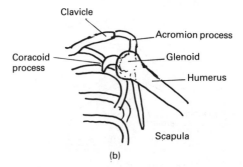

Clavicle

Acromion process

Coracoid process

Glenoid

Humerus

Scapula

(b)

Figure 21.3 *Lateral X-ray of shoulder joint*
(a) Position for X-ray: horizontal or erect
(b) Lateral X-ray of shoulder joint

continuing traction. Adduct the arm across the chest. Internally rotate the arm. Reduction is usually accompanied by a clunk. (Figure 21.5.)

Hippocratic method: Use this technique if there is an associated fracture of greater tuberosity or head — but not if head is completely separated from the shaft. The stockinged foot is placed in the axilla and longitudinal traction applied to the arm. Apply gentle outwards pressure with your toes and the head will be replaced in the glenoid. (Figure 21.6.)

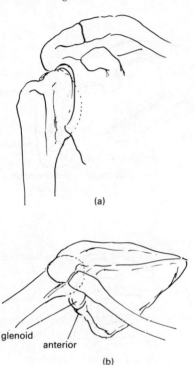

(a)

glenoid   anterior

(b)

Figure 21.4 *Post dislocation of shoulder*
(a) Antero-posterior X-ray. Note medial overlap and medial rotation of humerus
(b) Axial X-ray

If the patient's hand can be placed on opposite shoulder reduction is complete.

Hold in position with sling. Re-x-ray — 2 views.

Reduction — posterior

Apply traction with the arm at 90 degrees to the trunk. Externally rotate the arm, push on humeral head from the back.

Post reduction apply sling and re x-ray.

If reduction is unstable, plaster with the arm held in abduction.

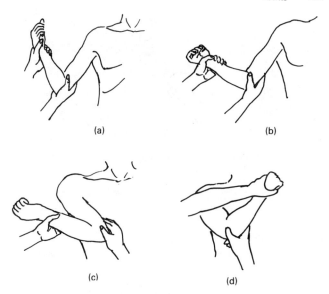

Figure 21.5 *Kocher's technique*
(a) Hold the elbow
(b) Externally rotate and abduct slowly and gently
(c) Adduct point of elbow
(d) Internally rotate adducted elbow

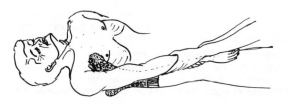

Figure 21.6 *Hippocratic technique. Apply traction over stockinged foot in axilla. Gentle inversion of foot will ease the head of the humerus laterally*

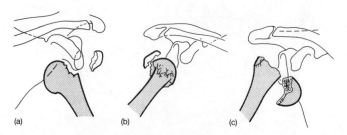

Figure 21.7 *Fracture dislocation of shoulder*
(a) Fracture of greater tuberosity
(b) Impacted fracture of surgical neck
(c) Separated fracture of surgical neck.

Fracture dislocation

Fracture of greater tuberosity and dislocation: reduce as for simple dislocation.

Treatment As for simple fracture.

Fracture neck humerus and dislocation

If head is in continuity with the shaft reduction by Hippocratic technique, simple traction and manipulation of the head in the axilla by the stockinged foot may be successful.

If the head and shaft are not in continuity, closed reduction is likely to fail. Therefore refer to Orthopaedic Surgeon. (Figure 21.7.)

Painful shoulder

Many people present with a painful stiff shoulder. The pain results from tendonitis or capsulitis and may radiate to the outer aspect of the upper arm. If there is a painful arc on movement then tendonitis is the cause. (Figure 21.8.)

Treatment — sling, NSAID, physiotherapy.

Shoulder pains from frozen shoulder are often severe with fluctuating intensity levels and may take 6–18 months to settle.

Always check in case the pain is referred from cervical spondylitis in the neck.

Acromio-clavicular joint

This is situated above the shoulder. The very strong coraco-clavicular and acromio-clavicular ligaments hold the joint in place.

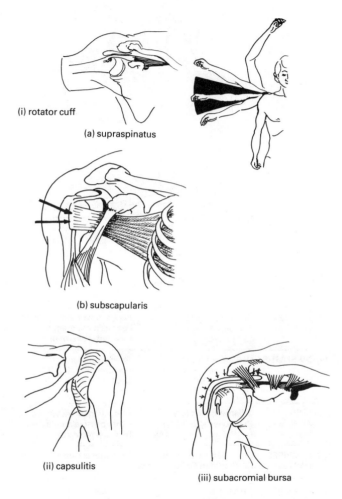

(i) rotator cuff

(a) supraspinatus

(b) subscapularis

(ii) capsulitis

(iii) subacromial bursa

Figure 21.8 *The painful shoulder*

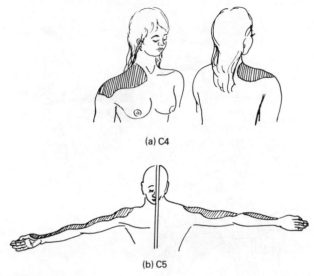

(a) C4

(b) C5

(iv) referred pain

(i) ROTATOR CUFF	Overuse, repeated strain. Supraspinatus — painful arc.	Active movement decreased. Passive movement full. Resisted movement painful.
(ii) CAPSULITIS	45+, minor trauma Pain spreads to wrist 4/12 Pain recedes 4/12 Full movement returns 4/12	Lateral rotation ↓ 60° Gleno-humeral ↓ 45° Medial rotation ↓ 15°
(iii) SUB-ACROMIAL BURSA	Inflamed, no injury. Pain to wrist 2–3 days. Painful arc as improves.	Abduction restricted. Other passive movts present. Resisted movts painless.
(iv) REFERRED PAIN	Cervical dermatomes: C4 shoulder, C5 lateral arm.	Neck movts cause pain.
(v) ACROMIO-CLAVICULAR JOINT PAIN	Strain, osteoarthritis. Localised tenderness.	Scapular rotation painful.

Figure 21.8 *(continued)*

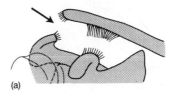 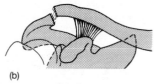

Figure 21.9 *Acromio-clavicular joint*
(a) Dislocation
(b) Subluxation

Examination

Look at the outline of the joint. The end of the clavicle may protrude subcutaneously. Tenderness is present under the outer end of clavicle.

X-ray

Widening of space between the end of clavicle and the acromium. If doubtful repeat with patient holding a weight, taking comparison view of other side. (See Figure 21.9.)

Dislocation

Usually a sling will suffice. *Refer* to fracture clinic as open repair may be necessary.

Sterno clavicular joint

If the sterno clavicular joint is injured, the medial end of the clavicle may be displaced either in front of or behind the manubrium. Anterior dislocations are usually minor and, apart from cosmetic defect, function well. They are treated with a sling.

Posterior dislocations can cause compression of the great vessels in the neck. They need immediate referral for reduction under general anaesthetic. In high-speed accidents look for cardiac contusion: patient needs ECG and monitoring.

X-rays are difficult to interpret: the diagnosis is clinical.

Elbow

The elbow is a hinge joint with strong collateral ligaments allowing articulation between the humerus and ulna. The radius is held in place by the annular ligament.

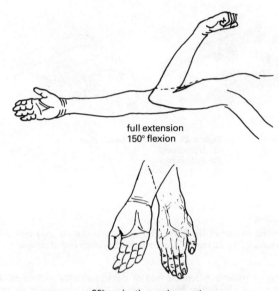

full extension
150° flexion

80° supination and pronation

Figure 21.10 *Movement of elbow*

Examination

Check range of movement. If diminished, the block may be due to either pain or bony obstruction. Swelling of joint is more noticeable on posterior inspection. Check pronation and supination of the forearm. Is the triangle between medial and lateral epicondyles and the olecranon equal sided?

Check distal sensation and pulses.

Feel for bony pain.

X-ray

Look closely at bony outline. In addition know the positions of the epiphyses. (See Figure 21.11.) Look for fat-pad sign anterior to humerus; this denotes a fracture (usually of radial head). Check position of proximal radius on lateral film. (It should be partially overlapped by humerus, see below.) *If you have any doubts compare with x-ray of normal elbow. Refer.*

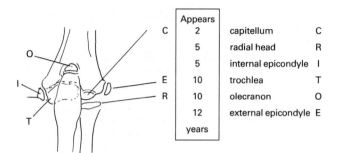

Appears		
2	capitellum	C
5	radial head	R
5	internal epicondyle	I
10	trochlea	T
10	olecranon	O
12	external epicondyle	E
years		

Figure 21.11 *Epiphyses at elbow*

Injuries

Usually caused by fall on outstretched hand, fall on point of elbow, or pulling of the arm.

Dislocation

Needs to be defined in terms of position of humerus. Usually anterior dislocation. The coronoid process may be fractured, which increases the chance of recurrent dislocation. The equilateral triangle between the olecranon and 2 epicondyles will be disturbed. Check distal sensation and pulses.

Reduction: Good relaxation. Hold elbow flexed, distract forearm and upper arm until reduction obtained. A clunk indicates reduction.

Post-reduction x-ray: Examine for fat pad sign, coronoid or condylar fracture. If present, fixation may be necessary. *Refer*.

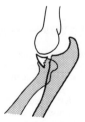

Figure 21.12 *Dislocated elbow (coronoid fracture)*

Post reduction: Apply plaster back slab (well padded) and sling with elbow in 90 degrees of flexion.

Fracture head of radius

Treat as soft tissue injury. Sling and gentle mobilisation as pain allows.

If head is comminuted or has gross irregularity of joint surface — *refer*.

Dislocated radial head

(Pulled elbow: Sunday afternoon elbow.)

In children the head of the radius does not develop sufficiently to be held firmly by the annular ligament until the age of 4 years. If a child is swung or is falling and catches hold of something, the head of radius can be dislocated. Parents often think the child has hurt its wrist because it will not pronate or supinate the forearm.

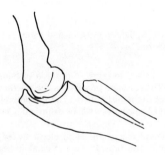

Figure 21.13 *Dislocated radial head of child. Note that the head of the radius is not visible but radius does not point to capitulum*

X-ray: Interpretation is difficult — two good lateral views of both elbows are essential.

Treatment: Is by pronating the forearm — a reasonable amount of force is needed. A click is felt. The child will begin to use the arm within 5–10 minutes. If unsuccessful, arm should be supinated — *refer* for re-manipulation.

Once reduced, no further treatment is necessary.

In adults, dislocation head of radius without a fracture is *rare*. Lateral x-ray shows proximal radius is not overlapped by the ulna. *Refer* to Orthopaedics with a full-length lateral x-ray.

Pain around elbow

Various types of tendonitis (see page 286) occur around the elbow, including Tennis elbow (lateral epicondyle) and Golfer's elbow (medial epicondyle). Pain may radiate down forearm. There is tenderness over the condyle with pain on stretching the muscles. Rest from activity, NSAI, and physiotherapy.

Olecranon bursitis occurs over the olecranon (see Bursitis for treatment).

Wrist and hand

The wrist is an ellipsoidal-shaped joint. It allows for flexion, extension, abduction, adduction, and circumduction. The proximal row of carpal bones articulate with the radius and the triangular radio-ulna cartilage. Also note carefully on the x-ray how the carpal bones articulate with each other.

Examination

Test movement, look for deformity. Check any local tender points. Check distal blood and nerve supply, particularly the median.

X-ray

AP and lateral x-rays are most useful. Check for fractures. Note — a tiny fracture of the ulnar styloid can cause severe pain. Look at the lateral x-ray: the pisiform normally stands out on its own. The lunate sits with its concave surface in contact with the capitate. If the lunate is clearly visible anteriorly (like the pisiform) then it is dislocated. If it is clearly visible but in normal relationship with the radius, a perilunate dislocation is present.

Look at the AP x-ray. Note that all the bones are congruous and in close proximity to each other with no holes or gaps.

The proximal row of carpals forms a curved articulation with the distal row. The distal row forms a straight articulation with the metacarpals. The bases of the metacarpals overlap each other.

Injuries

Lunate dislocation

See x-ray. The lunate will press on the median nerve and cause nerve damage if not reduced. Reduction (under GA). Apply longitudinal traction for several minutes. Supinate the wrist. Apply traction and dorsiflex the wrist. Press on the lunate with your thumb. The lunate should be felt to slip into place. Plaster in slight flexion is applied. If unable to reduce, open reduction is mandatory. *Refer.* (Figure 21.14.)

Perilunate dislocation

Reduce by traction. Treat as for lunate dislocation. Open reduction and stabilisation are often necessary.

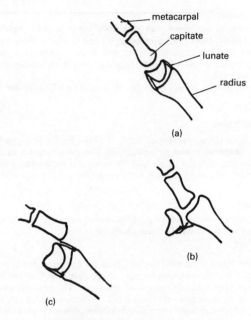

Figure 21.14 *Lateral views of carpal X-ray*
(a) Normal
(b) Dislocated lunate
(c) Perilunate dislocation

Other dislocations of the carpus occur. Closed reduction can be attempted but fixation may be necessary. (Figure 21.14.)

Thumb

Examination

Check movements: the thumb should be able to run down little finger to the distal palmar skin crease. Check for laxity of joints especially collateral instability following damage to metacarpo-phalangeal joint.

Injuries

Fracture dislocation

Of the carpo-metacarpal joint is a Bennett's fracture. Dislocation should be reduced by traction and stabilised in a plaster spica or admitted for

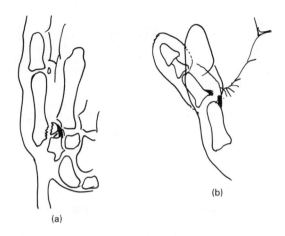

Figure 21.15
(a) Bennett's fracture dislocation of thumb
(b) Gamekeeper's thumb. Ulnar collateral ligament torn or avulsion fracture

percutaneous wire fixation. (See Figures 21.15 (a).)

Metacarpo-phalangeal joint (Gamekeeper's thumb). This may be injured in ski accidents. Check the ulnar collateral ligament. If the joint is unstable refer to Orthopaedic Surgeon for repair. If stable but painful (ligament sprained but intact) apply a thumb spica and review in 10 days. Avulsion fractures around joint are indications for Orthopaedic referral.

Fingers

Check flexion and extension. Inspect for rotational deformity. Test for lateral ligament instability.

X-ray

Check for fractures into the joint. Check for avulsion fractures — these are attached to ligaments. Check bone alignment.

Injuries

Dislocations of carpo-metacarpal joints

These are usually posterior. Reduction is by traction. Apply POP back slab. Thumb carpo-metacarpal dislocations reduce easily but are very unstable and may require internal stabilisation with a Kirschner wire.

Dislocation PIP joint

Digital nerve block. Reduce by extending the joint and apply traction whilst manipulating the base of middle phalanx around the head of proximal phalanx. If reduction is not possible by this means, open reduction is indicated. Apply a splint in extension as flexion tends to occur post-traumatically and is very difficult to overcome.

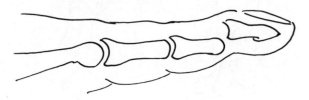

Figure 21.16 *Dorsal dislocation of DIP joint*

Dislocation of distal interphalangeal joint

Again is usually posterior. Reduction is usually easy with thumb pressure on base of the distal phalanx. Neighbour strapping not necessary.

Mallet finger (see page 353).

Hip

The hip is a ball-and-socket joint. It has a strong anterior ligament: movements: as Figure 21.17.

Examination

Is the patient able to walk? Look at position of the leg. Examine movements and compare with the other side. Are there any tender points?

X-ray

Antero-posterior (AP) and lateral. Look at Shenton's Line. Is there any disturbance of the trabecular pattern in the bone? Look at the pubic rami.

N.B. Pain may be referred from the hip to the knee and vice versa as they share a common nerve supply.

Injuries

Central dislocation

This is caused by a direct injury in the long axis of the femur. The head of the femur is driven through the acetabulum. This is a serious injury. IV fluid replacement should be commenced and blood cross-matched. Immediate referral to Orthopaedic department is mandatory. There may be other associated internal injuries.

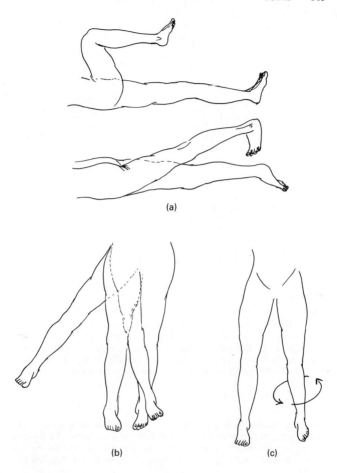

Figure 21.17 *Range of movements of hip joint*
(a) 110° flexion and 30° extension
(b) 50° abduction and 30° adduction
(c) 45° internal rotation 45° external rotation

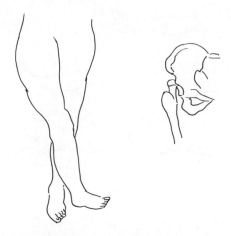

Figure 21.18 *Dislocation of hip*

Posterior dislocation

The leg is shortened, adducted, and internally rotated.

X-ray: Check for associated acetabulum fracture. (See Figure 21.18.) Reduction under general anaesthetic as soon as possible. The hip is flexed to a right-angle. Correct the adduction. Lift the entire leg forward while the pelvis is stabilised by an assistant. It clunks into place; then extend. *Refer* to Orthopaedic department for admission for traction. Ischaemic necrosis of head of femur occurs in 20 per cent of cases.

Check sciatic nerve for neuropraxia.

Slipped femoral epiphysis

This is commonest in fat male adolescents. It is associated with pain and a limp. X-ray in two planes to show slip. If the knee cannot be brought across to the opposite shoulder then slipped epiphysis should be suspected. *Refer* to Orthopaedic department. (See Figure 11.6, page 160.)

Pains around hip

Pains on the medial side of hip with tender point on pelvis may be due to adductor tendonitis. Pain below the joint anteriorly may result from psoas tendonitis (see tendonitis, page 286). Pain on lateral aspect of joint over great trochanter may be caused by a bursitis. In patients complaining of pain around the hip, check for herniae. (Also pressure from the inguinal ligament on the lateral cutaneous nerve of thigh can cause pain on upper lateral thigh and mimic hip pain.) Frequently hip disorders cause pain in the knee.

Children

See page 158.

Knee

The knee transmits all the body weight. Its stability is largely dependent on its ligaments, but well-developed quadriceps muscles help to stabilise it. It has a collateral ligament on each side. The anterior and posterior cruciate ligaments prevent sliding of the femoral condyles on the tibia. The menisci lie on top of the tibia. The medial meniscus is attached to its corresponding collateral ligament. (See Figure 21.19.)

Examination

Look for an effusion. A rapidly developing effusion usually indicates a serious joint problem: *refer* today.

- Test the ligaments. The knee needs to be flexed to 20 degrees in order to test the collateral ligaments.
- Test for cruciate ligament stability by pushing (posterior) and pulling (anterior) the tibia with the knee flexed to 90 degrees and the foot stabilised. Compare with other knee. (N.B. in posterior cruciate tear, the tibia may have fallen backwards and so give a false positive for anterior cruciate tear.)
- Check for tender points at the collateral ligament insertions and on the joint line.
- Check range of movements — see Figure 21.20.

  A 'springy block' to full extension is characteristic of an acute meniscal injury: *refer* for EUA and arthroscopy.

X-ray

In injuries, the lateral x-ray should be taken with the patient lying down and a shoot-through film taken.

Lateral x-ray

Look for fat–fluid interface in suprapatellar pouch. This indicates a fracture in the joint and orthopaedic referral is mandatory. Check the joint line. Check for depression of tibial plateau. Check the patellar cortex and the patella tendon insertion.

Anteroposterior (AP)

Check the tibial spines. Check the joint line. Check the body of the patella.

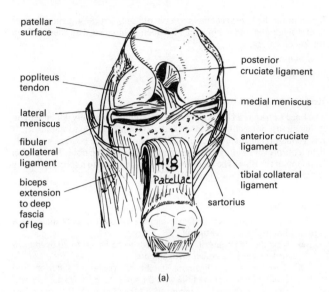

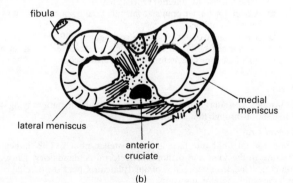

Figure 21.19 *The knee joint*
(a) Ligaments,
(b) Articular surface

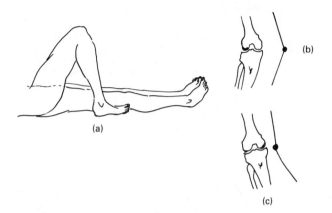

Figure 21.20 *Range of movements of the knee*
(a) The knee has 135° flexion
(b) Deformities pointing inwards (medially) are called VALGUS
(c) Deformities pointing outwards (laterally) are called VARUS

Injuries

- Usually by direct or twisting force on the knee with the foot fixed. If the patient says the knee twisted or uses clenched fists to demonstrate rotation suspect a ligament rupture. Any disruption of ligaments must be *referred* to the Orthopaedic department immediately.
- If an effusion has come up rapidly there is internal damage — *refer*.
- A late effusion is usually a sympathetic effusion and so bodes less ill.
- Effusions should not be tapped unless septic arthritis (see page 346) is suspected.
- Non-ruptured ligament injuries should be treated with NSAID, tubigrip support, and if necessary — crutches. Early quadriceps exercises should be instituted. 'Rest and exercise.' (Figure 21.21.)
- Vascular damage is likely with knee dislocations. Refer and reduce early.

Dislocation patella

Dislocation patella is more common in females. The patella jumps out laterally. It can be replaced by gentle pressure along its lateral border and

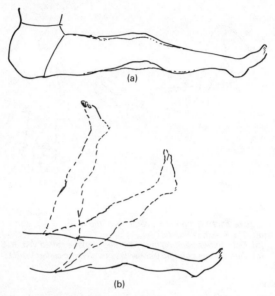

Figure 21.21 *Quadriceps exercises*
(a) Tighten quadriceps muscle, pushing knee flat on couch. Hold for two seconds: relax. Do 25 times. Repeat every hour. Can be done sitting or standing whilst waiting
(b) Tighten quadriceps muscle, pulling up the knee cap to make the leg straight. Lift and hold. Slowly lower on to bed. Repeat 10 times, three times daily

extension of the leg. X-rays are mandatory as there is an incidence of bone changes in patella or lateral femoral condyle (10%). A POP cylinder is applied, quadriceps exercises started, and the patient referred to the fracture clinic.

Pains around knee

Pain at insertion of patella tendon: the epiphysis at the insertion of the ligamentum patellae can be pulled by heavy use in pre-pubertal adolescents (Osgood-Schlatter's disease). Lateral x-ray will show widening and irregularity of the apophysis.

Treatment — is rest. Patients should not partake in the activities (e.g. sports, cycling or football) that produced the pain. The condition is self-limiting as the apophysis fuses between the ages of 15 and 16 years.

Pain behind the knee

Swelling in the popliteal fossa (Bakers cyst associated with OA and RA) may cause pain down the leg.

Treatment — is rest. Referral to the Orthopaedic Clinic. Excision is necessary only if the swelling obstructs knee flexion.

The hamstrings can develop tendonitis.

Pain in front of the knee pre-patella bursitis.

Pain beneath the knee cap: This is chondromalacia patellae. The pain is worse on going downhill and cycling. It is caused by roughness on the back of the patella.

Treatment — is by physiotherapy to develop the vastus medialis. It can be self-limiting. Persistent pain: *refer* to Orthopaedic department.

Clicking at lateral side knee: The ileo-tibial band slips across the lateral side of knee causing a click. The click is not significant. It may become painful. If painful, treat as tendonitis.

Ankle and foot

The ankle is a hinge joint. The talus is held between the malleoli. The ligaments are: the strong deltoid on the medial side, three small strands on the lateral side, and the inferior interosseus tibio-fibular ligament.

Flexion and extension take place at this joint.

The foot bones articulate with each other.

There are many small ligaments holding these together. A strong fascial band from the calcaneus (plantar fascia) with the dynamic support of the peroneus longus, anterior and posterior tibial and intrinsic muscles, holds the longitudinal arch of the foot in position. Inversion and eversion of the foot takes place at the subtalar joints.

Examination

- Look: swelling of the ankle is more noticeable from behind. In particular look for swelling above the malleoli. Look for swelling in the foot. Check all movements of ankle and foot.
- Feel for tenderness behind the malleoli, the fibula up to knee, at insertion of the talo-fibular ligament and at the base of the fifth metatarsal.
- Check for continuity of Achilles' tendon. (The foot should plantar flex when the calf is squeezed with the patient lying prone.) Test for active plantar flexion against the resistance of your hand.

X-ray ankle

If patient

1 Is over 60
2 Cannot weight bear

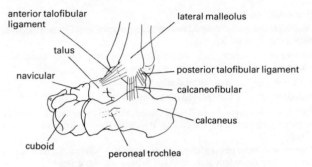

Figure 21.22 *Lateral side of the left ankle joint*

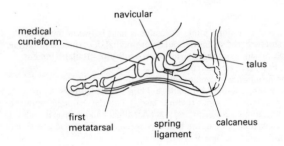

Figure 21.23 *Longitudinal arch of foot*

3 Has pain or swelling above malleolus
4 Fell down steps
   (a) *Antero-posterior* (AP): check for fractures of the tibia and
       fibula. Check joint line. Check distance between medial
       malleolus and talus (any increase in diastasis is significant).
   (b) *Lateral*: check the posterior border of the tibia. Look at the
       lateral malleolus. Look for small avulsions off the navicular.
       These indicate ligament damage.
   (c) *Foot*: Check the alignment of the bones with each other. *N.B.*
       The talus and calcaneus form a continuous joint with the
       navicular and cuboid. The navicular articulates with the three
       cuneiform bones. The cuboid and the cuneiforms articulate
       distally with the metatarsals.

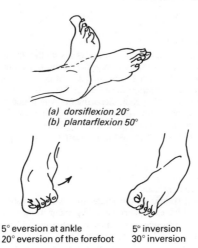

(a) dorsiflexion 20°
(b) plantarflexion 50°

5° eversion at ankle
20° eversion of the forefoot

5° inversion
30° inversion

Figure 21.24 *The ankle joint movements*

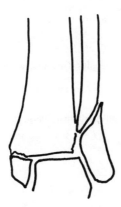

Figure 21.25 *X-ray: Potts fracture of lateral and medial malleoli with diastasis*

Injuries

Fractures — dislocations

Lateral or posterior fracture — dislocations of the ankle joint must be reduced immediately, ideally before x-ray, as the skin is pulled tightly over the distal edge of the tibia and is in danger of necrosis. The foot is often avascular and the circulation must be checked after manipulation. Then x-ray and refer to Orthopaedic department. Any dislocation of the fore foot can be unstable and may need fixation, therefore refer to Orthopaedics. If avascular you may have to manipulate.

Dislocation of toes — treat as for metacarpals (see Chapter 23).

Sprains

- Beware of diagnosing sprained medial ligament of the ankle without an x-ray. The medial malleolus breaks more readily than the ligament tears.
- Lateral sprains of the ankle are common, usually the anterior band of the external collateral ligament. Immediate swelling with marked bruising is diagnostic of tearing of the ligament and recovery will be much longer. Stress x-ray to demonstrate any talar tilt. Young athletes require operative repair. There is often associated tarsal ligament strain.
- Sprained ankles should be mobilised from day 1 as this gives quicker recovery. If there is also pain in the foot, recovery takes 2–3 times as long. In such cases strong support strapping, non-steroidal anti-inflammatory drugs, and physiotherapy help. Plasters may cause long-term stiffness.
- Small avulsion fractures should be treated as sprains.

Pains around ankle

Tendonitis

(See Chapter 20.) q.v. Tendonitis of the muscles in front and behind the ankle is common.

The plantar fascia on the sole of the foot may become painful.

Treatment

As for tendonitis, but add a sorbothane insole to the shoe.

22

Fractures and bone infections

Fractures

It should always be possible to diagnose a fracture by clinical methods alone and use x-rays only to confirm the position of the bone fragments, but alas this ability often comes only with the experience that a new casualty officer has not had in his previous training.

Listen carefully, assess the amount of trauma, the type of injury, onset and severity of pain, swelling, bruising, and interference with function from the patient's history.

Look to determine limb position, deformity, swelling, condition of skin and circulation: if any wounds are present do they connect with the fracture from within or without?

Feel gently along the bone for tenderness, irregularity, and distally for skin circulation, temperature, pulses, and tenseness of the soft tissues. Palpate the ligaments of adjacent joints with fingertips and try to assess stability. Test for skin sensation and muscle action beyond the fracture.

X-ray to confirm the diagnosis, but more importantly to determine the correct treatment. Two views at right-angles (antero-posterior and lateral), are needed always. If you are confident, after a careful clinical examination, that there is no fracture there is no need to x-ray unnecessarily; tell the patient your diagnosis and treatment but always record your findings in the notes. (See Figure 22.1).

Treatment

Basic principles of first aid should be applied to all fractures on entering the department to avoid pain, further damage to the skin or circulation, and shock. Wounds are dressed, limbs are straightened and splinted. Give adequate analgesia, intravenously for severe injuries.

Multiple fractures, even if not compound, will cause shock; so measure blood pressure and pulse rate, then start an intravenous infusion of normal saline (see Multiple Injuries, page 15).

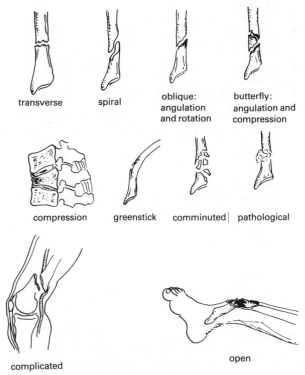

transverse   spiral   oblique:
angulation
and rotation

butterfly:
angulation and
compression

compression   greenstick   comminuted| pathological

complicated   open

Figure 22.1 *Types of fracture*

Limb ischaemia

Limb ischaemia following a fracture is a dangerous complication which if not recognised and treated swiftly can lead to compartment syndrome, muscle ischaemia, necrosis followed by fibrosis and Volkmann's contracture or gangrene.

● *Pain*, severe and often agonising, is the dominant feature, with a pale, tense limb often with paraesthesia. Nailbed circulation is absent. Passive extension of the fingers in supracondylar fractures, or flexion of the toes in upper tibial fractures, is restricted and painful.

- *Urgent treatment is required: refer.*
- Correction of the deformity in an unreduced fracture by gentle longitudinal traction, under IV pethidine, will often improve the distal circulation.
- If a fracture has been reduced and held in POP this must be divided down to skin and opened along its full length.
- Restricting dressings, often hard with blood, must be cut.
- An arm held in flexion after reduction for a supracondylar fracture should be extended until the distal circulation returns. It does not matter if the reduced position of the fracture is lost; the arm is elevated, in extension with a padded posterior splint, until the swelling decreases and it is then remanipulated.

Pathological fractures

Minimal force will cause fractures in bone weakened by osteoporosis in old age, infection, cysts, and either primary or secondary tumours. There may be a history of previous treatment but often the pathological fracture is the presenting sign.

Transverse shaft fractures in the old are particularly suspicious.

Stress fractures

Repetitive minor trauma, such as occurs in training for competitive sports, marathon or long-distance running, or marching in military recruits, will often cause a stress or fatigue fracture. The patient will give a history of repeated hard exercise followed by pain and limping. This worsens with the pain occurring sooner in the activity and eventually without it.

On examination there is bone tenderness, often localised with slight swelling. X-ray in the early stages often is normal. Later x-rays show slight rarefaction of the cortex, a linear fracture, followed by callus formation (see Figure 22.2). If the diagnosis is unclear a technetium bone scan is useful as it shows a 'hot spot' at the fracture site.

The common sites are the second or third metatarsals, fibula, tibial shaft, patella, neck of femur, and less commonly the shaft of femur.

If you suspect this diagnosis, firmly advise the patient to stop further training and rest the limb: re-x-ray in 2 weeks.

Battered baby syndrome

Multiple fractures, of different ages, with varying amounts of callus, in long bones and ribs should make you suspicious. A careful examination of the naked child may often reveal bruises of varying colours, blue to green then yellow, cigarette burns, and finger marks. *Refer* See NAI (page 161).

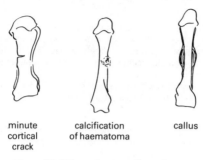

minute   calcification   callus
cortical   of haematoma
crack

Figure 22.2 *Stress fracture: X-ray changes*

Fractures of the arm

Clavicle

Listen: A fall on the outstretched arm.

Look: The arm has dropped down and the bone causes a swelling under the skin.

Feel: The bone end may threaten to penetrate the skin. Check brachial pulse and plexus, particularly if associated with abrasions of face and shoulder from a motorcycle accident.

X-ray: Fracture usually in middle third of shaft, often comminuted. (See Figure 22.3.)

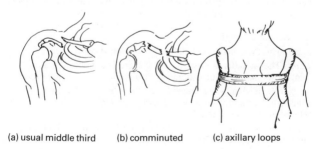

(a) usual middle third   (b) comminuted   (c) axillary loops

Figure 22.3 *Fractures of clavicle*

Treatment

1 Initially support the weight of the arm with a St John's sling.
2 Patients often feel happier with a figure-of-eight bandage (or axillary loops), bracing the shoulders back for the three weeks it takes for union: the fracture unites with overlap and abundant callus, 1% go on to non-union.
3 Check supports daily until comfortable, then less frequently until stable (10–14 days). Support for 21 days.

Scapula

Listen: A direct blow may fracture the blade, and often the underlying ribs as well. A fall onto the outstretched hand may fracture the glenoid articular surface or neck. Painful injuries.

Look: A varying amount of swelling occurs. Carefully check for chest trauma, arterial or brachial plexus injury. May be source of bloodloss.

Move: Movements are restricted.

X-ray: If comminution of the body is seen, x-ray the chest for signs of haemo- or pneumothorax. In fracture of the scapular neck depression of the glenoid by the weight of the arm is seen. Occasionally the fracture involves the articular surface.

Treatment

1 Support the weight of the arm as for fracture of the clavicle.
2 Review following day in fracture clinic.

N.B. If you have any doubts about intrathoracic injury *refer* for admission.

Humerus

Head and neck

Many of these injuries are associated with dislocation of the shoulder — hence the need to x-ray the joint before attempting manipulation. Fracture dislocations are difficult and should be referred if possible.

3 and 4 part fractures of head also need *referral*? ORIF in young or replacement in elderly.

Listen: Has there been a fall onto the outstretched arm?

Look: The shoulder is swollen, and if there is a dislocation as well, the joint shows characteristic flattening with a prominent acromion process.

Feel: The head may be palpable in the subcoracoid region. Test the axillary nerve; motor — deltoid muscle, sensory — small area over the infero-lateral part of deltoid.

X-rays: Fracture of the greater tuberosity is often seen in a dislocation, the periosteum usually holds the fragment, with supraspinatus insertion, in contiguity with the humerus; post-reduction films show it in its normal position. Lateral view is essential.

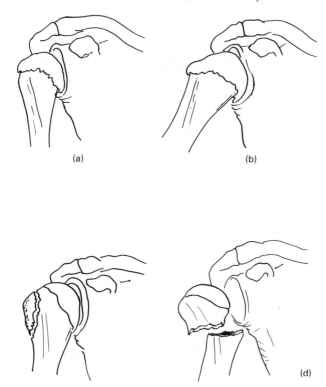

Figure 22.4 *Fractures of proximal humerus*
(a) Impacted adduction fracture of neck
(b) Impacted abduction fracture of neck
(c) Fracture of greater tuberosity
(d) Displaced fracture of surgical neck

Neck of humerus

This is a transverse fracture; the shaft is frequently abducted and impacted and this is a stable injury (see Figure 22.4). If the shaft is displaced medially and anteriorly it is less stable. When associated with dislocation the head may be completely separated. This is *a very serious injury* because of the risk of avascular necrosis.

Treatment

1 Fracture of the greater tuberosity alone needs support with a collar-and-cuff sling for two to three weeks. If displaced ORIF.
2 Fractures of the neck of the humerus with little displacement should be treated in the same way.
3 Start physiotherapy early in an impacted fracture.
4 Displaced fractures should be treated in a collar-and-cuff sling and *referred* early particularly 3 and 4 part fractures.
5 Fracture dislocations of the shoulder joint are best referred, but if this is not possible, the Hippocratic method of reduction is recommended unless the humeral head is already completely separated from the shaft.

Shaft of humerus

Fractures of the shaft following a fall are usually spiral in configuration: a direct blow will produce a transverse fracture. (Figure 22.5.) Damage to the radial nerve producing wrist drop is not uncommon and should always be tested for. Involvement of the radial nerve is an indication for exploration, so refer the patient.

Treatment

Collar-and-cuff sling; a well-padded POP U slab or cast brace will add further weight to the arm and provide some protection from knocks.

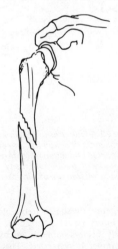

Figure 22.5 *Fracture shaft of humerus*

Supracondylar

These fractures usually occur in children following a fall onto the arm. In 90 per cent of cases the lower fragment is posteriorly displaced. (See Figure 22.6.)

There is a considerable risk of vascular and nerve involvement so this patient should *always* be admitted for treatment and post-reduction observation of the distal circulation, finger movements — particularly of extension, pain, and sensation. Reduction of this fracture requires considerable skill to obtain a good carrying angle and correct rotation so patient should be *referred*.

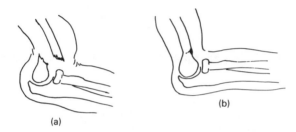

(a)

(b)

Figure 22.6 *Supracondylar fracture*
(a) Displaced
(b) Greenstick

Fractures of the elbow

Medial epicondyle

This is often displaced with damage to the ulna nerve. Operative reduction may be necessary. *Refer.* (See Figure 22.7.)

Capitellum

This fracture is best seen in the lateral x-ray and is frequently displaced proximally; operative treatment is required. *Refer.*

Trochlea

If displaced, open reduction is required. *Refer.*

Olecranon fracture

This fracture follows a fall on the elbow and is frequently displaced or comminuted. *A fissure fracture without displacement can be easily missed.*

Feel: In displaced or comminuted fractures the separation in the olecranon may be felt and active extension of the arm is not possible. The arm should

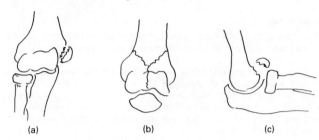

Figure 22.7 *Fractures of the elbow*
(a)   Medial epicondyle fracture
(b)   Intercondylar fracture
(c)   Capitellum fracture

be held in extension with a padded POP slab and the patient referred for open reduction.

Head of radius

This results from a fall on the outstretched hand. Movements of the elbow are restricted and painful; particularly pronation and supination.

X-ray: will show a minimal fissure fracture, comminution or depression of the articular surface.

Treatment

Fractures involving the articular surface, with comminution of the neck (or in a child with displacement of the epiphysis of the neck) need skilled reduction: *refer*. Undisplaced fissure fractures require a collar-and-cuff sling for three weeks with early mobilisation.

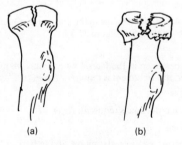

Figure 22.8 *Radial head fractures*
(a)   Fissure fracture
(b)   Comminuted fracture

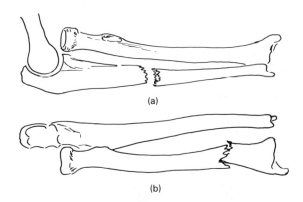

Figure 22.9 *Fractures of radius and ulna*
(a) Monteggia fracture dislocation
(b) Galeazzi fracture dislocation

Fractures of the shafts of radius and ulna

Fractures of both bones at the same level are common following a direct blow, but following rotational injury the fractures will be at different levels. Fractures in children are frequently rotational and greenstick.

Fracture of the shaft of ulna is often solitary and transverse following a blow with a baton. However, an ulna fracture may be associated with dislocation of head of radius (Monteggia fracture) and a fracture of the midshaft of the radius may be associated with dislocation of the head of ulna (Galeazzi fracture dislocation). (See Figure 22.9.)

X-ray: The whole of the forearm. The elbow and wrist joints must be seen on the film to exclude fracture dislocations.

Treatment: These fractures should be *referred* for further treatment. A padded POP backslab should be applied as an interim measure.

Colles fracture

This results from a fall on the outstretched arm: there is posterior and radial displacement of the lower end of the radius with a fracture of the ulnar styloid. (See Figure 22.10.) A characteristic dinner fork deformity of the forearm is present. Inmediate pain and swelling occur. In severely displaced and comminuted fractures injury to the median nerve may occur. In simple fractures involving Lister's tubercle damage may occur to the extensor pollicis longus causing later rupture and a drooping thumb.

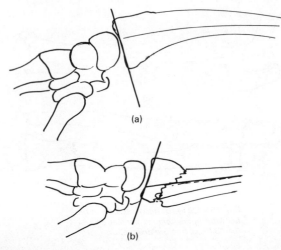

Figure 22.10 *Colle's fracture*
(a) In the normal wrist, the angle of the lower articular surface with the shaft of the radius is less than 90°. If this angle is greater than 90°, MUA is required.
(b) Radial inferior fragment
    (i)   is impacted
    (ii)   dorsal displacement and angulation
    (iii) rotated dorsally and radially
    (iv) displaced laterally
    (v)   avulsion of ulnar styloid

Treatment

In impacted fractures with minimal displacement, or where the angle between the inferior articular surface and the shaft is only slightly less than 90 degrees, a padded POP posterior slab is sufficient; manipulation is not required. Younger patients should be *referred* ?ORIF.

Manipulation. Correction of the deformity is obtained in the following ways:

    (a) By traction which disimpacts the fracture.
    (b) Reduction is achieved by gripping the lower fragment in the hand.
    (c) Ensuring that disimpaction is complete by extending the lower fragment.

(d) Pronating the wrist.

(e) Correcting any posterior angulation and displacement by pressure with the ball of the thumb on the lower fragment whilst achieving a fulcrum action above the fracture, on the shafts of the radius and ulna, by the other hand.

(f) Traction on the thumb and middle, ring and little finger is maintained whilst the arm is held in pronation, neutral flexion and ulna deviation.

(g) A plaster of paris U slab is applied over padding ensuring that a gap is left on the ulnar border; the plaster slab is held by a wet cotton bandage.

(h) An X-ray is necessary to check the reduction.

(i) The arm is elevated and the patient should be discharged wearing a high sling with instructions to exercise the fingers, elbows and shoulder regularly.

(j) The reduction and splint should be checked the following day and the plaster is completed in the following week. (See Figure 26.17.)

Smith's fracture

This is a fracture of the lower radius above the wrist joint with forward and volar displacement — a reverse Colles fracture. Look carefully in lateral film for inferior radio/ulna dislocation. (Figure 22.12.)

Treatment

MUA, an above elbow splint in neutral position.

Barton's fracture

The fracture extends from the articular surface upwards and forwards, carrying the carpus with it — i.e. a fracture dislocation. Operative fixation is required: *refer*. (Figure 22.12.)

Fracture of radial styloid

These fractures are often impacted with minimal displacement but as they are intra-articular the wrist should be splinted until the fracture is united. (Figure 22.12.)

Scaphoid fractures

History of a fall on the outstretched dorsiflexed hand, followed by pain and swelling in the antomical snuff box, with weakness of the grip. (See Figure 22.13.)

Feel: There is tenderness and often swelling in the anatomical snuff box over the scaphoid.

X-ray: Extra oblique views are essential, so do make a specific request for scaphoid views. The fracture may be of the tuberosity, the proximal pole, or the waist of the bone.

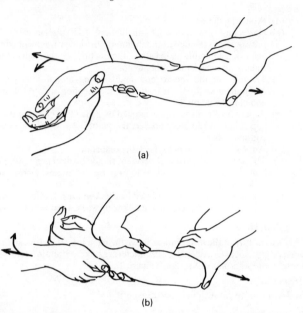

Figure 22.11 *Manipulation and reduction of Colle's fracture*
(a) Disimpaction by traction and increasing the backward angulation. Traction maintained. No undue force is required as it may increase comminution in elderly
(b) Robert Jones grip applied with 'reducing' hand on distal fragment against the counter-pressure on the proximal fragment from the 'anvil' hand. Traction maintained
(c) Locking the reduction by pronation. The 'anvil' hand remains stationary while the pronation is done entirely by the 'reducing' hand. The wrist is forced into ulnar deviation by this same manoeuvre
(d) Plastering position. Extend elbow holding wrist pronated and main-taining traction by holding thumb in one hand and index, middle and ring fingers in the other. See Fig. 26.17 for application of POP. (After Sir John Charnley.)

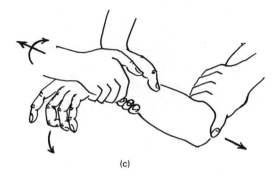

(c)

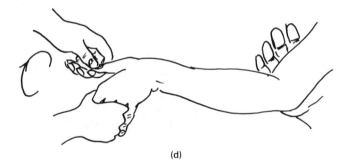

(d)

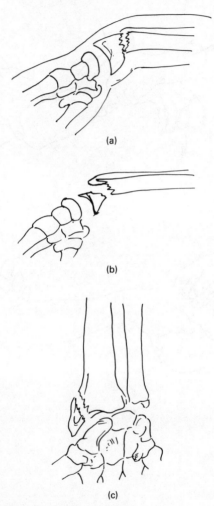

Figure 22.12 *Fractures of the lower radius*
(a) Smith's fracture
(b) Barton's fracture-dislocation
(c) Radial styloid fracture

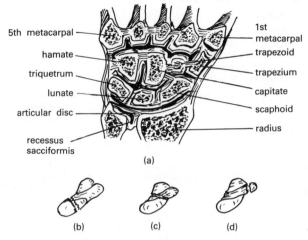

Figure 22.13 *Scaphoid fractures*
(a) Normal relations and ligament in wrist
(b) Proximal fracture
(c) Waist fracture
(d) Tuberosity fracture

Treatment

1. In the established case, with a visible fracture, a scaphoid POP is applied in the position of function which allows the patient to hold a glass. *Refer*. If displaced fractures *refer* early.
2. If the fracture is not visible in the original x-rays but you think that clinically the bone has fractured, apply a scaphoid POP; review the patient in 10 to 14 days for removal of the POP and re-x-ray.
3. If your clinical diagnosis is a sprain of the radial collateral ligament of the wrist joint, apply a support bandage and review the patient in 14 days if tenderness is still present.
4. Small flake fracture tip of radial styloid indicates ligament injury.

Carpal bones

Other carpal bones are less commonly fractured, but avulsion fragments from the dorsum of the joint are often seen in severe sprains of the wrist. Less frequently the triquetral or pisiform may be fractured. These should be treated according to the clinical severity by a bandage or POP back slab and reviewed after two weeks. Beware history of high velocity trauma: carpal dislocations are common.

Fractures of the pelvis and leg

Pelvis fractures

    (a) isolated fracture with an intact pelvic ring
    (b) stable fracture of pelvic ring
    (c) unstable fracture of pelvic ring
    (d) fracture of acetabulum
    (e) fracture of sacrum/coccyx

Fractures of the pelvis are usually associated with severe trauma, often involving a crushing force. There is frequently heavy hidden blood loss when the patient is severely shocked. (See Multiple Injuries, page 15.) The pelvic ring may be unstable, and in fractures of the pubic and ischial rami there is a danger of rupturing the pelvic urethra. In crush injuries careful attention must be paid to the abdomen for the signs of intra-abdominal injury, particularly to bladder, rectum, or rupture of the diaphragm. Disruption of the pelvic ring is frequently accompanied by opening of the sacro-iliac joint. However, they are not uncommon after falls in the elderly.

Listen: There is usually a fall or crushing injury.

Feel: The iliac crest, the ischial tuberosity, the rami of the pubis and its symphysis are palpated; the stability of the pelvic ring is tested by springing. The levels of the great trochanters and the position and length of the legs are estimated to avoid missing, as frequently happens, dislocations of the hips. Muscle power and sensation in the legs are tested to check for signs of sciatic nerve neuropraxia. PR may reveal a displaced prostate: check tip of penis for urethral blood; if patient is unable to pass urine retrograde or suprapubic urethrography is required.

Treatment

If the patient is shocked, start an intravenous infusion with normal saline, group and crossmatch blood, follow with dextran; *refer* for surgical opinion and peritoneal lavage. Fractures without intra-abdominal injuries should be referred to the orthopaedic surgeon for admission.

Fracture of the coccyx

Is very painful and follows a direct fall onto the 'tail'. Diagnosis is made by PR, not by x-ray. Reassure patient and start a high-fibre diet to render the stools soft. Prescribe NSAID to relieve pain.

Neck of femur

These may be basal, transcervical or subcapital (see Figure 22.15).

Listen: The injury is often quite trivial, e.g. tripping over a rug. The hip is painful and there is inability to lift the leg. The patient is usually elderly.

Look: The leg is shortened; the foot is exterally rotated.

Feel: There is tenderness over the joint line and attempted movement,

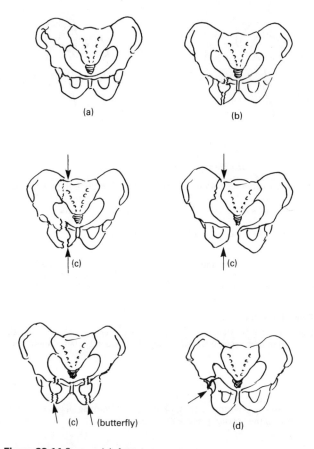

Figure 22.14 *Some pelvic fractures*
(a) Isolated fracture with stable pelvic ring
(b) Stable fracture of pelvic ring: ring broken in one place
(c) Unstable fracture of pelvic ring: ring broken in 2 places. Note that the sacro-iliac joints or symphysis pubis may be disrupted
(d) Fracture of acetabulum. Central dislocation may occur.

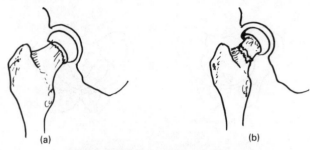

Figure 22.15 *Fractures of neck of femur*
(a) Subcapital impacted abduction
(b) Transcervical

especially rotation, is painful. Occasionally the fracture is impacted when, apart from pain and a limp, the physical signs are minimal and confusing. Arrange review and re-x-ray if you suspect a fracture but initial films do not confirm.

X-ray: Must be in two planes to make the diagnosis.

Treatment

Definitive is operative. Immediate care consists of placing the patient on a mattress to avoid pressure on the sacrum, then applying skin traction to stabilise the limb, as the lateral peroneal nerve (at the neck of the fibula) is at risk while the leg is externally rotated.

Trochanteric fractures

These frequently occur in the elderly. In younger people they usually result from more severe trauma. They are frequently comminuted. (See Figure 22.16.)

Listen: There is more pain.

Look: The hip is swollen and bruised over the greater trochanter and the leg is short and externally rotated.

X-ray: Shows a pertrochanteric fracture with varying degrees of comminution of the greater and lesser trochanters.

Treatment

Apply traction and admit for operative treatment.

Shaft of femur

- Fractures in the upper third: the upper fragment is flexed and abducted (see Figure 22.17).
- Middle third fractures are often spiral, transverse or comminuted.

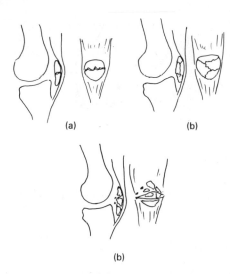

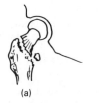

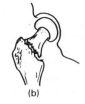

Figure 22.16 *Pertrochanteric fractures*
(a) Comminuted
(b) Spiral

Figure 22.20 *Fractures of patella*
(a) Transverse
(b) Comminuted stellate

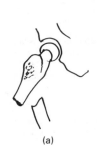

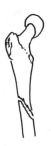

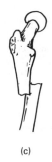

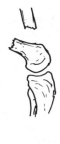

Figure 22.17 *Fractures of shaft of femur*
(a) Upper third
(b) Spiral mid third
(c) Transverse mid third
(d) Supracondylar

X-ray: Postero-anterior and lateral views are required to demonstrate fracture. In fissure fractures a skyline view should be taken to as articular surface damage or irregularity.

Treatment

1 Fissure fractures without displacement require aspiration of haemarthrosis and Robert Jones' compression splinting band for a week, followed by a POP cylinder.
2 Comminuted or transverse fractures will require operative tre ment: *refer*.
3 Early quadriceps exercise is sufficient in cases where the knee been strained or contused.

N.B. Congenital bi-partite patella is not uncommon and should not confused radiologically with a fracture. There is a well-defined separat line in the upper outer quadrant which is usually bilateral. In addition knee does not show the clinical attributes of a fractured patella so treatment following injury need not be restrictive.

● Fractures of the lower third (supracondylar), are often flexed at the knee joint and may be associated with injury to the popliteal artery or sciatic nerve.

Listen: The trauma is usually severe except in the pathological fracture.

Look: The thigh is usually bruised and swollen, the leg is short and angulated if efficient first aid has not been rendered. The limb distal to the fracture must be carefully assessed for nerve or arterial damage.

X-ray: Must demonstrate both the hip and knee joints as there may be associated damage.

Treatment

These patients are often shocked, so an intravenous infusion must be started, skin traction and a Thomas splint applied, preferably before x-rays are taken.

(See application of Thomas splint, Figure 26.21, page 416.)

Supracondylar fracture

The lower fragment is flexed at the knee joint, when in this position there is a risk of compression of the femoral artery with ischaemia of the lower leg.

Look: There is gross shortening and swelling of the lower thigh.

Feel: Carefully examine the popliteal, posterior tibial and dorsalis pedis pulses.

X-ray: Will demonstrate the position of fracture but is best taken after a Thomas splint has been applied. (See Figure 22.18.)

Treatment

Skin traction is applied after gentle traction with the knee flexed. When applying a Thomas splint it may be necessary to use a Pearson's flexion attachment to the splint. To reduce the fracture satisfactorily it may be necessary to insert a Steinmann's or Denham's pin in the tibia, particularly if there is vascular involvement. *Refer*.

Fractures in the knee

Intra-articular fractures involving the knee joint always produce a painful haemarthrosis which develops soon after the injury. The position of the

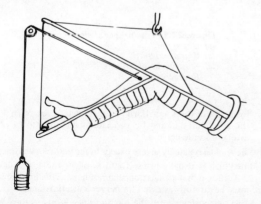

Figure 22.18 *Thomas splint with Pearson flexed knee attachment*

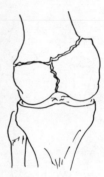

Figure 22.19 *Intercondylar fracture of femur*

leg below the knee should be compared with the opposite limb and any valgus or varus deformity noted, see Figure 22.19.

X-rays will demonstrate the extent of the distortion of the articular surface. Effusions of the knee joint which are aspirated and contain blood and fat globules are diagnostic of a fracture, so the x-rays should be re-assessed and the fracture identified.

Fractures of the femoral condyles

X-rays: In 2 planes — fractures of (a) single condyle; (b) both condyles resulting in a T fracture or (c) comminuted fracture of both condyles.

Treatment

Aspiration of the knee joint; application of a Robert Jones bandage, or traction on a Thomas splint, is adequate for an undisplaced single condyle fracture but the others will require operative treatment. *Refer* to the orthopaedic surgeons.

Fractures of the patella

Listen: The fracture may be caused by direct trauma such as a fall, or in a car accident when the knee hits the dashboard. *N.B.* always examine the hip joint carefully to exclude a fracture dislocation. A traction injury will fracture the patella with separation of the fragments. This is particularly likely to happen in osteoporosis due to age or steroids. (See Figure 22.20.)

Look: Clinically a haemarthrosis is present.

Feel: A palpable gap may be felt between the two fragments. Contraction of the quadriceps may be inhibited, and extension of the knee or straight leg raising painful or not possible, depending on the degree of damage.

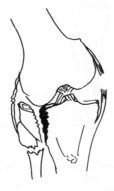

Figure 22.21 *Bumper fracture of tibial plateau*

Upper end of tibia

Fracture of the tibial plateau

This fracture, the Bumper fracture, commonly follows a blow on the outer aspect of the knee. There is depression of the upper tibial surface in the lateral compartment with a sprain or tear of the medial collateral ligament of the knee joint. (See Figure 22.21.)

More severe injury will separate the lateral tibial condyle with avulsion of the tibial spine or tear the cruciate ligaments as well as the medial collateral ligament. This is *a severe injury* and should be *referred* to the orthopaedic surgeons for operative treatment. A posterior POP splint should be applied to stabilise the unstable knee.

Fractures of the tibia and fibula

Fractures of the shaft of the tibia and fibula may be either transverse, oblique or comminuted and usually involve both bones. (See Figure 22.22.)

Fractures are usually at the junction of the middle and upper third, or midshaft or junction of the middle and lower third.

As most of the shaft of the tibia is subcutaneous, this fracture is frequently compound, if not from without, then as a result of a spike of bone penetrating the skin from within. The leg is swollen, bruised, shortened, and frequently angulated. The foot may be rotated either internally or externally. The circulation of the foot may be at risk because of rotation and angulation.

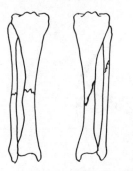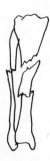

Figure 22.22 *Fractures of shaft of tibia*
(a) Transverse
(b) Spiral
(c) Double (Segmental) fracture (upper oblique)

● *First aid treatment is urgently required on admission to the depart-
    ment. This should consist of (a) analgesia (b) effective splintage,
    with either a pneumatic splint, box splint, or well-padded POP
    back slab and U slab, applied after the position of the fracture has
    been corrected by gentle traction under Entonox. In compound
    injuries, wounds should be dressed, antibiotics and booster
    tetanus toxoid should be given. This should all be instituted as an
    emergency procedure before x-rays are taken. This injury is a
    severe injury so there will be blood loss and shock.*

In road traffic accidents other injuries, to head, chest and abdomen,
should be carefully looked for. A tense limb, even if the fracture does not
appear to be grossly displaced, may result in muscle ischaemia and compartment syndrome.

X-ray: These should always be done after the limb has been splinted and
will confirm the extent and comminution of the fracture.

Fractures of tibia

Fractures of the tibia may occur without fracture of the fibula. However, if
there is a fracture of the lower tibia or medial malleolus the neck of the
fibula must be x-rayed as well to exclude fracture, and the common
peroneal nerve tested to exclude neuropraxia. Treatment in the A & E
department is similar to above: *refer* to orthopaedic department after
splintage and x-ray.

Fractures of fibula

Fractures of the fibula are usually associated with fractures of the tibia: in
ligamentous damage to the ankle with separation of the interosseus and

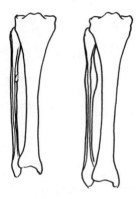

Figure 22.23 *Stress fracture of fibula*
(a) Fine linear fracture: calcification
(b) Callus formation

medial ligaments there may be a spiral fracture of the shaft or neck of the fibula. Shaft fracture may result from a direct injury, as from a kick in football. The fibula is frequently involved with stress fractures in marathon and long-distance runners. (See Figure 22.23.)

X-rays: Should include the knee and ankle joint to exclude trauma at these sites.

Treatment

● A solitary fracture of the shaft of fibula requires minimal support as this bone is not weight-bearing but merely controls rotation. Often a viscopaste bandage from toes to tibial tubercle will give comfort and support.

● Stress fractures of the fibula may be treated in similar fashion, but in this case the important thing is to stop the active training which has caused the injury.

● The limb is re-x-rayed after three weeks to assess progress.

Fractures of the ankle

Fractures of the ankle joint are commonly referred to as 'Pott's fractures' which is not strictly correct but is universally understood. The mechanism of the injury is described as if the inverted or everted foot is moved in relation to the tibia. In fact the foot is usually fixed on the ground and the body moves in the opposite direction. (See Figure 22.24.)

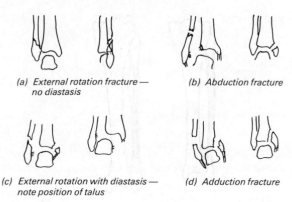

*(a) External rotation fracture —
no diastasis*

(b) Abduction fracture

*(c) External rotation with diastasis —
note position of talus*

(d) Adduction fracture

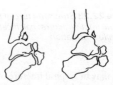

(e) Vertical compression fracture

Figure 22.24 *Fractures of the ankle (after Lauge-Hansen)*

Classification of ankle fractures

Classification of ankle fractures:
(Figure 22.24)

(a) External rotation, foot inverted,	→	external rotation fracture, no diastasis,
(b) Abduction, foot everted,	→	abduction fracture,
(c) External rotation, foot everted,	→	external rotation fracture with diastasis.
(d) Adduction, foot inverted,	→	adduction fracture.
(e) Dorsiflexion, foot everted,	→	vertical compression fracture.

First degree; one malleolus fractured,
Second degree: two malleoli fractured,
Third degree: two malleoli are fractured. In addition (i) the posterior or anterior margin of tibia may be fractured; (ii) the inferior tibio-fibular joint may be divided or (iii) the ankle is dislocated.
Uncommon fractures result from either a transverse or a vertical force.

Listen carefully and obtain an exact history of the mechanism of injury as this will simplify the technique of reduction.

Look: The ankle is usually swollen immediately after the injury and bruising may appear early. The degree of swelling is usually proportional to the severity of the injury, but may be aggravated by damage to the medial and lateral collateral ligaments or the inferior interosseus ligaments with diastasis or dislocation.

Feel: Examine carefully with the fingertips over the bony outline of the ankle and the ligaments and define the exact sites of tenderness. This will help to clarify the diagnosis.

X-ray: Required in two planes. Must be carefully examined for signs of ligamentous injury as well as bone fractures. The joint space between the talus, the medial malleolus and the inferior tibial surface must be equal. Any widening of the gap between the medial malleolus and the talus is diagnostic of diastasis with rupture of the inferior interosseus ligament. An x-ray with 15° internal rotation will show the mortice. If lateral malleolus is intact x-ray neck of fibula.

Treatment

● *Fractures of the lateral malleolus alone* often can be treated by a supporting bandage and early movement in the absence of ligamentous injury. However, if there is marked swelling a weight-bearing POP cast can be employed.

● *Fractures of the medial malleolus* are best treated by operative reduction and fixation so *refer*.

● Second- and third-degree fractures may be treated by closed manipulation, correcting the displacement depending whether the fracture is adduction, abduction, or external rotation in type. A padded, below-knee POP cast is applied with the foot at right-angles. Many need open reduction and internal fixation so it is best to *refer*.

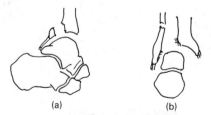

(a)   (b)

Figure 22.25 *Fracture dislocation*
(a) Posterior dislocation of talus: pressure on skin anteriorly
(b) Lateral dislocation of talus: pressure on skin medially

● *Third-degree Pott's fracture with dislocation* puts pressure on the anterior tibial vessels and the skin: this fracture requires urgent reduction and temporary splintage immediately on arrival in the department prior to x-ray. Intravenous pethidine is used to assist reduction. These fractures, best treated by open reduction and internal fixation, should be referred for orthopaedic opinion after provisional reduction, stabilisation, and x-ray. (See Figure 22.25.)

Fractures of the foot

Injuries of the foot may be associated with trauma to the ankle and it is important that these should be differentiated. The injury may result from a twisting force or from a fall from a height. Early swelling and bruising will occur as there is often an associated ligamentous injury. X-ray of the foot should be requested if an injury to the tarsal bones is suspected. If possible, specify special views of the talus and os calcis on request form.

Fractures of the talus

These usually result from motorcycle or head-on collision accidents. Fracture of the body or neck of talus, or of the neck, and talo-navicular dislocation may occur. On occasion these injuries may be compound. (There may be damage to the navicular in severe twisting or adduction injuries.) The risk of avascular necrosis is high in these fractures and painful osteoarthritic changes in the talo-navicular and sub-talar joints are common. These fractures should be *referred* for orthopaedic opinion. (See Figure 22.26.)

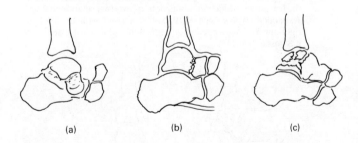

(a)   (b)   (c)

Figure 22.26 *Talus injuries*
(a) Dislocation of talus
(b) Fracture of neck
(c) Compression fracture of body

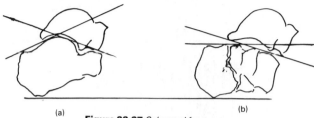

(a)

(b)

Figure 22.27 *Calcaneal fracture*
(a) Normal angle
(b) Note flattening of sub-talar joint

Fractures of the calcaneus

These are usually associated with a twisting injury or a fall from a height and may be bilateral. Minor avulsion injury or compression fractures may be seen. There is swelling, bruising, and localised tenderness over the fracture. X-ray confirms that the sub-talar joint is not involved. These fractures may be treated by wool and a supporting bandage, crutches for a few days, followed by progressive weight-bearing and exercise.

Fractures involving the sub-talar joint are usually associated with severe swelling and bruising of the foot, with marked flattening and loss of the normal longitudinal arch of the foot. Operative treatment is unnecessary, but in view of the painful swelling which will occur, the patient is best admitted, with a wool crêpe bandage dressing or ice packs, for elevation and early active non-weight-bearing exercises. *Refer.* (See Figure 22.27.)

As this bone is frequently injured by a fall from a height it is important to assess the thoraco-lumbar spine, from T 10 to L 5, as wedge fractures may occur.

Fractures of tarsal bones

Fractures of the cuboid, navicular, and cuneiforms are often associated with rotational or axial trauma to the foot, usually when vertical force is also applied: the cavalry fracture (Figure 22.28). (In the case of the cuboid there may be some subluxation of the lateral two metatarsals in motor-cycle injuries: *refer.*) Treat with wool and crêpe bandage, elevate then non-weight-bearing with early exercise. In view of the long-term risks of osteoarthritis, *refer* to the fracture clinic for follow-up.

Mid-tarsal fracture dislocation

This occurs at the talo-navicular and calcaneo-cuboid joints with damage to the cuboid and navicular bones. With bone displacement there is vascular involvement of dorsalis pedis and posterior tibial arteries. There is severe risk of forefoot ischaemia so the dislocation must be

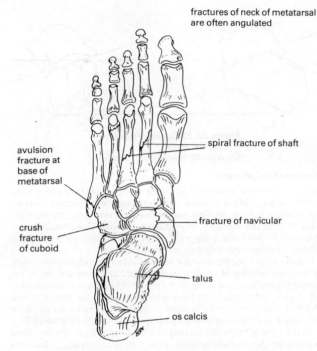

Figure 22.28 *Some fractures of tarsal and metatarsal bones*

reduced as soon as the diagnosis has been established radiologically. Further treatment will be required to stabilise the reduction, so *refer*.

Fractures of the metatarsal

Fractures of the metatarsal are often associated with rotational injuries or weights dropping onto the foot (Figure 22.28). The commonest injury is an avulsion fracture of the base of the fifth metatarsal and this should always be palpated for tenderness.

Treatment is a weight-bearing POP cast to relieve the patient of pain and restore confidence, although splintage is not really necessary.

Tarso-metatarsal fracture dislocations (Lisfrancs) are not uncommon — the foot is very swollen and ischaemia is a severe risk. The best x-ray is a true lateral.

Stress fractures

These frequently involve the shaft of the second or third metatarsals and follow repeated stress in training for long-distance running or marching. Pain is located to the mid-tarsal region and is aggravated by twisting the foot. There may be swelling and localised tenderness over the site of the fracture. (See Figure 22.29.)

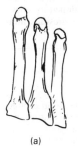 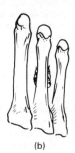 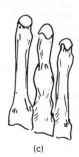

(a) (b) (c)

Figure 22.29 *Stages of stress fracture of metatarsal II*
(a) Minute cortical crack
(b) Calcification of fracture haematoma
(c) Callus

X-ray: Usually no evidence of fracture is seen on the initial x-ray so this is repeated after two weeks to confirm the diagnosis. Radio-isotope scan will demonstrate a hot spot, but this is not really necessary.

Treatment

- Stop all active training and support the foot with a cotton elastic bandage such as tubigrip.
- Confirm the diagnosis at two to three weeks: the x-ray shows, in sequence,? a crack, spots of calcium, finally callus.
- Advise the patient not to start training for four to six months.
- Other fractures of the metatarsals should be referred to the fracture clinic for treatment. Solitary fractures of the great toe metatarsal or multiple metatarsal fractures need urgent assessment: *refer*.

Fractures of the toes

Fractures of the toes follow weights dropping onto the foot, frequently an industrial injury — the toes being run over by trailers at work — or by kicking with bare feet.

Treatment

Single fractures of the phalanges of all toes can be treated by gaiter splinting of the adjacent toe for two to three weeks. These can be painful for a long time.

Fractures of the great toe are best treated by a walking plaster with a platform support to the toe if it is very painful or a metatarsal orthopaedic felt pad.

Crush injuries to the terminal phalanges with sub-ungual haematoma are technically compound injuries, particularly if the nail is drilled to relieve pressure. Treat with povidone iodine and non-adherent dressing, antibiotic cover and review in five days.

Bone infections

Acute osteomyelitis

Infection of bones and the medullary cavity result either from a direct infection from the wound of a compound fracture or are haematogenous from a septic focus. The latter type of spread occurs more so in children than in adults although trauma to an implanted hip can result in bone infection. (See Figure 22.30.)

Acute haematogenous osteo-myelitis

This is relatively uncommon but occurs in children during the growing phase. There is an infection in the metaphysis of long bones, particularly the femur and tibia. The end vessels beneath the epiphysis are involved. If the epiphyseal line is intra-articular then septic arthritis will follow. In neonates the infection may cross the epiphysis itself into the joint.

Clinical findings

There is an acute febrile illness with severe toxaemia, pyrexia, and nausea. During the septicaemia a bronchopneumonia may arise. The joint involved is painful and movements are severely restricted. The bone is tender and shows some superficial swelling and oedema.

X-ray is of no value in the early stages of the diagnosis but will exclude fractures. Later in the missed cases there will be subperiosteal new bone. Later a patchy osteoporosis or sequestrum will be seen.

Blood culture should be taken as soon as the clinical diagnosis is made and in the commonest infection will grow Staphylococcus aureus. Less commonly *H. influenzae* or streptococcus pyogenes will be found.

Treatment

The treatment of this serious infection is a combination of chemotherapy and early surgery so the patient should be *referred* to the Orthopaedic Surgeon as soon as the diagnosis is suspected. Antibiotics should be a combination of cloxacillin or flucloxacillin with sodium fusidate.

The affected limb should be splinted to make the patient comfortable.

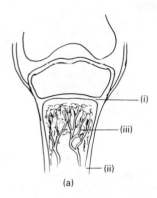

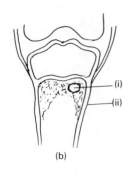

(a) Normal anatomy of epiphysis
    (i) plate
    (ii) thick periosteum
    (iii) metaphyseal end arteries

(b) (i) metaphyseal infection
     (ii) superiosteal pus

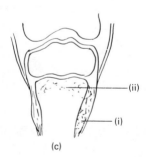

(c) Later signs
    (i) subperiosteal calcification
    (ii) metaphyseal mottling

Figure 22.30 *Acute haematogenous osteomyelitis*

NOTES

23

The hand

The hand

The hand has the power to grip, oppose thumb to fingers and pinch, or finely pick up. With its fine sensation and proprioception it is able to do delicate manipulative procedures. All injuries and infections should be treated promptly to avoid stiffness, lack of mobility, and interference with the patient's ability to live and earn.

Method of examination

Listen to the time and details of the accident; onset of symptoms and how movement and sensation have been affected. What is his job and favourite hobby?

Look at the position of rest and for obvious deformities; compare with the other hand. Contrast colour, temperature, shape, and size of the fingers and nails. Define the exact position of wounds and relate this to underlying anatomy.

Feel the temperature and texture of the digits and hand. A dry area on the skin indicates nerve damage. Gently define exact tender spots.

Feel swellings and abnormal lesions.

Movements, active and passive, at all joints, are measured and compared with the other hand. Test flexion, extension, abduction and adduction at the wrist and metacarpo-phalangeal joints. Measure flexion and extension of the interphalangeal joints of the digits: observe abduction and adduction of the thumb at right-angles to the palm, and its freedom of opposition. (See Figure 23.1.)

Check stability of collateral ligaments of all joints.

X-rays are required in two planes if a fracture or foreign body (FB) is suspected. Always note nature of FB and if possible x-ray a fragment to check if it is radio-opaque. A marker on the site of entry is essential.

Wounds

Clinically it may not be obvious that tendons or nerves have been divided, especially at the wrist. Such patients should have a gauze dressing applied, antibiotics started and be referred for a surgical opinion. (See Figure 23.2.)

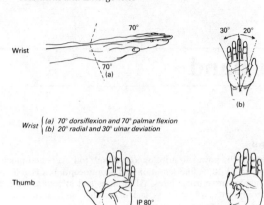

Wrist
- (a) 70° dorsiflexion and 70° palmar flexion
- (b) 20° radial and 30° ulnar deviation

Thumb
- (c) has 80° flexion at the IP joint, 50° at the MCP joint and 150° at the CMC joint
- (d) has 60° abduction

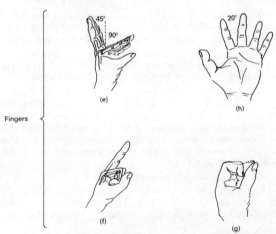

Fingers
- (e) The metacarpal joint has 45° hyperextension and 90° flexion
- (f) The proximal interphalangeal joint has 100° flexion
- (g) The distal interphalangeal joint has 10° hyperextension and 80° flexion
- (h) There is about 20° of abduction or adduction between each finger

Figure 23.1 *Range of movement of digits and wrist*

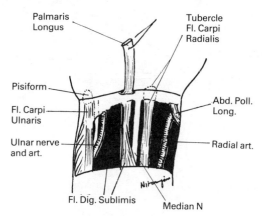

Figure 23.2 *Anatomical relations at wrist*

- The hand is gently washed at the sink with soap and water; use povidone iodine surgical scrub if hand is very dirty or greasy.
- Local anaesthesia: 1 per cent lignocaine *without adrenalin* is used for a digital nerve block for fingers.
- Excision of dead and contaminated tissue, conserving skin, is meticulous. Skin must be treated gently and conserved — there is none to spare.
- Carefully inspect the deeper structures for damage.
- The wound edges are closed using an atraumatic cutting needle with size 4.0 black silk, nylon or prolene. Crush or bursting injuries, or those over 24 hours old are not sutured because of the swelling or infection that will occur. These wounds are dressed with povidone iodine or silver sulphadiazine and inspected 3 days later for delayed primary suture. Flaps of skin often have a precarious blood supply which can be cut by a suture: these should always be replaced using Steristrips, Histoacryl glue without tension.
- Apply a non-adherent Melolin pad; dress the finger with tubegauze.
- Larger wounds of the hand are bandaged in the functional position and elevated in a high sling for 48 hours (Figure 23.3). If the hand is not hurting the wound is left undisturbed until healed: sutures are removed at 8 days.
- Skin loss should be replaced: on the dorsum or volar surface of hand or finger with split skin; on the pulp with a full thickness

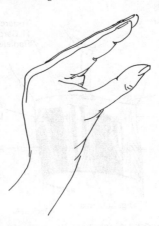

Figure 23.3 *Position of function (left hand)*
Wrist: extended
Metacarpo-phalangeal joint: flexed
Interphalangeal joints: extended
Thumb: abducted

skin graft. For a tip injury see page 363. If you are not able to do these: ask, or if help is not readily available use a synthetic skin such as Omniderm or granuflex as a temporary dressing.

A very useful method of applying a tourniquet to a finger is:

Put on a surgeon's glove.
Make a small hole in the tip of the glove of the finger.
Roll back the glove on the finger.
This forms a tourniquet and gives a sterile field. (See Figure 23.4.)

The anatomical functional position for dressing the hand (Figure 23.3)

The hand should be allowed to move whenever possible, but if you have to immobilise it always do this in the functional position: the fingers are extended at the interphalangeal joints and flexed at the metacarpo-phalangeal joints. The thumb should lie opposite the index finger in abduction.

Tendon injuries

Extensor tendons

The finger lies partially flexed at the affected joint and the patient is unable to extend against resistance. Be careful that a flicker of movement is not

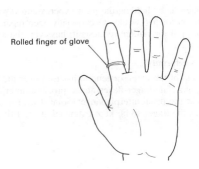

Rolled finger of glove

Figure 23.4 *Applying a finger tourniquet*

confused as an intact tendon. Repair is done with a fine 4.0 non-absorbable suture. The digit is kept extended for 14 days then gently mobilised in the physiotherapy department.

Mallet finger

The extensor tendon has been torn off its insertion to the base of the distal phalanx, often with a small fragment of bone, see Figure 23.5. Forced flexion of the distal joint by a blow on the tip, e.g. by a cricket ball, is the

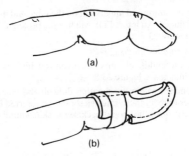

(a)

(b)

Figure 23.5 *Mallet finger*
(a) Drooping distal interphalangeal joint
(b) Frog splint — tape over middle segment of digit: hyperextended distal interphalangeal joint

cause: treatment is by holding the joint hyperextended with a frog splint which is kept on for 6–8 weeks. Occasionally open repair is required for persistent droop if the patient requests it: however, the joint is often left stiff and extended.

Boutonnière's deformity

The middle slip of the extensor tendon has torn over the proximal interphalangeal joint. The finger flexes at the proximal interphalangeal joint and extends at the distal interphalangeal joint. (See Figure 23.6.) Treatment requires the finger to be kept extended at the PIP joint, e.g. by a Zimmer splint.

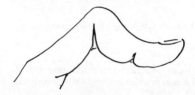

Figure 23.6 *Boutonnière's deformity*

Flexor tendons

Either or both of the flexor tendons may be divided.

(a) Flexor digitorum superficialis (FDS)

Test by holding the uninjured fingers flat on the table and make the patient flex the injured finger. An intact FDS will flex the proximal IP joint against resistance, see Figure 23.7.

(b) Flexor digitorum profundis (FDP)

Test by holding the middle phalanx down and watching the DIP joint flex if the tendon is intact, see Figure 23.8.

Repair of the tendons within the sheath is difficult and the results are poor because of adhesions: all these injuries should be referred immediately to a hand surgeon. If this is not possible close the skin wound only then *refer* later.

Digital nerves

These are often divided but, because of pain and general upset, not diagnosed: examine carefully for loss of sensation and sweating distal to the wound before anaesthetising the finger. A nerve divided proximal to the pulp should be repaired with 6.0 prolene, using magnification.

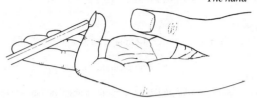

Figure 23.7 *Testing flexor digitorum superficialis (FDS). Hold uninjured fingers flat: see flexion at PIP joint*

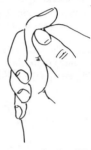

Figure 23.8 *Testing flexor digitorum profundus (FDP). Hold middle segments flat: see flexion at DIP joint*

Fractures in the hand

Metacarpal

The neck of the little finger (5th) metacarpal is most frequently fractured, by fighting, with forward angulation. Most of these fractures are impacted, stable, and only require garter strapping of the little and ring fingers for 10 days to avoid accidental pulling of the joint. If the fracture is angulated more than 30 degrees or has a rotational deformity, then manipulate holding the metacarpo-phalangeal joint at 90 degrees; immobilise little and ring fingers in functional position for 14 days; follow with physiotherapy.

Shaft of metacarpal

A single bone fracture requires a supporting cotton tubegauze bandage and elevation only as it is splinted by the other metacarpals. Multiple fractures or thumb are best treated by internal fixation so should be elevated and referred.

Dislocation of base of metacarpal may occur after severe injury in motorcyclists — *N.B.* palpable base and short metacarpal.

Phalanges

Simple fractures require garter strapping to the adjacent digit and gentle movement.

Angulated fractures require manipulation under digital nerve block anaesthesia.

Fractures of the proximal phalanx are liable to angulate late so should be re-x-rayed in 10 days.

Multiple fractures, particularly if spiral or compound, will require operative treatment and should be referred.

Spiral fractures with shortening require traction or internal fixation. *Refer.*

Avulsion fragments are attached to the collateral ligaments so the joint may become unstable.

Intra-articular fractures of the base or head of the phalanx often lead to instability or ugly angulation of the finger with painful osteoarthritis later: they should be *referred*. (See Figure 23.9.)

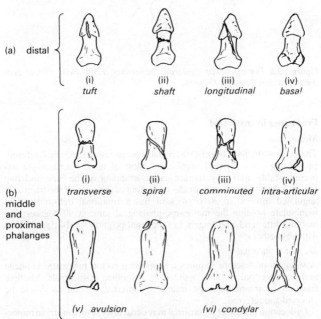

Figure 23.9 *Fractures of phalanges*

The thumb

The general principles discussed above apply to the thumb but special care is essential because of its unique role in the function of the hand. Angulation, rotation, and shortening are more disabling and must be avoided.

Bennett's fracture

The fracture of the base of thumb metacarpal is intra-articular so reduction is best done by open reduction and fixation by an AO screw or Kirschner wire. Failing this, Charnley's technique of traction, abduction and POP fixation is advised. (See Figure 23.10.)

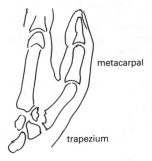

metacarpal

trapezium

Figure 23.10 *Bennett's fracture of thumb*

Gamekeeper's thumb

More often results from a ski-stick injury. Damage occurs to the ulnar collateral ligament with instability. (See Figure 23.11.) *Refer.*

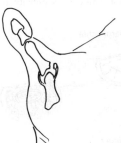

Figure 23.11 *Gamekeeper's thumb — ulnar collateral ligament torn or avulsion fracture*

Infections of the hand (Table 23.1)

The majority are caused by staphylococcus pyogenes and respond to treatment with ampicillin and flucloxacillin or erythromycin. However, in 15 per cent, streptococcus is involved by itself or mixed: the spread of infection is more rapid and the complications — lymphangitis, cellulitis and septicaemia — must be looked for and avoided: benzylpenicillin is the drug of choice but is best given by injection in severe spreading infection.

Diagnosis and treatment

- The cardinal signs of infection — redness, swelling, heat, tenderness, and loss of function — must be looked for and noted.
- Another fact to be asked about is loss of sleep: inability to sleep 48 hours after the onset of symptoms with the cardinal signs indicates that pus is present and must be released by an adequate incision. Pus will not clear with antibiotics alone.
- In many hand infections a collarstud abscess is seen: failure to evacuate the deep cavity leads to failure to cure the patient.

Paronychia

The nailfold is infected: if treated early, before pus formation, it will resolve with antibiotics. Pus must be let out by de-roofing the nailfold, probe and drain. See Figures 23.12 and 23.13.

Chronic infection is due to fungal infection and is treated with nystatin cream or Castellani's paint twice daily for 6 weeks or potassium permanganate solution. The fingers must be kept dry.

Pulp space infections (Figures 23.12 and 23.13)

Early infection within 48 hours will respond to antibiotics. If 4 to 5 days after onset of symptoms, a sleepless night, a tense, throbbing, swollen pulp is seen then it should be incised at the site of maximum tenderness. Often the skin blister has a small track leading to a cavity in the pulp space. The blister is excised, the track is probed, and the pus and slough curetted from the cavity. A bacteriology swab is sent for culture and sensitivity; to start give flucloxacillin.

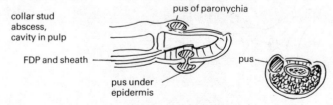

collar stud
abscess,
cavity in pulp

pus of paronychia

FDP and sheath

pus

pus under
epidermis

Figure 23.13 *Infections of finger*

TABLE 23.1

Differential Diagnosis of Hand Infection

	Paronychia	Terminal pulp infection	Acute cellulitis
Time of presentation from onset	2–5 days	4–5 days	12–24 hours
Cause	Nail biting Manicuring	Puncture wound	Prick or not known
Organism	Mixed	Staphylococcus	Streptococcus
Symptoms	Tender swelling round nail fold	Throbbing pain confined to the end of the finger increasing daily and preventing sleep	Hot red finger. Malaise, shivering and tenderness up arm to axilla
Physical signs	Fluctuant swelling of nail fold. Often subcuticular pus.	Hot red *tense* and tender pulp. Often subcuticular pus. Rest of the finger normal	Hot red finger. Not very swollen
Movements	Full. Painless	Full. Painless	Practically full. Painless
Temperature	Normal	Normal	Raised
Lymphangitis	No	No	Yes
Differential diagnosis	1. Early acute cellulitis 2. Lateral pulp infection 3. Late subungual haematoma	1. Acute cellulitis 2. Early paronychia 3. Haematoma of pulp following trauma	Early pulp infection especially apical infection

Acknowledgement: Joan Sneddon.

Tendon sheath infection	Boil or carbuncle	Palmar and web infection	Infective arthritis
6–36 hours	2–3 days	2–3 days	1–3 days from onset infection. Up to 3 weeks from time of original injury
Mid-line injury with sharp instrument	Often not known	Puncture wound — often splinter	Cut or puncture over dorsum of the joint
Streptococcus	Staphylococcus	Staphylococcus	Mixed
Hot red swollen finger. Extremely painful especially on movement. Malaise. Tenderness up arm to axilla	Painful swelling on the back of the hand or fingers History of previous boils	Throbbing pain in the palm and gross swelling of the back of the hand	Painful swelling all round the infected joint and discharging wound on the dorsum
Whole finger hot, red and swollen. Maximal on dorsum. Tenderness along course of the sheath maximal in proximal compartment in the palm	Cellulitis and oedema of dorsum, with triangular spread to the wrist. Later discharging lesion	Infected puncture wound in palm brawny, red and tender. Swelling and pitting oedema of dorsum. In web infections fingers separated. Best seen from the dorsum	Cellulitis of whole finger. Swelling tenderness maximal all round the infected joint. Discharging wound on dorsum
Extremely painful especially extension	Full	Slight limitation by pain in fingers	Flexion and extension limited and painful. Lat. movement increased and crepitus present
Raised	Slightly raised	Slightly raised	Normal
Yes	Sometimes	Sometimes	No
1. Acute cellulitis 2. Middle or proximal space infection 3. Fascial infection	Palmar or web infection	1. Early carbuncle 2. Tendon sheath infection involving proximal compartment	1. Infected laceration not involving the joint 2. Neglected acute paronychia 3. Mallet finger

Boils

Occur on the hairy dorsum of the hand or fingers. Test urine for sugar. Apply povidone iodine, give flucloxacillin.

Interdigital web infection

If pus has formed de-roof the blister, gently probe the cavity to evacuate pus. Any incision should be 1 cm proximal to edge of web to avoid the tendon sheath and use Hilton's technique.

Tendon sheath infection

The finger is very painful, held in slight flexion, and attempted movement causes severe pain. *This is a dangerous infection* so the patient is admitted for surgical drainage and systemic antibiotics.

Septic arthritis

Usually follows a neglected infection close to the joint or, not uncommonly, a blow against human teeth. Movement is painful, the joint is swollen with an effusion. Admit for surgical treatment; fusidic acid and flucloxacillin should be started.

Osteomyelitis

This complication is seen in neglected pulp infections when incision and drainage is too delayed or inadequate. The pulp is swollen considerably, is throbbing despite a discharging sinus. Early x-rays may be normal; later loss of bone texture or a sequestrum is seen. A pulp infection which does not improve after a few days of antibiotics requires x-ray, culture, exploration, curettage, and a long course of fusidic acid.

Important miscellaneous injuries

Injection injury

A severe injury which is seen more frequently with accidents from high-pressure grease or paint guns. Only a small deceptive puncture wound, surrounded by boggy swelling, is seen. *Urgent admission* for exploration and removal of foreign material is essential.

Oil-based veterinary vaccines

These contain mineral oil and can cause intense vascular spasm. Prompt surgical attention is required: early incision and irrigation, especially in pulp or tendon sheath involvement. *Refer.*

Subungual haematoma

Evacuate with a drill or hot paperclip. X-ray to exclude a fracture which, present in 60 per cent, is open so requires antibiotics.

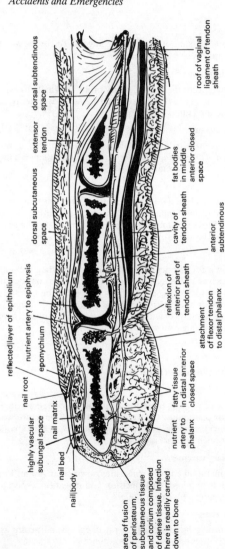

Figure 23.12 *Surgical anatomy of finger*

Nailbed lacerations

The nail should be replaced if possible and the suture is placed through the nail. A badly damaged or dirt-ingrained wound needs the nail to be removed. If part of the bed is lost replace with a fine Thiersch graft, sutured through the nail. The nail will grow over the graft.

Splinters

Superficial visible splinters are easily removed with a hypodermic needle. Larger, deeper, or fragile ones require a ring block, splinter forceps and maybe an incision to expose properly.

Fingertip injury

To cut a small slice off the tip is a common injury. Smear the wound with

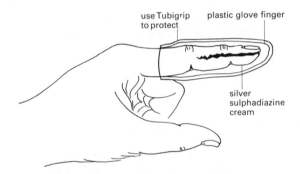

Figure 23.14 *Burst or fingertip injury of finger*

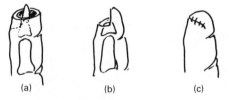

Figure 23.15 *Terminalisation of partially amputated finger*
(a) Excise, trim skin edges
(b) Fashion flaps, nibble bone end
(c) Suture without tension

flamazine, place the finger in a fingerstall or surgical glove finger, change after 4 days. The tip soon epithelialises. (See Figure 23.13.)

Larger loss of skin and pulp with exposure of bone needs a small full-thickness skin graft or terminalisation (see Figure 23.14) after the insertion of a lignocaine LA ring block. The bone end should be nibbled down first.

Thumb or index pulp and multiple injuries may require cross-finger or other skinflaps: this should be done by an expert: *refer*.

Burns of the hand

These should always be treated in a plastic Bunyan bag, elevated and movement encouraged. See page 239.

NOTES

24

The hostile environment

Heat and cold

Thermal injuries

Maintaining normal body temperature requires that heat loss equals heat gain. Heat is produced by metabolism or gained from the environment. Thermoregulation is dependent on cutaneous thermal receptors and hypothalamic centres.

Effects of heat on the body

In a hot environment thermal receptors in the skin initiate reflex vaso-dilatation and sweating through cholinergic sympathetic nerves; these responses are reinforced by the hypothalamus as core temperature rises.

Acclimatisation is a term defining cardiovascular, endocrine, exocrine, and other physiological adaptions to heat stress: it requires one or two weeks to develop allowing the individual to work comfortably and safely under conditions of heat stress. Sweat can be formed in larger amounts and with lower salt content in those acclimatised to heat than in those unacclimatised. If heat loss is insufficient the consequent rise in body temperature leads to hyperventilation, cerebral dysfunction and ultimately cardiovascular collapse with a rapid rise in body temperature and death. As body temperature rises above 41°C, heat denaturation of protein causes damage to large cells of cerebellum and cerebral cortex, and later to vascular endothelium, hepatic and renal cells, and striated muscle.

Causes of heat illness include failure of adequate heat transfer to the environment due to high environmental temperature or humidity, lack of air movement, excessive clothing, vigorous exercise, age, poor acclimatisation, alcohol abuse, obesity, febrile illness, drugs which depress sweating (anti-cholinergics, Tricyclic antidepressants, beta blockers) or promote heat production (amphetamines, neuroleptics), plus drugs that alter the response of the hypotholamus (dopaminergic blocking effect) e.g. phenothiazines and finally inadequate fluid intakes.

Disorders due to heat

Minor disorders

Heat oedema is a transient benign disorder that occurs during initial exposure to hot weather. It disappears spontaneously and seldom requires treatment.

Miliaria (heat rash) is caused by sweat gland occlusion; it may impair sweat function and evaporative heat loss.

Heat syncope: Salt and water loss induced by sweating and heat-induced vasodilatation of the superficial blood vessels may induce syncope in unacclimatised individuals. Beside syncope there is a slight tachycardia and moist skin; fever is absent. Recovery is rapid if patient is kept supine.

Heat cramps

Workers in hot climates sweat profusely and replace sweat losses with water but inadequate salt. Cramps tend to occur in muscles used for working but often do not appear until after work or until cooled rapidly in the shower. They are common in acclimatised and physically fit men whose bodies produce vast quantities of sweat. Mild hyponatraemia is a consistent finding.

- *Salted liquids* (one-half teaspoon of salt per litre of water) or merely increasing dietary salt intake leads to improvement.

Heat exhaustion

Common disorder occurring after sustained heat stress: it may be due to water or salt depletion or both.

Primary water loss heat exhaustion

This is dangerous as it increases the risk of heat stroke. It is seen most commonly in the elderly, very young, or the infirm or active persons who take salt supplements without adequate water.

Symptoms include thirst, fatigue, weakness, anxiety, and impaired judgement.

Signs include dehydration, hyperventilation paraesthesia, tetany, and muscular inco-ordination. Body temperature may rise to 39°C. Frank heat stroke may occur in advanced cases. Investigations show haemo-concentration, hypernatraemia and oliguria.

Salt depletion heat exhaustion

Occurs mainly in unacclimatised persons who replace sweat losses with water but inadequate salt. Sweating and urinary output remain normal.

Prominent symptoms include weakness, fatigue, headaches, giddiness, and muscle cramps.

Signs include pale, clammy skin, hypotension and tachycardia; fever is notably absent.

Treatment

- Most patients with heat exhaustion can be treated with lightly salted fluids, rest, and elimination of heat stress. Hypernatraemic dehydration should be treated with isotonic dextrose. Most patients recover within 48 hours.

Heatstroke

This describes a clinical syndrome produced by overheating of the body core. The syndrome comprises rectal temperatures greater than 41°C in association with severe confusion, unconsciousness, hypotension, or peripheral circulatory failure. It can be produced in normal people by several hours' physical exercise in a hot, humid environment close to or above body temperature. Otherwise heat-stroke in sedentary people is usually associated with impairment of sweating and vasodilatation either by drugs or disease.

Classical heatstroke

This occurs in the elderly, the chronically ill, patients with advanced heart disease, the obese, and alcoholics. Hot, humid weather of three or more days' duration usually precedes epidemics of this disorder. The patient may be on certain drugs (anti-cholinergics, neuroleptics). General autonomic hypofunction in diabetics is also a common cause. The patients usually stop sweating, and body temperature mounts and collapse follows. Typical findings include rectal temperature greater than 41°C, hot, dry, flushed skin, profound cerebral dysfunction, bizarre behaviour, and coma. Hypotension is common.

Exertional heatstroke

Develops in labourers, military recruits, long-distance runners. They display the same physical findings except about half of these patients continue to sweat; if this occurs the skin may be deceptively cool, despite a very high core temperature.

In exertional heatstroke lactic acidosis is the rule, whereas in the classic form respiratory alkalosis is usual. In exertional heatstroke major rhabdomyolysis may occur with its associated complications of hyperkalaemia, hyperphosphataemia, hypocalcaemia, hyperuricaemia, myoglobulinaemia, and acute renal failure.

Both forms of heatstroke may be complicated by clotting abnormalities due to hepatic injury or even disseminated intravascular coagulation. Thrombocytopenia due to bone marrow injury and mild leucocytosis occur. Jaundice, acute renal failure, pancreatitis, brain damage, peripheral neuropathy, myocardial necrosis and arrhythmias and adult respiratory distress syndrome may all occur.

Investigations include: PCV, WCC, electrolytes, urea, blood sugar, PT + LFT, CPK, blood gases, pH, thick film for malaria parasites, ECG and CXR.

Treatment

- Early aggressive treatment may avoid permanent neurological damage.

- The speed of cooling the patient is more important than the method. Cases of heatstroke need admission to ITU.
- The patient should be stripped, then active cooling with fanning and sponging or covering the patient with wet sheets. Active cooling must be stopped when core temperature drops below 39°C to prevent progressive hypothermia. Active cooling also produces undesirable shivering which may be abolished by IV chlorpromazine 25 mg up to 75 mg (with care of BP). This should be delayed until good IV rehydration has been established to prevent hypotension.
- Chilled IV normal saline may be given for patients who continue to have hyperpyrexia. All unconscious patients should be catheterised. Hypotension not responding to saline suggests myocardial injury. The stomach should be emptied by passing an NG tube as vomiting and aspiration occur often during cooling. Glucose may be needed for hypoglycaemia. Lactic acidosis usually responds to volume expansion. The patient should be transferred to ITU as soon as possible.

Effects of cold on the body

In a cold environment cutaneous thermal receptors and later hypothalamic centres bring about reflex vasoconstriction in the skin through noradrenergic sympathetic nerves.

If the mean skin temperature of the adult falls below 33°C there are also reflex increases in muscle tone and shivering brought about by somatic motor nerves which increase heat production by five times. The neonate does not shiver but increases heat production by metabolising its brown fat stores. Most healthy and well-fed adults may maintain their body temperature for a long time with skin temperature as low as 12°C if the individual is fat but only as low as 25–30°C if the individual is thin. Children are at a disadvantage because of their larger surface area in relation to body mass.

Immersion in water below 12°C leads to rapid loss of heat, even in obese people, as the cold paralyses the peripheral blood vessels and leads to cold vasodilation.

Disorders due to cold

Frost bite

This is caused by temperature below freezing and is confined to the extremities and exposed areas of the body.

The first stage, frostnip, is the 'white spot' most often seen in the face or on ears. At this stage this can be re-warmed by skin-to-skin method.

In the next stage the injured area has a marbled white frozen appearance and is insensitive. It feels cold and firm and moves freely over underlying bony points.

In deep frost bite penetration occurs through skin and subcutaneous tissues into deeper structures; the frozen surface is pallid, yellowish, and waxy. It feels cold and solid and will not move over bony prominences — in warm atmosphere condensation may occur on the skin.

Extreme cases which are not rapidly rewarmed result in loss of tissue. The skin becomes grey and remains cold due to vascular thrombosis. Blisters with proximal oedema may mark the line of demarcation. Dry gangrene follows and the tip becomes black and mummified. Reliable definition of the line of demarcation occurs at about ten weeks. Moist gangrene, the result of added infection, extends the tissue damage.

Treatment

- Rewarming should be started as soon as possible; firm pressure of a warm hand, hot breath and immersion in water 41–44°C (tolerant to the normal hand) should be instigated until normal colour returns. This may soon be followed by blister formation, oedema, and an intense burning pain.
- *Friction and rubbing of any kind increases tissue damage and is contra-indicated.* A booster dose of tetanus toxoid should be given and some authorities recommend administration of broad-spectrum antibiotics.

Hypothermia

Is defined as a core temperature of less than 35°C and is a medical emergency. Its prompt recognition is critical to avoid serious morbidity or death. As hypothermia develops cerebral blood flow declines resulting in a reflex lowering of the brain's metabolic needs. This allows successful cerebral resuscitation of hypothermic patients even after prolonged periods of anoxia or circulatory arrest.

Approximately 3 per cent of patients admitted to British hospitals in winter have rectal temperatures below 35°C. The great majority of these have cooled as a result of the effects of drugs or disease in cold surroundings. Ethanol, barbiturates, malnutrition, insulin hypoglycaemia, myxoedema, and anoxia due to carbon monoxide poisoning also reduce heat production in cold conditions. Other patients cool after collapsing, and being immobilised as a result of injuries, strokes, heart attacks or pneumonia. In these patients provided rewarming is carried out at a moderate rate the hypothermia has little effect on the outcome and mortality is eventually that of the underlying condition. In the elderly, hypothermia, hyperventilation, hypotension, and thrombocytopenia are common signs of bacteraemia and sepsis. (See Figure 24.1.)

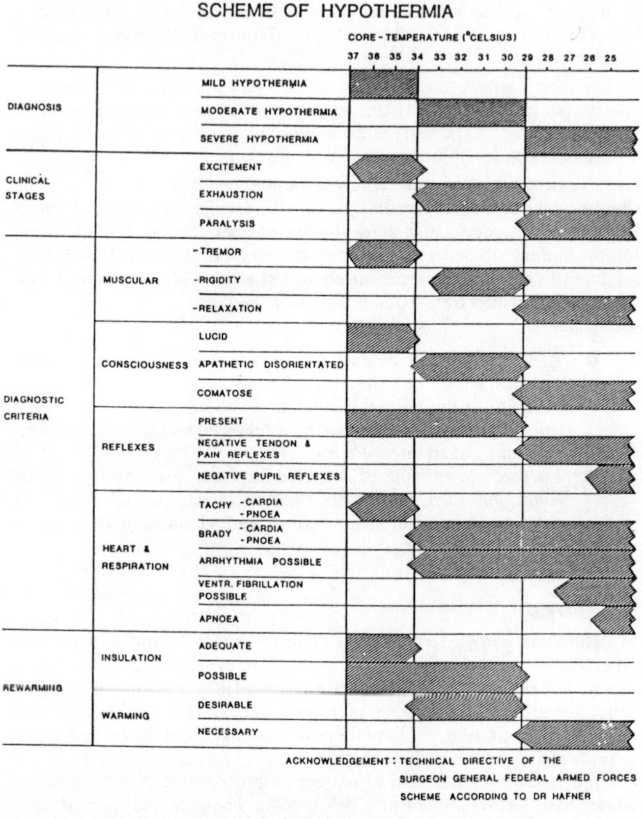

Figure 24.1 *Scheme of hypothermia*

Clinical manifestations appear as temperature falls to 32°C: these include a decline in the mental status, ataxia, tremulous speech, and hyperreflexia. At lower temperatures hyporeflexia, stupor, dysarthria, and sluggish pupillary responses appear. Shivering usually drops below 32°C and muscle rigidity becomes prominent. Heart rate falls as does the blood pressure, peripheral vascular resistance, cardiac output, and central venous pressure. Cardiac arrhythmias are very common — characteristic ECG changes include prolongation of QRS and J waves, atrial fibrillation is common at temperatures 28–35°C. Ventricular fibrillation may occur at temperatures below 28°C. Depression of respiration results in mild respiratory acidosis but lactic acid build-up during shivering causes metabolic acidosis. Glucose metabolism is depressed and blood glucose and potassium rise as body temperature falls. Gastric erosions and haemorrhage and pancreatitis occasionally follow severe hypothermia.

Acute heat loss, as occurs in immersion in icy sea water, leads to a rapid fall in core temperature which can be fatal if rescue is not achieved in a few minutes. Once shivering ceases, at about core temperature 30°C, muscle spasm flexes the body and impairs respiration, voluntary muscle spasm, and power is lost — death results from cardiac arrest or ventricular fibrillation.

Less acute heat loss as occurs on land, i.e. exposure to hill walkers, climbers and skiers, is usually associated with severe fatigue and gives rise to progressive deterioration in central nervous functions. At 30°C these patients are usually unconscious and often pulseless but tendon and pupillary reflexes persist. These patients are also susceptible to local cold injuries (frost bite).

Management of hypothermic patients

This is difficult and depends upon predisposing factors and previous or predisposing illness. They are best managed in intensive care units. Airway patency must be ensured in comatose patients and steps taken to prevent aspiration of gastric contents. Blood pressure, pulse, core temperature, ECG, neurological status, and urine output should be monitored frequently during rewarming. IV access should be considered and the following investigations performed — PCV, WCC, E+ U, blood glucose, TFT, amylase, CXR and blood gases.

- *For the haemodynamically stable and mildly hypothermic patients* passive rewarming with blankets is ideal. A warming rate of about 0.5°C per hour is generally accepted as optimal.

- *Active rewarming becomes necessary in patients with severe hypothermia of short duration or cardiopulmonary arrest*, or both. This is especially important in patients with ventricular fibrillation or asystole because the hypothermic myocardium is resistant to mechanical or pharmacologic intervention until temperatures are above 28°C to 30°C. It is therefore important to remember that core temperature measured on the rectum is usually 1°C higher and lags behind myocardial temperature.

- *After prolonged exposure* slow rewarming without external heat is better. Active external rewarming techniques (i.e. immersion in hot water, direct heat to body surface) lead to 'rewarming shock' and accentuated lactic acidosis. To avoid this, rapid re-warming of blood has been attempted by administration of warm intravenous fluids and heated oxygen. Peritoneal and myocardial lavage with solutions warmed to about 40°C have also been shown to be effective.

● *Supportive measures.* Due to wide diversity of electrolyte derangements in hypothermic patients no general recommendations regarding fluid management are made — except warming the fluid to 37–40°C before administration. As patients are warmed, metabolic acidosis may worsen as lactate is washed out of previously hypoxic tissues. Severe respiratory impairment with significant CO_2 retention should be treated with assisted ventilation. Hyperglycaemia should be suspected especially as patient is rewarmed. As noted previously hyperglycaemia occurs with falling temperature; the hyperglycaemia should be treated only if severe and life threatening.

With people of any age admitted to hospital with hypothermia it is usually a secondary consequence of their main disease. Excess mortality occurring in cold weather is due mainly to deaths from coronary insufficiency and other cardiovascular disease, usually not precipitated by hypothermia but by reflex effects of sudden exposure to cold. However, it is a serious complication and affects the morbidity and mortality of the primary lesion.

Drowning and near-drowning

Drowning is one of the commoner causes of accidental death. A high percentage of the victims are children under the age of four. In accidents outside the home there is a higher percentage of male victims. Predisposing factors include inadequate supervision, trauma, alcohol, drugs, epilepsy, and over-estimation of swimming capability.

Pathophysiologically, drowning can be of four sorts:

1 Wet drowning

There is initial laryngospasm but early relaxation and subsequent aspiration of water or gastric contents that are vomited after swallowing water. This accounts for the majority of drownings.

Theoretically the initial pathophysiologic events should be different in freshwater (hypotonic) submersion and saltwater (hypertonic) submersion. In freshwater submersion the fresh water entering the lung is rapidly absorbed into the circulation and results in hypervolaemia, dilution of electrolytes and lysis of red blood cells with a consequent increase in serum potassium and hence ventricular fibrillation. In saltwater drowning, calcium and magnesium ions are absorbed resulting in ventricular fibrillation. The difference is mainly academic as patients arriving at hospital have usually swallowed too little water to induce the complete syndrome, and in either case the immediate treatment of a victim without a pulse or respiration is to clear the airway and start external cardiac massage and artificial ventilation.

2 Dry drowning

Asphyxiation secondary to intense glottic spasm which persists beyond the point of apnoea so no water is aspirated. This accounts for 10–20 per cent of drownings. This is essentially a post-mortem description of death.

3 Secondary drowning

Death occurs 15 minutes to 72 hours after extraction from water and is due to the adult respiratory distress syndrome. Anyone who has inhaled significant amounts of water should therefore be admitted to hospital at least 24 hours for CXR and observation, no matter how quickly or how well they appear after initial resuscitation.

4 Immersion syndrome

Cardiac arrest is rare but may occur secondary to an intense noradrenergic reflex drive to the ventricular muscle (resulting in fibrillation) and peripheral vasoconstriction; sometimes assisted by vagal slowing from sudden cooling of the face and body surface in water.

Submersion victims can be classified as drowning and near-drowning victims. Drowning victims die within 24 hours while victims of near-drowning survive at least 24 hours. The most important consequences of near-drowning are severe hypoxaemia and metabolic acidosis. Cardiac arrhythmias and central nervous system injury with cerebral oedema can occur as a result of this. Outcome in near-drowning is best judged by the neurological status. The shorter the interval between extraction from the water to first spontaneous gasp the better the prognosis. The effect of hypoxia on the CNS may be significantly reduced if the water is cold, so more time must be given for resuscitation. In the case of children whose smaller size (and relatively larger surface area) allows more rapid cooling the chances of successful resuscitation with no chronic neurological sequelae are higher.

Cardiovascular derangement includes arrhythmias and shock. Renal failure may ensue from hypoxia, acidosis, hypoperfusion, myoglobinuria, or haemoglobinuria secondary to haemolysis. Disseminated intravascular coagulation may also occur.

Both freshwater and saltwater lead to surfactant loss resulting in atelectasis and ventilation perfusion mismatch. ARDS is always a threat.

The initial appearance of the patient

This can vary from coma to agitated alertness. Cyanosis, coughing, and the production of pink frothy sputum are common. Tachypnoea and tachycardia, rales and rhonchi may be detected. Neurological signs vary. Signs of associated trauma (e.g. cervical spine injury) should be sought.

Treatment

- This begins with establishment of an airway and if necessary immediate cardiopulmonary resuscitation.
- The stomach is often distended with swallowed water so should be emptied with a naso-gastric tube.
- High-concentration oxygen is necessary and the patient may need ventilation on positive end-expiratory pressure if $PaO_2 <$ 10 kPa.
- Hypovolaemic shock must be treated with colloid administered cautiously because of damaged pulmonary capillaries and monitoring of cardiac rhythm is essential.
- Cerebral oedema, if present, should be treated with hyper-ventilation to lower $PaCO_2$ and mannitol 50 ml 20 per cent + frusemide 10–20 gms given together.
- Initial investigations include Hct, Electrolyte and Acid/base status arterial blood gases, ECG, and CXR. Core temperature using low temperature thermometer.
- In A & E even patients who quickly become normal should be hospitalised for 24 hours to watch for subsequent picture of adult respiratory distress syndrome.

Barotrauma and decompression sickness

Breathing air under pressure forces nitrogen (inert gas) into the tissues. On decompression these nitrogen bubbles reform in the body tissues. Normally the lungs filter these bubbles and expel them in expiration but if decompression occurs too quickly the lungs cannot cope and pulmonary hypertension develops. Normal physiological shunts open up and bubbles now on the left side of the heart become air emboli. These commonly occlude coronary, cerebral, and especially spinal arterioles. The results are, therefore — sudden death, myocardial infarction, cerebrovascular accident, paraplegia, or hemiplegia.

During descent, the pressure increases 1 atmosphere for every 33 feet (10 m) of descent.

Decompression Sickness

This is a more subtle form of barotrauma and air embolism. It involves the liberation of inert bubbles from the soluble phase into tissue or blood. Clinically it can mimic almost every medical condition known. Asymptomic bubbles are termed 'silent' and may precede overt manifestations in many cases. They may also be the foundation on which decompression sickness develops during subsequent dives.

Type I 'Pain Only': limb or joint pains, itch, skin rash, localised swelling.

Type II 'Serious': CNS disorder, inner ear (vestibular), lungs, cardiac, type I symptoms under pressure.

Onset: 50 per cent within one hour, 90 per cent within six hours, 1 per cent after twenty-four hours. *Any patient who presents immediately after ascent with any neurological signs or symptoms, no matter how subtle, needs immediate O$_2$ treatment and recompression because they have an air embolus.* Treatment involves immediate recompression followed by gradual decompression. Patient should be lying semi-prone on the left with the buttocks raised. 100 per cent oxygen should be administered as immediate first aid and continued whilst transporting to recompression facilities.

1 Skin bends: treat with 100 per cent oxygen alone.
2 Joint bends: depends on symptoms onset interval and time of presentation.
3 All others: treatment ideally is recompression.
4 Low molecular weight Dextran, heparin, steroids, aspirin.

If you have a patient with a diving medical problem telephone:

(a) Portsmouth (0705) 822351
(b) In emergency (0705) 818888

NOTES

25

Travellers' diseases

Travellers' diseases

Exotic diseases are now frequently seen in A & E departments with the increase in travel and the advent of the high-speed jet. Movement from areas where disease is endemic to home can take a day or less. The patient may be an immigrant, newly arrived or one who has recently visited the old country, or someone who has been on a holiday, or a young person making the journey of a lifetime, living rough and exposed to infection. Always ask about recent travels, country, town, village, and movement within the country; what innoculations were taken; what prophylactics in malarious areas were used, and if they were continued after return home. (See Table 25.1.) Other diseases beside malaria which may cause symptoms only after return are amoebic dysentery, filariasis, leishmaniasis, schistosomiasis, trachoma, trypanosomiasis, typhoid, typhus, venereal disease, and viral hepatitis.

Presentation

Cough

Consider pneumonia — atypical, legionnaires' microplasma, viral or the secondary infection of AIDS.

Diarrhoea

Traveller's diarrhoea is the commonest: 'Tripoli trots', 'Gyppi tummy', 'Montezuma's revenge' are all common to new arrivals in an area and usually are short-lasting. If symptoms persist, then other causes such as shigella or amoebic dysenteries should be sought for. Giardiasis is fairly common, as are parasitic infestations. Cholera is uncommon but not unknown.

Fever

Always consider malaria first in patients returning from any malarial area even if the stop was only a short aircraft staging stop. (See Figure 25.1.) Lassa fever and VHF are rare but dangerous and may arise from the country areas of West Africa, Senegal to Nigeria. Typhoid may have been caught in India, Pakistan or the Mediterranean countries. River abscess, amoebic or tropical, may be a late manifestation of the diseases.

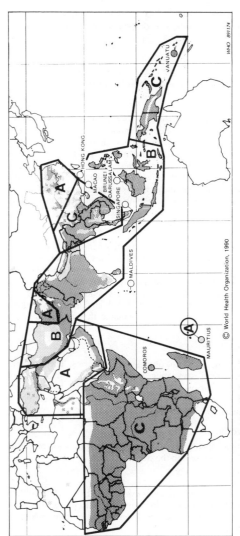

Acknowledgement: World Health Organization.

Figure 25.1 *Recommendations for malaria drug prophylaxis by area 1990.* **A:** *In zone A, risk generally low and seasonal; no risk in many areas (for example urban areas).* **B:** *Low risk in most of the areas of zone B. Chloroquine, with or without proguanil, will protect against P. vivax; it may fail to prevent infection with P. falciparum, but may still alleviate the severity of disease.* **C:** *In Africa, risk high in most areas of zone C; except in some high-altitude areas. Risk low in most areas of this zone in Asia and America, but high in parts of the Amazon basin (colonization and mining areas). Resistance to sulfadoxine-pyrimetham common in zone C in Asia, variable in zone C in Africa and America.*

Legionnaires' disease may follow a stay in modern hotels or hospitals where the water supply to showers or droplets entering the ventilation system are infected.

Jaundice

The commonest causes are hepatitis A or B but falciparum malaria, infectious mononucleosis or yellow fever may be responsible.

Skin rash

The most frequent cause may be insect bites, fleas, mosquitoes, sandfly, or tsetse fly depending on country visited and mode of travel. Acute rashes are usually from the common infectious fevers such as measles or chicken pox but the more sinister haemorrhagic rash of the viral, Lassa, or yellow fevers must be thought of. The rose-red, raised maculopapular rash of typhoid; the lymphangitis of filariasis with a transient urticarial erythematous rash; or the rash of secondary syphilis are less common. Chronic rashes may result from leishmaniasis, creeping eruptions of cutaneous lava migrans or, to be seen rarely, the nodules or plaques of leprosy.

Traveller's diarrhoea

The acute signs and symptoms of this condition are well known to travellers and fortunately are short-lasting. The cause is a change in the bowel flora and the presence of a bowel pathogen, an enterotoxinogenic *E. coli*. If the disease does not settle quickly, stool cultures should be taken to exclude Shigella or Salmonella dysentery, Campylobacter jejuni. If the patient has been more ill with raised TPR, high fluid loss, vomiting, and bloody diarrhoea with mucus then amoebic dysentery should be considered.

Typhoid fever

This is a septicaemic illness and not only a gastro-enteritis. The temperature is elevated, the patient is sweating, has headache, constipation, and develops rose-red spots on his trunk. TB and brucellosis have a more insidious onset with an evening raise in the temperature and sweating. A blood culture should be taken and *refer*.

Giardia lamblia infection

This causes abdominal discomfort and loose stools with a lot of flatus. Cysts or trophozoites are present in the stools.

Amoebic dysentery

This may be of acute or chronic onset. Freshly passed stools will contain motile amoebae which must be seen to establish the diagnosis. The antibody titre is raised in liver disease so the diagnosis can be confirmed by a fluorescent antibody test.

No infective agent

Normal stool cultures suggest that the cause of abdominal pain and diarrhoea is an exacerbation of a pre-existing condition such as diverticulitis, irritable bowel syndrome, Crohn's disease or ulcerative colitis. The patient need not have had overt symptoms or signs of these conditions which may have been aggravated by a severe attack of traveller's diarrhoea. Many antibiotics disturb the normal gut flora and super-infections can cause quite severe diarrhoea. Large doses of antidiarrhoeal drugs can themselves cause nausea and vomiting.

Helminth infections

Bowel parasites should be looked for in the stools of patients with vague abdominal symptoms, particularly those who have been travelling and living rough. Eosinophilia is usually present. Thread worms often cause *pruritus anti* whilst hookworms often cause anaemia. Tapeworms will be accompanied by some degree of weight loss.

Haematuria following an exposure to fresh water in Africa, Egypt, South America and the Caribbean area should make you think of the possibility of infection by the freeswimming larvae of Schistosoma. The illness develops 4 to 6 weeks after exposure with fever, cough, abdominal pain and an urticarial rash. An intestinal form is accompanied by a bloody diarrhoea.

Viral haemorrhagic fever (VHF)

Patients returning from the rural areas of West Africa, south of the Sahara, presenting with an undiagnosed fever must be placed in an isolation room and the possibility of VHF considered. The infections of Lassa, Marburg, Ebola and Congo/Crimean haemorrhagic fevers have an incubation period up to 21 days. The onset of the illness is insidious with fever, malaise, and headache. Pyrexia may last 16 days with temperatures up to $41^{\circ}C$.

The virus is spread by contact with infected blood, urine or semen. *Protective clothing (gloves and a plastic apron) should be worn. If the patient is bleeding then plastic gowns and operating gloves are necessary.* The possibility of infection is then graded and the patient is placed in an index of suspicion according to the DHSS Memorandum on the control of VHF.

(a) Strong: A patient who has left a known endemic area, urban or rural, in the previous 3 weeks; contacts of confirmed cases; laboratory workers who handle VHF viruses.

(b) Moderate: A patient from tropical Africa within 3 weeks of leaving a rural area or small town not generally considered endemic; or where the onset and course of the fever are consistent with VHF.

(c) Minimal: A patient who left tropical Africa in the previous 3 weeks but from a major city where the risk of VHF is considered negligible.

Special precautions have to be taken with blood from these patients so do not take any specimens until the case has been discussed with the duty physician and microbiologist. Only in moderate and minimal risk cases can you examine the blood for malarial parasites and that must be done at the bedside, in isolation, taking precautions as described above.

Diphtheria

A toxic patient with a sore throat must have the membrane on the tonsil lifted off. If it leaves a bleeding surface the diagnosis of diphtheria must be suspected and excluded. The washleather membrane, dirty white or greyish, is adherent and when swabbed bleeds. The tachycardia in diphtheria is out of proportion to the pyrexia, the onset is insidious, the pharynx is dull red with moderate oedema. There may be a blood-stained nasal discharge, husky voice and high-pitched cough. Laryngeal obstruction may develop when intubation, cricothyroid stab or tracheostomy is life-saving.

Treatment

By antitoxin which must be given on a clinical diagnosis; the swab will only confirm.

Dosage:

small membrane, tonsils   40,000 units IM;
larger, pharynx   80,000 units IV in 200 ml N saline;
severe, pharynx, larynx   120,000 units IV in 200 ml N saline.

Always test for sensitivity to horse serum.
A course of erythromycin is started.

Legionnaires' disease

This often presents in small epidemics with a relatively high mortality rate. There is a high fever, prostration, confusion and hallucinations, dysarthria, chest pain, increased respiratory rate and other signs of pneumonia culture; antigens in the urine. The serum creatine level is raised but the serology is not diagnostic until later. Unusual presentation of pneumonia should be asked for details of their activities during the previous week or so. If the patient has been in a building where water droplets are produced from showers, humidification or jaccuzis, etc., then this diagnosis should be thought of early so that urgent measures can be taken to halt the spread.

Poliomyelitis

This is an enteroviral infection which, with modern efficient oral vaccine available, is a disease which should not be seen. Unfortunately it may occur in visitors from warm areas where it is endemic; they have been infected from carriers. Early signs are of a viral illness with sore throat, headaches, malaise, pyrexia; muscle pains become more severe and are followed by muscle weakness and paralysis. *Refer* for isolation and check on the vaccination state of all who have been in contact. A booster dose of oral vaccine is advised.

Rabies

A viral infection which follows a bite from an infected animal — dog, cat, fox, bat, wolf. Rabies is common in tropical countries and is slowly spreading across Europe. It is necessary to take an accurate history about the bite — was the animal ill, savage, rabid or was it provoked? Did it live or was it killed and examined? The spread is by saliva so that a scratch from the tooth of the rabid animal is sufficient to infect; people 'trekking' in high-risk areas should have pre-exposure vaccination.

The incubation period is 2 to 9 weeks and is dependent on the distance from the brain; facial bites are more dangerous. Anxiety and apprehension start suddenly, followed by pyrexia, headache and malaise. Swallowing can cause spasm of the throat muscles and inability to drink water — hydrophobia. The spasms spread to the chest and body muscles. The patient becomes more excitable, even maniacal, and is unable to swallow his saliva.

Prophylaxis is post exposure and consists of giving a course of human diploid cell vaccine and anti-rabies serum (equine). These vaccines are obtainable only from the Public Health Laboratory Service at London, Birmingham, Cardiff, Exeter, Leeds, Liverpool, Newcastle and Edinburgh. The PHLS must be contacted and the case discussed with them (telephone 071-200-6868). Enquiries about suspected rabid animals should be made to the District Veterinary Officer for animals in UK, and to the Rabies Doctor of the International Relations Division of the DHSS at Alexander Fleming House, Elephant and Castle, London SE1 (071-407 5522) about rabid animals overseas.

If the animal lives for 15 days after there is little risk of infection — this is why it is most important to find out what happened to it.

Malaria

Any patient who has ever lived in, or travelled through a malarious area should be suspected of having malaria if a fever develops. Antimalarial prophylaxis is not always effective, since chloroquine and proguanil resistance is common.

Of the four species of malaria parasite (p. falciparum, p. ovale, p. vivax and p. malarial) p. falciparum is the most dangerous and can lead to rapid death. *P. vivax* and *p. malarial* can remain dormant in the liver for years.

On examination: temperature, ? anaemia, ? splenomegaly, ? hepatomegaly, ? conscious level (cerebral malaria) ? dehydration. Investigations: FBC, U+E, LFT, creatinine (? renal failure), blood cultures, viral

WHAT YOU NEED WHERE: WHAT MAY BE CAUGHT WHERE

Below we give the DHSS recommendations. Wherever you're travelling make sure your polio and tetanus immunisations are up to date. None of the precautions listed below is recommended for Europe and North America.

Africa — north

Algeria	MCT
Burkina Faso	MCTY
Cape Verde Islands	MT
Chad	MCTY
Egypt	MCT
Gambia	MCTY
Guinea	MCTY
Guinea-Bissau	MCTY
Libya	MCT
Mali	MCTY
Mauritania	MCTY
Sierra Leone	MCTY
Somalia	MCTY
Tanzania	MCTY
Togo	MCTY
Uganda	MCTY
Zaire	MCTY

Africa — south

Angola	MCTY
Botswana	MCT
Lesotho	CT
Malawi	MCT
Mozambique	MCT
Namibia	MCT
South Africa	MCT
Swaziland	MCTY
Zambia	MCTY
Zimbabwe	MCT

Caribbean

Anguilla	T
Antigua and Barbuda	T
Antilles	T
Bahamas	T
Mexico	MT
Nicaragua	MT
Panama	MTY

South America

Argentina	MT
Bolivia	MTY
Brazil	MTY
Chile	T
Colombia	MTY
Ecuador	MTY
Falkland Islands	T
French Guiana	MTY
Guyana	MTY
Paraguay	MT
Peru	MTY
Suriname	MTY
Uruguay	T
Venezuela	MTY

Burma	MCT
China	MT
Hong Kong	T
India	MCT
Indonesia	MCT
Japan	T
Kampuchea	MCT
Korea	CT
Malaysia	MCT
Mongolia	T
Nepal	MCT
Pakistan	MCT
Philippines	MCT
Singapore	CT
Sri Lanka	MCT
Taiwan	CT
Thailand	MCT

Indian Ocean Islands

Madagascar	MCT
Maldives	MCT
Mauritius	MT
Reunion Islands	T
Seychelles	T

Morocco	MCT
Niger	MCT**Y**
Senegal	MCT**Y**
Sudan	MCT**Y**
Tunisia	CT

Africa — central

Benin	MCT**Y**
Burundi	MCT**Y**
Cameroon	MCT**Y**
Central African Republic	MCT**Y**
Congo	MCT**Y**
Ethiopia	MCT**Y**
Gabon	MCT**Y**
Ghana	MCT**Y**
Ivory Coast	MCT**Y**
Kenya	MCT**Y**
Liberia	MCT**Y**
Nigeria	MCT**Y**
Rwanda	MCT**Y**
Sao Tome and Principe	MCT**Y**

Malaria corrected WHO 1990

Barbados	T
Cayman Islands	T
Cuba	T
Dominica	T
Dominican Republic	MT
Grenada	T
Haiti	MT
Jamaica	T
Montserrat	T
Puerto Rico	T
St Christopher-Nevis	T
St Lucia	T
St Vincent	T
Trinidad, Tobago	T
Virgin Islands	T

Central America

Belize	MT
Costa Rica	MT
El Salvador	MT
Guatemala	MT
Honduras	MT

Middle East

Bahrain	CT
Cyprus	—
Iran	MCT
Iraq	MCT
Israel	CT
Jordan	CT
Kuwait	CT
Lebanon	MCT
Oman	MCT
Qatar	CT
Saudi Arabia	MCT
Syria	MCT
Turkey	MCT
Yemen	MCT

Asia

Afghanistan	MCT
Bangladesh	MCT
Brunei	CT

Australasia

Australia	—
Fiji Islands	T
Kiribati	T
New Caledonia	T
New Zealand	—
Papua New Guinea	MCT
Solomon Islands	MT
Tahiti	T
Tuvalu	T
Vanuatu	MT

Key

M anti-malarial
C cholera
T typhoid (and infectious hepatitis)
Y yellow fever (in **bold** if a certificate usually required for entry)

Acknowledgements to the Consumers' Association.

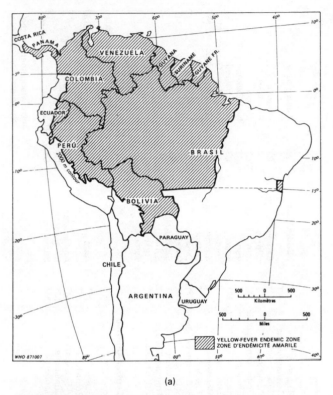

(a)

Acknowledgement: World Health Organization.

Figure 25.2 *(a) Yellow fever endemic zone in the Americas, (b) Yellow fever endemic zone in Africa*

Note: Although the 'yellow fever endemic zones' are no longer included in the International Health Regulations, a number of countries (most of them not being bound by the Regulations or bound with reservations) consider these zones as infected areas and require an international certificate of vaccination against yellow fever from travellers arriving from those areas. Maps (a) and (b) are therefore included in this publication for practical reasons

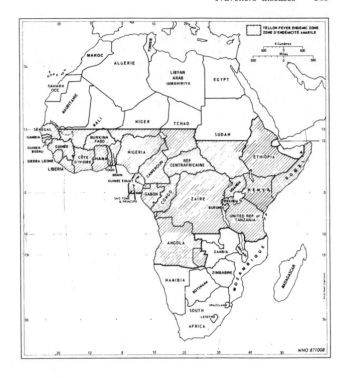

(b)

Acknowledgement: World Health Organization.

Source: *Vaccination certificate requirements and health advice for international travel: Situation as on 1 January 1988*, Geneva, World Health Organization, 1988.

titres, blood for thick + thin films, (in same bottle as FBC). Urine — colour black? Bilirubin — lab for microscopy.

Initial Management: Rehydrate, cool (paracetamol + fan = tepid sponging), refer medics (for chloroquine or quinine if malaria confirmed).

Different Diagnosis: Flu, UTI, chest infection, all causes of pyrexia, both local and tropical if recently travelled.

Advice: Malaria Reference Laboratory: 071-387 4411 (at the National Hospital for Tropical Diseases).

NOTES

26

Practical procedures

Wound management

The aim is to promote healing by primary intention without infection, so that there will be minimum scarring and normal function.

Management of wounds depends on:

- The nature of the wound.
- The time after the injury that the wound is presented.
- Wounds fall into the following major categories
  1 Abrasions
  2 Incised wounds
  3 Flaps
  4 Lacerations
  5 Crush wounds.

1 Abrasions

May be small or very large in area; in RTAs they often result from sliding contact of the patient's skin with the ground. Consequently, the abrasion may be full of dirt, clothing, paint from vehicles or the like. They are usually only superficial in depth, and so heal quickly. They must be cleaned thoroughly at the time of presentation or new epithelium grows over the foreign material resulting in a 'traumatic tattoo', which will be unsightly and permanent.

Cleaning should be under adequate anaesthesia — GA in children, or in adults if the area is large. A soft scrub-brush and Savlon solution should be used to remove the dirt. Hydrogen peroxide (half strength) will aid the cleaning process. It is also styptic and stops ooze. An antibacterial cream should then be applied.

2 Incised wounds

Cleanly cut edges do not require excision. Anaesthetise with 1 per cent lignocaine and suture or use steristrips in short wounds. Histoacrylic glue is useful in children and wounds not under tension.

3 Flap lacerations

When a flap of skin is lifted the most vulnerable point is the apex of the flap, as it is furthest from the blood supply. Distally based flaps are more at risk than proximally based flaps. The management of the flap tends to depend on the anatomical position. Because of the good blood supply to the head and neck, it is possible to suture those on the face safely. However, as few sutures as possible are inserted, especially near the tip which needs a special suture. (See Figure 20.1, page 269.)

If a pre-tibial flap is raised, it is better not to suture it, but to close it as far as possible with steristrips and allow spontaneous healing. It is better to leave a slight defect than to put tension on the flap.

4 Wound excision of lacerated wounds

Wounds seen within 8 hours of injury (up to 12 on face where the blood supply is good) may be excised and sutured.

Before anaesthetising wound, carefully examine the affected part, especially in fingers, so damage to nerves or tendons is discovered or excluded. (Sensation loss cannot be tested after anaesthetic is given.)

The wound is usually anaesthetised by 1 per cent lignocaine solution infiltrated around the wound, or a digital block for digits (see Figure 26.8). Clean the wound thoroughly and gently irrigate with saline if required. Examine the deep structures for damage using a swab to absorb blood. Any devitalised deeper tissue must be excised. Next examine the wound edges — any obviously dead tissue must also be removed, but be as conservative as possible. Convert irregular wound edges to a tidy wound. If the wound edges are approximately 90°, then the wound may be sutured directly. If the edges are oblique, they should be excised to 90°, using either a scalpel or sharp-pointed scissors. (The one exception is the eyebrow which should not be excised.) The wound is then sutured in layers.

Undermining of the skin edges may be required to prevent closure under tension — undermining enables the tension to be spread throughout the wound and so decreases the likelihood of necrosis at a given spot. Undermining is carried out through the upper subcutaneous tissues. If it is too superficial the flap will be devitalised.

5 Crush-type wound

These cause severe tissue damage and oedema. Obviously devitalised tissue should be excised. In general sutures should be avoided, though sometimes a few may have to be placed at strategic points of the wound to prevent complete dehiscence. They should have a flamazine dressing applied and be reviewed at 48 hours and 5 days when delayed primary closure can be considered. The affected part should be elevated for 48 hours to reduce swelling. (See Figure 20.3. Burst injury of finger, page 270.)

High energy release missile injury

A combination of laceration and crush injury — Figure 26.1.

The temporary cavity expands and contracts, foreign bodies, dirt and

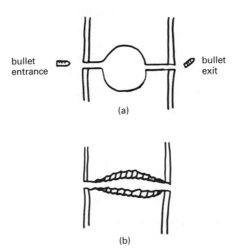

Figure 26.1 *High energy release missile injuries*
(a)   Temporary cavity in limb
(b)   Permanent cavity in limb

bacteria are sucked in. The permanent cavity is surrounded by a band of dead muscle.

Treatment

All HVMI need exploration, fasciotomy, excision of all dead tissues — particularly muscle that does not bleed or contract. The wound is dressed and left open. Delayed primary suture or graft is done after 4–5 days.

Wounds seen late

If the wound is over 12 hours old clean it thoroughly, after fasciotomy excise dead and contaminated tissues, prescribe antibiotics and review 2–3 days later. If it is still clean and not infected, it may then be sutured: delayed primary suture. Further excision may be required: review again 2–3 days later.

Excision biopsy

Aim of excision biopsy is to excise the lesion in total — both laterally and in the deep plane. The margin of clearance required depends on the nature of the lesion. If the lesion is benign, 2 mm clearance is adequate, but at least 0.5 cm is required for potentially malignant lesions.

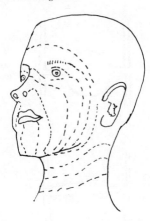

Figure 26.2 *Langer's lines of the face. Incisions and lacerations along these lines heal with finer scars*

Therefore ASSESS:

    1 Nature of lesion
    2 Is primary closure possible?
        (a) Is incision biopsy appropriate?
        (b) Should excision and reconstruction, e.g. skin grafting, be carried out?

Technique of excision biopsy

The vast majority of lesions can be excised satisfactorily under local anaesthesia.

    (a) Plan incisions to fit into the skin creases or natural lines on the face. (See Figure 26.2.)
    (b) Mark the area and planned incisions with ink prior to injection of local anaesthetic.
    (c) Inject LA — as little as is commensurate with adequate anaesthesia as it distorts the area. Adrenaline may be used on face but is not a substitute for satisfactory haemostasis.
    (d) Excise lesion — usually in the centre of an ellipse.
    (e) Reconstruct the wound, it may be necessary to undermine the skin edges — insert a layer of deep absorbable sutures if necessary, then a subcutaneous layer of inverted sutures, and then close skin. Interrupted sutures are easiest but a continuous subcuticular suture may be used if wished.

(f) Review at 8–10 days for suture removal.
(g) Send lesion for histology in formaline and make sure you check results.

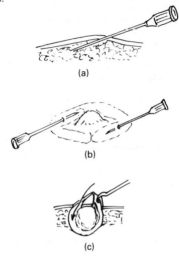

Figure 26.3 *Excision of sebaceous cyst*
(a) Subcutaneous infiltration
(b) LA block
(c) Dissection close to wall of cyst

Excision of sebaceous cysts

If the cyst is infected and pointing, it should be incised and drained as described for abscesses.

N.B. Patients often present with moderately inflamed cysts, etc., especially on faces and necks. Antibiotics may abort the infection, the patient should be reviewed after a few days to check that pus has not formed.

When the inflammation settles, the cyst should be excised in about 6 weeks.

Elective removal of uninfected cysts (Figure 26.3)

1 Mark the incision lines (around the punctum) prior to the injection of local anaesthetic. This should preferably follow the lines of skin tension or be placed in a natural fold line, especially on the face.

2 Anaesthetise the area, using 1 per cent lignocaine, though lignocaine with adrenalin may be useful on the face. Adequate anaesthetic must be injected into the surface of the skin, and both around
  and beneath the cyst. Try to avoid injection into the cyst — it
  usually leads to a messy rupture and makes the subsequent procedure more difficult.

3   (a) Incise skin where planned and raise a small ellipse (0.5 cm)
         attached to the superior surface of the cyst and use this for
         handling purposes.
     (b) Now carefully define the outline of the cyst, preferably by
         blunt dissection, though sharp dissection using scissors may
         be necessary, especially if the cyst has been inflamed.
     (c) Keep the scissors close to the cyst wall — it is preferable to
         damage the cyst rather than any underlying structures.
     (d) The cyst should shell out, hopefully all in one piece.

4 Haemostasis must be meticulous, and then the 'dead space' (space
  left by the removal of the cyst) is closed by subcutaneous absorb-
  able sutures.

5 If cyst is punctured, attempt to close puncture with artery forceps.

6 If the material is too friable and this is not possible, evacuate the
  cyst contents and then dissect out all of the cyst wall.

7 Once the cyst wall has been completely removed close the wound
  in layers as above.

8 The skin is then closed, usually with interrupted sutures.

Abscesses

If a patient presents with a throbbing, red, tense, or fluctuant abscess it
must be incised and drained at that time. Antibiotics at this stage are
ineffective.

In A & E departments, small abscesses may be satisfactorily dealt with
under local anaesthetic, but larger abscesses will require a general anaesthetic. Ethylchloride should not be used as the analgesia provided is not
adequate to allow the necessary debridement of the abscess cavity.

Procedure

1 Inject a sufficient quantity of lignocaine around the abscess and
  deep into it, and allow adequate time for it to be effective.

2 Incise the abscess where it is pointing or the site of maximum
  tenderness and fluctuation.
  A small incision (approximately 1 cm) is large enough to start with
  and can be enlarged as necessary.

3 Take a swab for C & S.

4 Clean liquid pus away.

5 Open cavity with sinus forceps (Hilton's method). (See Figure
  26.4.)

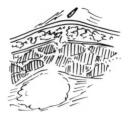

(a) 1 cm incision over point of
maximum tenderness

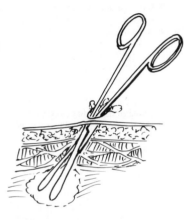

(b) Insert sinus forceps deeply in search for pus. If located open forceps and
withdraw

Figure 26.4 *Hilton's method of draining an abscess*

6 Curette cavity thoroughly.
7 Pack with proflavine wick — packing is not intended to be haemostatic but to prevent the abscess closing at the skin, so should be
   loose.
8 Remove any necrotic skin around incision site.
9 Change packs daily under analgesia until wound is clean and
   showing evidence of granulation.

Breast abscess

Breast abscess is seen less frequently in the puerperium. A subareolar
abscess with anaerobic bacteria probably results from duct ectasia and
these patients may need further surgery. *Refer.*

Peripherally sited abscesses are predominantly *Staph. aureus* in origin.
Incision and drainage is the effective treatment under a general anaesthetic when all the loculi can be opened.

Acute paronychia

The finger tip is swollen, painful and pus is usually visible around the nail base. (Figure 26.5.)

Procedure

1 Anaesthetic with digital nerve block (see Figure 26.8).
2 Incise cuticle over the pus.
3 Release pus and then de-roof the cavity.
4 If the nail-bed does not have any pus underneath, then it can be left intact. If you're not sure, push the cuticle along its width and inspect the nail bed. If the base of the nail is firmly attached and the bed looks healthy, do no more.
5 If, however, pus is seen coming out from under the nail and the nail itself is loose, lift the nail and excise the base with scissors. If there is a lot of pus present the nail will effectively be floating free and the whole of it should be removed.
6 If the paronychia follows a crush injury and infected haematoma, inspect the base for broken spicules which should be removed if found.

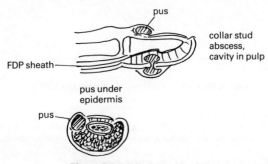

Figure 26.5 *Infections of the finger*

Chronic paronychia

This usually results from the hands continually being wet — e.g. in housewives. The causative organism is often monilia.

Surgery is only rarely indicated — usually to deal with secondary bacterial infection.

Treatment

1 Nystatin orally and as a cream topically.
2 Keep the hands dry.

3 Castellani's paint.
4 Potassium permanganate 1–2 per cent solution soaks can be useful in persistent cases.

Incision of finger pulp abscess

The history is of three or four days of increasing pain in the tip of the finger, which has become swollen and tender to the touch. If pain has kept the patient awake at night then I & D (incision and drainage) is mandatory.

On examination, the pulp is obviously swollen and very tense. There may be visible pus but if not, it does not mean that the area can be left. If the pulp is hot, red, very tender and tense, incision and drainage must be carried out as the abscess is deep and has not been able to decompress itself by tracking to the surface.

Procedure

1 Mark the most tender spot prior to anaesthesia.
2 Anaesthetise using a digital nerve block unless the finger is swollen. *NEVER USE ANY ADRENALIN WITH THE ANAESTHETIC IN THIS REGION.*
3 Allow adequate time for the onset of anaesthesia — usually some 5 minutes or so.
4 De-roof any obvious blister with pus, or incise over the previously marked tender spot.
5 Open the cavity and probe with sinus forceps — this will reveal the deep fibrous connections and release the deeper pus. (See Figure 26.5.) Send pus for C&S.
6 Excise the wound edges.
7 Insert a small wick —usually ribbon gauze soaked in betadine. An adequately padded dressing is then applied.
8 High arm sling.
9 Review daily — improvement should be rapid. If things do not resolve quickly, a further drainage procedure may be required.
10 X-ray the distal phalanx to exclude osteomyelitis.
11 Follow-up routinely to check on finger function.

Tendon sheath infections

Tendon sheath infections usually arise from a midline finger puncture injury, though they may occur without obvious recent trauma.

Diagnosis

1 There may be a midline wound on finger.
2 The finger is swollen, red and hot, and held in mid-flexion.
3 It is tender to the touch, the tenderness being maximal along the surface markings of the sheath (midline of finger) and often extends into the palm (proximal compartment).
4 Any attempt to extend the finger meets resistance as it is very painful.

Management

1 If the finger is seen in the early stages, antibiotics (ampicillin and flucloxacillin) in high doses may be tried and the hand elevated in high arm sling (HAS). If this is done the patient must be reviewed daily to monitor progress.

2 If the patient is seen with an established tendon sheath infection, or there is failure to respond to antibiotics, then the patient should be referred to the Orthopaedic Surgeons for surgical incision and drainage. Depending on the severity of the infection, the wound site, each end of the sheath, or the total length of the sheath may have to be explored under GA with a tourniquet.

Aspiration of the knee joint

Joint aspiration is performed

1 To establish the diagnosis in a swollen knee.
2 To reduce the tension in an effusion and so relieve pain following trauma.

Joint aspiration must always be carried out under full aseptic conditions.

Procedure

1 Position the patient lying down so that the knee is as straight as possible or only slightly flexed. The leg should also be slightly internally rotated.

2 The knee joint may be aspirated via the supra-patellar pouch which communicates with the knee joint proper. The supra-patellar pouch may be approached from either the medial or lateral side of the patella, though the lateral approach is preferred to avoid vastus medialis muscle. Locate the mid point of the lateral side of the patella and the retro-patellar groove. Mark this spot on the skin with an indelible marker. (See Figure 26.6.)

3 Clean the skin thoroughly with povidone iodine — never forget that you are opening a possible route for infection into the joint.

4 Towel up with sterile towels.

5 With a small needle raise a small skin weal with local anaesthetic at the previously marked point. Change to a larger needle and advance thus in a posteromedial direction (to allow for the slope of the patella), injecting anaesthetic as you go.

There should be some resistance when the joint capsule is reached — inject more local (this may be quite painful for the patient), and then advance the needle a little further and attempt to aspirate the fluid that is in the joint. Continue until fluid is drawn into syringe. If you hit bone, withdraw the needle, realign it and try again.

6 Remember to apply pressure with your other hand over the supra-patellar pouch to express fluid.

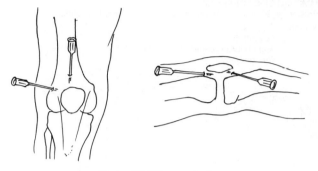

Figure 26.6 *Knee aspiration*

7 The fluid collected should be sent:
   (a) For culture and sensitivity
   (b) For serology
   (c) For microscopy for crystals and cells

If the fluid is heavily blood stained, examine it for fat globules which indicates a fracture of one of the bones in the joint. *Refer*.

If the fluid is turbid consider infective arthritis and treat appropriately. *Refer*.

8 Seal the needlestick with a small sterile dressing and apply a Robert-Jones bandage.

Crico-thyrotomy

IF IMMEDIATE RISK OF CHOKING
(simple emergency airway before expert tracheostomy is available)

Indications: Trauma
Epiglottitis
Angioneurotic oedema
Foreign body

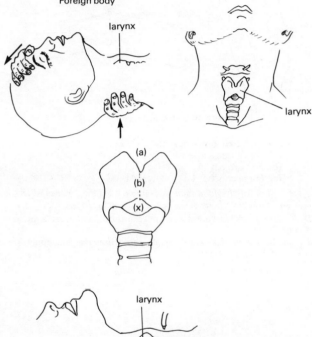

Figure 26.7 *Crico-thyrotomy*
* *Lie patient flat on back*
* *Tilt head well back*
  * *—place one hand under neck*
  * *—place other hand on forehead*
  * *—tilt head well back as shown by arrows*
* *Find the 'Adam's Apple'*
* *Find notch of upper edge (a)*
* *Run finger down ridge (approx. 2 cm) (b)*
* *Find dip at (x)*
* *Insert large-bore cannula at (x) at 45°*
* *Puncture Cr-Th membrane in lower half to avoid Cr-Th arteries*

Ring block

This is used to anaesthetise a digit. The digital nerves run anterolateral to the bones. The nail is usually the last part of the digit to become anaesthetised. (Figure 26.8.)

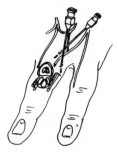

Figure 26.8 *Ring block of digital nerves*

Method

1 Use 1 or 2 per cent plain lignocaine.
2 (a) Insert needle from dorsum. inject 0.5 ml over dorsal digital nerve
   (b) Inject 2.0 ml LA over the volar branch — 2.5 ml should be used on each side of the digit. It normally takes about 5 minutes to work.

Thoracocentesis

Remember that the nerves and vessels run just below the ribs.

Equipment needed

1 Local anaesthetic
2 Scalpel
3 Trocar and cannula
4 Tubing and clamp
5 Underwater seal
6 0 silk suture

Method (Figure 26.9)

● Choose the position of the drain — it should be in the midaxillary line at the nipple level.
● Infiltrate local anaesthetic into the skin and down as far as the pleura.
● Make a 2 cm incision in the skin.
● Use blunt dissection to dissect down to and above the rib.

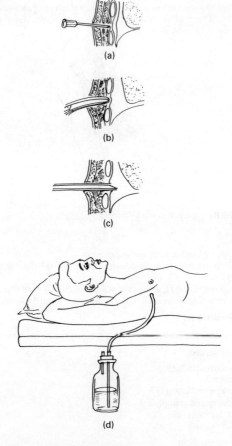

Figure 26.9 *Thoracocentesis*
(a) Infiltrate LA
(b) 2.5 cm skin incision, blunt dissection to pleura
(c) Insert Argyle trocar cannula
(d) Connect to underwater seal

- Divide the intercostal by blunt dissection.
- Insert trocar and cannula. Use non-dominant hand for insertion of trocar holding the trocar firmly with the dominant hand approximately 5 cm from the end. A give will be felt on entering pleural space.
- Withdraw the trocar, attach the cannula to clamped tube: connect to the underwater seal drain. Release clamp.
- Suture in place, tie, tie double loop around tube.

Notes

1 The bottle must always be below the site of the drain.
2 Ensure there is no leakage around the drain insertion site.
3 When moving the patient the tubing should be clamped.

Peritoneal lavage

Equipment needed

- Scalpel
- Peritoneal lavage cannula
- 1 litre of normal saline and local anaesthetic

Method (Figure 26.10)

1 Catheterise patient
2 Inject local anaesthetic to an area 5 cm below the umbilicus in the mid line. Anaesthetise down to and including the linea alba.
3 Make a small incision.
4 Insert the cannula through this incision and through the linea alba.
5 Withdraw the trocar.
6 Attach the normal saline to the cannula and allow 1 litre to run into the abdomen.
7 Leave for about 5 minutes.
8 Place the bag lower than the abdominal cavity: this will cause the fluid to flow out of the abdomen by siphonage.
9 The fluid can then be sent for analysis: RBC, WBC, bile.
10 Frank blood or RBC count greater than 100,000 is positive. (If the *Daily Telegraph* cannot be read through the fluid there is a positive result.)

Central line insertion

Central lines may be inserted into either the internal jugular or subclavian veins.

Internal jugular (Figure 26.11)

1 The patient is put lying with slight head-down tilt in order to engorge the vein.
2 Turn the head to the left (for right internal jugular).

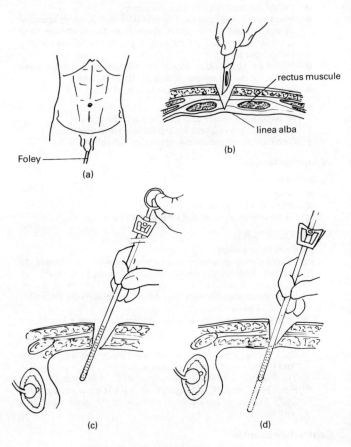

Figure 26.10 *Peritoneal lavage*
(a) Incision in midline below umbilicus
(b) Incise into linea alba
(c) Insert trocar and cannula, withdraw trocar
(d) Advance cannula

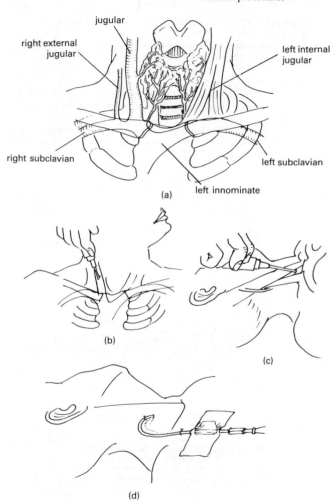

Figure 26.11 *Insertion of internal jugular central line*
(a) Anatomy of the veins at the root of the neck
(b) Insertion of needle
(c) Pass cannula into vein, withdraw needle (See Figure 26.12b)
(d) Connect to IV saline or manometer

3 Insert the needle on the medial side of the sternoclavicular muscle at its mid point.
4 Aim slightly lateral and downwards at an angle of about 35°.
5 The vein should be entered in less than 5 cm.

Subclavian (Figure 26.12)

1 The patient is put lying with a head-down tilt.
2 Enter the skin just lateral to the mid-point of the clavicle. Aim for the sternal notch.
3 The vein should be entered at about 5 cm. *Note*: after insertion of central line cannula the chest should be x-rayed to exclude a pneumothorax.

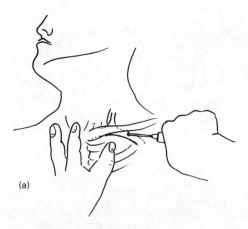

(a)

Figure 26.12 *Insertion of subclavian CVP line*
(a) Needle inserted approximately 5 cm
(b) Insert cannula, withdraw needle
(c) Attach to manometer or IV saline

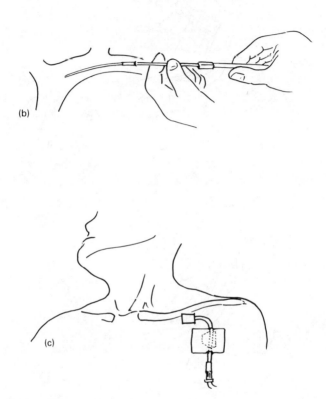

(b)

(c)

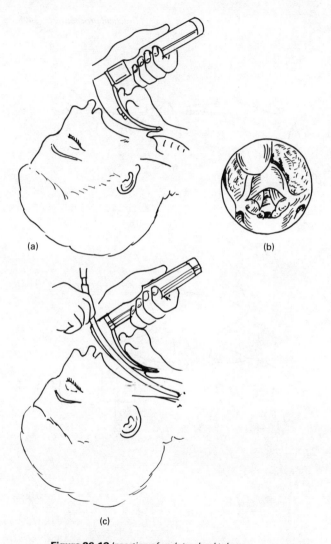

Figure 26.13 *Insertion of endotracheal tube*
(a) Position of laryngoscope — be careful of incisor teeth
(b) See the vocal cords
(c) Insert endotracheal tube

Insertion of endotracheal tube

ET tube (Figure 26.13)

1 Select the tube size, size 8 for a large male, size 7 for a female.
2 Have the patient lying flat.
3 Hold the laryngoscope in your left hand.
4 Slide the 'scope down the right side of the mouth, pushing the tongue over to the left. The tip of the laryngoscope should reach to the base of the epiglottis.
5 Lift the jaw forward. Be careful of the teeth.
6 If there is fluid in the pharynx obstructing your view to the trachea, remove it by suction. The cords should be seen.
7 Insert the tube into the trachea using your right hand.
8 Inflate the cuff of the tube.
9 Attach the ventilation system to the tube.
10 Check that each side of the chest has been inflated: if each side has not been inflated reposition the tube and check again.
11 When the correct position is achieved tie the tube in place.

Plasters and splints

The normal type of plaster used in the A & E department is plaster of paris. This comes ready impregnated into a roll. After setting, the plaster sets to form a hard cast. The rate of setting is dependent on the temperature of the water, the warmer the water the shorter the setting time. Water of about hand temperature is probably the best to use.

There are a number of newer synthetic types of casting material on the market but these need experience to put on and so are not really suitable for use by the SHO in the emergency situation.

The object of applying plaster is to immobilise the injured site. In order to do this adequately the joint above and below the injured bone must be immobilised. This is not necessary if the injury is very close to a joint. In fractures of the forearm and lower leg in order to stop rotation the knee/elbow must be bent slightly when the plaster is applied.

Application plaster

Plaster may be applied either as a back slab or a cylinder. In acute injuries the injured part swells; when a cylinder plaster is applied it should be both well padded and split to skin after application in order to allow for expansion of the injured tissue. A cylinder is necessary if rotation of the bones is a possibility, as a back slab is usually not sufficient to stop rotation, e.g. mid forearm fractures. Back slabs are preferable for Colles fractures.

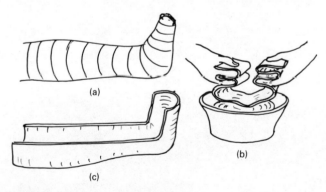

Figure 26.14 *Application of POP back slab*
(a) Apply adequate wool
(b) Immerse slab in water. Smooth on flat surface, pressing layers together
(c) Apply smoothed POP slab to limb and hold in place with a wet crêpe bandage

Equipment needed

Before starting to apply the plaster make sure all the materials necessary are available and ready. You will need padding, plaster, water and a bandage. There should also be an assistant who can hold the limb in the correct position while you are applying the plaster.

Apply adequate padding around the limb making sure that the bony points are well protected.

1 Back slab
    (a) Take 8 layers of plaster folded over.
    (b) Cut it to slightly longer length than the final plaster required as the plaster tends to shrink slightly when wet.
    (c) Immerse the plaster completely in the water until bubbles stop emerging.
    (d) Squeeze the plaster gently to exude excess water and lay on the padded affected part.
    (e) Smooth it carefully to remove wrinkles.
    (f) Wet a crêpe bandage and strap around the limb; hold in position until set which is about 5–10 minutes. (See Figure 26.14.)

2 *Cylinder-type plaster*
    (a) Hold the limb in the correct position. Apply generous padding.
    (b) Unwrap the first 10 cm of the plaster roll (when wet the end can be very difficult to find).

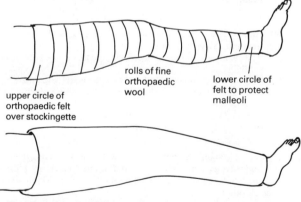

    upper circle of orthopaedic felt over stockingette
    rolls of fine orthopaedic wool
    lower circle of felt to protect malleoli

    (i) Apply 15 cm POP bandage smoothing each layer gently
    (ii) Turn over ends of stockingette
    (iii) Avoid pressure on the tendo achilles insertion by shaping POP

Figure 26.15 *Application of POP cylinder*

<table>
<tr><td>

**ORTHOPAEDIC
DEPARTMENT**

Please read the following
instructions carefully:

DO NOT WET, CUT, HEAT OR
OTHERWISE INTERFERE WITH
THIS PLASTER

Report at ONCE
(1) If it cracks, becomes loose or
    otherwise uncomfortable.
(2) If there is any pain.
(3) If there is any discharge.
(4) If the fingers or toes become
    numb or difficult to move.
(5) If the fingers or toes become
    swollen or blue.

The plaster may feel tight for some
time after application. This can
usually be relieved by lying down
and elevating the arm or leg on one
or more pillows and by constantly
moving those joints of the arm and
leg that are not covered by plaster.

</td><td>

**NOTICE TO PATIENTS
WEARING
PLASTER CASTS**

For the first twenty-four hours keep
the limb raised as much as possible,
keep the arm in the sling provided,
and the foot raised on a pillow or
cushion protected with a waterproof
cover.

Keep the fingers and toes moving.

If any of the following are noticed,
report to the Accident Room or
Plaster Room, **at once, day or night:**

(1) Swelling of the fingers or toes.
(2) Blueness of the fingers or toes.
(3) 'Pins and needles' in the fingers
    or toes.
(4) Coldness of the fingers or toes.
(5) Any real pain in the limb.

**Please report to the Plaster Room
at (for example, 9 am) next morning.**

</td></tr>
</table>

Figure 26.16 *Instructions to patients wearing POP casts*

    (c) Immerse the plaster completely in water until bubbles cease
        emerging. Squeeze gently.
    (d) Roll evenly around the limb making sure that it is not applied too
        tightly.
    (e) Rub the layers together with palm of the hand (never use fingers
        or thumb as these will cause indents in the plaster which leads to
        pressure sores).
    (f) Further layers of plaster can be applied gently massaging the
        layers together. (See Figure 26.15.)

Notes

    1 In acute trauma the limb always swells for 48 hours, therefore
      cylinder-type plasters must be split down to skin. After splitting a
      crêpe bandage may be wrapped round the plaster. The limb must
      be elevated.
    2 When applying plaster to hands and feet spread the metacarpals
      (metatarsals) as they may be bunched together when the plaster is
      being applied. This can cause pain in the hand/foot.
    3 Count the toes/fingers after applying plaster. Make sure that the
      little toe is not covered.

4 Give plaster instructions orally and give the patient written instructions. (See Figure 26.16.)
5 The patient must be reviewed the next day to assess any problems.
6 If the patient complains that the plaster is too tight then it is too tight and must be split; then elevate the limb.

Type of plaster

Colles plaster

This is applied from just below the elbow to just proximal to the heads of the metacarpals. The thumb is left free to move. When applying spread the metacarpals by holding the fingers apart. (See Figure 26.17a.)

Scaphoid plaster

This is similar to the Colles plaster but incorporates the thumb up to the interphalangeal joint. The distal phalanx is left free. The thumb and hand are held in the position of holding a pint glass. (See Figure 26.17b.)

Plaster for Smith's fracture

The hand is supinated. The wrist is dorsi-flexed. The plaster is applied to above the elbow. The elbow is placed at right-angles. (See Figure 26.17c.)

Above-elbows plasters

These are used for fractures of the radius and ulna. The plaster extends from the hand to 3/4 of the way from the elbow to the shoulder; the elbow is placed at right-angles. The degree of pronation or supination of the forearm depends on the exact position of the fracture.

Below-knee plasters

For fractures around the ankle joint a below-knee plaster is applied. It extends from distal metatarsals to just below the knee so that it does not impinge on the thigh when the knee is flexed. The ankle should be at right-angles unless otherwise indicated. It is important to remember that while the plaster will set in 5–10 minutes it does not gain its full strength for 24 hours, therefore weight-bearing should not commence before this time. (See Figures 26.18a and b.)

Full leg plaster

This is used for fractures of the tibia and fibula. The knee must be flexed to about 10° when this is being applied. The plaster extends from the head of the metatarsal to 3/4 way between knee and groin. The ankle is held at a right-angle. (See Figure 26.18b.)

Cylinder pop

This is to hold the knee in extension. It extends from the ankle to the upper thigh. Before applying the plaster, orthopaedic felt is applied to the area of the malleoli. This stops the plaster rubbing on the malleoli and causing pressure sores. (See Figure 26.15.)

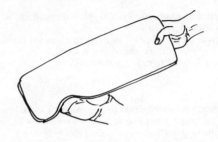

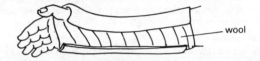

Figure 26.17 *(a) Application of Colles POP slab*

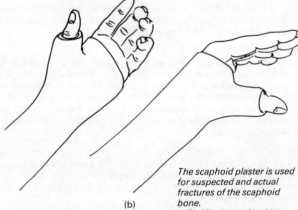

(b)

The scaphoid plaster is used
for suspected and actual
fractures of the scaphoid
bone.
The final cast should
result in full supination
of the forearm, a
dorsiflexed wrist and the
thumb held in opposition to
the index finger.

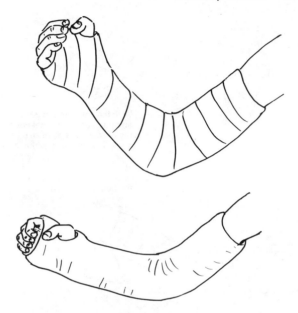

(c) Above-elbow POP. The upper limit of the POP must be below the insertion of the deltoid. Avoid tight bands of plaster forming across the elbow crease – they may press on the arteries

Acknowledgements to Smith and Nephew
Pharmaceuticals Ltd.

Complications

1 Circulation impairment. Injured limbs always swell. This can cause vascular impairment if an unexpanding cast is applied. In order to minimise the risk, cylinder cast on limbs in acute trauma should be split down to skin but not through it. If any circulatory problems are discovered then the cast should be removed or split and opened. Dressings may harden with dried blood, so make sure that these are not constricting.

2 Nerve problems. Pressure on nerves can cause palsies. Early pressure on the nerves causes pins and needles. At this stage the cast should be released or removed and re-applied.

3 Pressure sores. If insufficient padding is applied over bone prominences the plaster will rub and cause pressure sores.

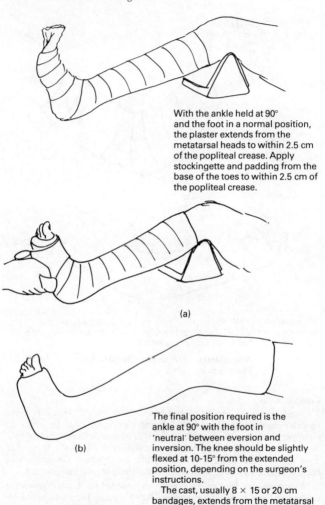

With the ankle held at 90°
and the foot in a normal position,
the plaster extends from the
metatarsal heads to within 2.5 cm
of the popliteal crease. Apply
stockingette and padding from the
base of the toes to within 2.5 cm of
the popliteal crease.

(a)

(b)

The final position required is the
ankle at 90° with the foot in
'neutral' between eversion and
inversion. The knee should be slightly
flexed at 10-15° from the extended
position, depending on the surgeon's
instructions.

The cast, usually 8 × 15 or 20 cm
bandages, extends from the metatarsal
heads to within 2.5 cm of the gluteal fold.

Figure 26.18
(a) Below-knee POP
(b) Full-leg POP

Acknowledgements to Smith and Nephew
Pharmaceuticals Ltd.

4 Wasting and stiffness. When a limb is held immobile the muscles waste and the joints become stiff. In order to minimise this risk, active mobilisation of fingers or toes should be encouraged. Proximal unsplinted joints must also be exercised. Movements such as straight leg raising for the leg can be encouraged. Active physiotherapy is needed immediately after removing the cast.

Splints

There are a number of splints on the market which hold parts of the body in position to allow healing. The following are common ones you will find:

Mallet splint

This splint is used when there is a mallet deformity of the finger. It holds the terminal phalanx of the finger in hyperextension and is strapped on with zinc oxide plaster. It usually has to remain on 6 to 8 weeks after the injury. (See Figure 26.19.)

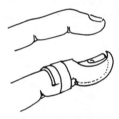

Figure 26.19 *Mallet finger splint*

Cervical collars

Cervical collars are used in neck injuries. They must fit around the neck so that the head rests on the top of the collar and the bottom of the collar rests on the upper chest. Many types are available commercially. Remember that it is the length of the neck that determines the size of the collar. A lady with a swan neck will require a larger collar than a 20-stone man with a short bull neck.

Futuro splint

This splint is designed to hold the wrist in dorsi-flexion. It consists of a stiffened palmar part which is applied to the front of the wrist and the palm of the hand. It is held in place by velcro straps and is used for painful tendonitis around the wrist. It can be easily removed and re-applied by the patient. (See Figure 26.20.)

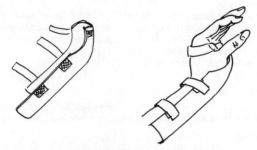

Figure 26.20 *Futuro splint*

Thomas's splint (Traction splint, Hares splint) (Figures 26.21 and 26.22)

These splints are designed to hold a fractured femur in traction, so reducing movement of the fragments, pain and shock. They consist of a buttress applied to the ischial tuberosity with metal arms extending distal to the foot. Between the metal bars, bandage is applied to support the weight of the limb.

Figure 26.21 *Application of Thomas splint (courtesy of Johnson and Johnson and RAMC)*

(a) One person applies continuous traction to the leg
(b) Prepare Thomas splint with non-stretch support
(c) Apply foam traction kit or improvise with non-stretch 7.5 cm strapping
 (i)   With the right foot flexed at a right-angle, position the spreader plate 7–10 cm from the sole of the foot and at right-angles to the leg. Ensure that this position is held and that the foam padding covers the malleoli
 (ii) Measure the length of the strapping required and cut or fold each strip to this length
 (iii) Beginning at the ankles, apply one or two turns to hold the foam padding securely in position. Next, using firm but even tension, apply the bandage in a 'figure of eight' style from without inwards to retain the leg in a neutral position. It is important that no wrinkles should occur in the bandage at this stage, as pressure sores may develop. If too much tension is applied, then constriction of the blood flow to the foot and ankle may occur. Use the other bandage for the above-knee section
 (iv) The traction cords can be used as a single or double cord depending on the type of traction required. The pull of the cord must be along the line of the foam extension piece
(d) Traction can now be applied by use of weights or fixed traction
(e) Check the condition of the skin daily and make sure that the patient has a full range of movement in his toes or ankles. Check that the foam extention piece has not slipped down the leg.

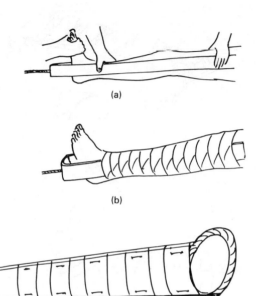

(a)

(b)

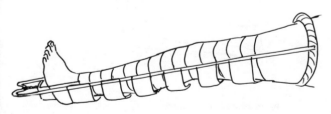

(c)

(d)

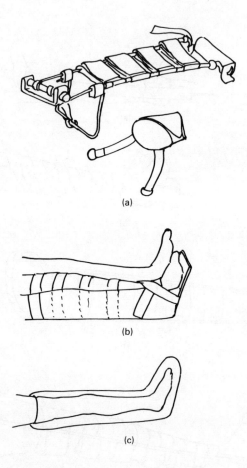

Figure 26.22 *Special splints*
(a) Hare traction splint
(b) Box splint (Courtesy of Loxley Medical)
(c) Inflatable splint (Courtesy of F.W. Equipment Co.)

The application of the splint

At least two people are required for proper application of the splint. One person holds the affected limb and applies traction to it which he maintains throughout the manoeuvre. The second person applies a traction bandage to the leg. In order to do this the leg should be shaved. A sticky bandage is applied on each side of the leg from the angle to the mid-thigh region. Make sure that the bandage is applied on the sides and does not go anteriorly or posteriorly. This is held in place by a crêpe or other bandage wrapped round the limb. The splint is applied to the leg so its buttress is against the ischial tuberosity. The limb is laid on the splint. The string from the traction is tied to the end of the splint. Use Spanish windlass to tighten. Only then is traction released. (Figure 26.21.)

Blow-up splints (Figure 26.22)

There are a number of splints on the market which conform to the shape of either an upper limb or lower limb and which can be placed on the limb while deflated. When in position they are inflated and form an efficient form of splintage. These are used by ambulance personnel but are useful in the A & E department to splint untreated fractures on arrival. Use for short duration only, look for adverse pressure effects.

All A & E staff should know how to apply the simple splints described above.

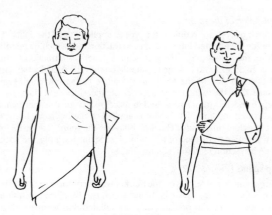

Figure 26.23 *Broad arm sling*

Slings

A sling is applied with either a triangular bandage or collar and cuff.

Triangular bandage — applications as a sling

Triangular bandage is a half of a square of 100–110 cm in length.

Broadarm sling

This is used when the arm and forearm need to be supported. (See Figure 26.23.)

Method:

1 Place one end of the unfolded bandage over the shoulder on the side away from the injury. Place the point of the triangle behind the elbow of the injured side. Bend the elbow to a right-angle, making sure the thumb is uppermost. Fold the loose end of the bandage in front of the injured arm and tie at the side of the neck. The triangle behind the elbow should be pinned to the bandage coming up the front of the elbow.
   Note: The hand should be supported as well as the forearm or else problems around the wrist can occur.

2 The finger nails should be left visible to observe changing colour.

3 There should be no wrinkles.

High sling

This is used when the hand is injured or infected and needs dependent drainage. (See Figure 26.24.)

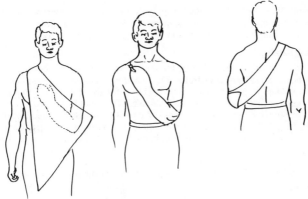

Figure 26.24 *High sling*

Method:
  1 Bend the patient's forearm so that the fingers touch the opposite clavicle.
  2 Apply the upper side of the bandage along and parallel to the upper border of the patient's forearm and hand so that the bandage extends to a little beyond the elbow on the injured side.
  3 Tuck the base of the bandage well under the injured forearm and hand. (See Figure 26.24.)
  4 Take the lower end of the bandage up across the patient's back and tie it to the end on the injured side.
  5 Tuck in at elbow.

Collar-and-cuff sling

Collar-and-cuff slings are made of foam surrounded by slightly stretchable soft material. It is used when elbow movement is not required but allows movement at the shoulder. A hitch is placed around the wrist. A further hitch is made around the neck. The hitches can be held in place with either the special clamps provided or safety pins.

Bandaging

Bandages are used to give support to an injured area or apply pressure to the area in order to limit swelling. Bandages fall into two categories: (a) tubular bandages; (b) rolls of bandages.

Tubular bandages

Tubular bandages usually are elasticated and come in varying sizes: they are applied to the limbs with a special applicator. They are designed to be applied in a double layer. Before applying, the correct size must be chosen using the manufacturer's recommendations. Bandage of correct size is applied with the applicator very much as one would put on a sock.

Roll bandages

Roll bandages are manufactured in various forms and sizes. They may be either stretchable or non-stretchable. In addition they may be adherent or non-adherent. Adherent bandages are better for giving support as they do not slip once applied. Non-stretch bandage should not be applied around an injured limb as any subsequent swelling will cause vascular impairment. When applying roll bandages round a limb you should always start distally and work proximally. Each turn of bandage should overlap the previous turn by 2/3rd.

For supporting new injuries elastoplast is preferred.

The following is the method of application to various parts of the body:

Ankle

Attach the bandage at the base of the toes. For a lateral sprain start on the outside and work medially; for a medial sprain start on the inside and work

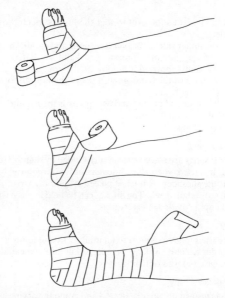

Figure 26.25 *Ankle strapping (courtesy of Smith and Nephew)*

laterally. Fix two turns around the foot and then bring the bandage up and around the ankle. Take a further turn around the foot and then a turn around the heel. One more turn around the foot and ankle is applied and then the bandage continued up the leg. (See Figure 26.25.)

Thumb spica

Place the hand and thumb in a safe position, which in the hand is the position of holding a pint glass. Place two turns of the bandage around the thumb just below the interphalangeal joint. On left thumb turn anti-clockwise, on the right thumb clockwise. Bring the plaster straight across the palm around the hand and over the base of the thumb. Continue into the cleft of the thumb around the thumb and back across the palm. Repeat 3–4 complete turns, overlapping each by at least a half. (See Figure 26.26.)

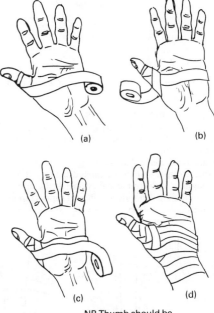

(a)

(b)

(c)

(d)

NB Thumb should be abducted in position of function — See Figure 23.3.

Figure 26.26 *Thumb spica (courtesy of Smith and Nephew)*

Neighbour (garter) strapping of fingers

Put a piece of gauze between the affected fingers. Apply a length of elastoplast around the proximal phalanges of the two fingers. Apply another length around the intermediate phalanges of both fingers. Make sure that the inter phalangeal joints can be flexed. (See Figure 26.27.)

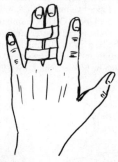

Figure 26.27 *Neighbour strapping of fingers (courtesy of Smith and Nephew)*

Support strapping to previously injured ankle

A previously injured ankle needs support on lateral aspect. For this a non-stretchable plaster strapping is applied running from the medial side just below the malleolus, under the sole of the foot and up the lateral side of the ankle anterior to the malleolus extending 3–4 inches above the malleolus. Two or three further lengths are applied like this. It is held in place with a further length of non-stretchable plaster at the upper end which goes 3/4 way round the leg. This gives sufficient support to the ankle for use in sport but further bandaging, as for injured ankle, may be applied if thought necessary. (See Figure 26.28.)

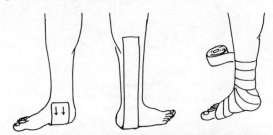

Figure 26.28 *Support strapping for ankle*

Bandaging for ulcers

Most ulcers on the lower limb are due to varicose vein problems. After ensuring that there is no vascular impairment the ulcer should be dressed with the appropriate dressing. An elasticated one-way stretch bandage (Dickson Wright) applied from toe to knee aids dispersal of any oedema. This bandage should be removed on getting into bed at night and applied before getting out again in the morning. Removal of oedema fluid is aided by frequent elevation of leg. (See page 282, Chapter 20.) Medicated paste bandages can be used as dressings on the wounds underneath the elasticated bandage. These gauze bandages are non-distendable, therefore should not be applied in a circular manner but rather applied around once and folded back on themselves to go round the other way. Thus when the bandaging is completed it is possible to peel them off by opening at the point of folding. (See Figure 26.29.) The bandages consist of:

(a) Zincaband which contains a zinc oxide paste. This is useful for clean wounds.
(b) Calaband which is zinc oxide with calamine lotion. This is used where there is slight irritation around the wound.
(c) Icthaband which is zinc paste with ichthammol. This is a coal tar base and it is good for eczema.
(d) Quinaband — this is zinc oxide with clioquinol. This masks smells and may be used for indolent ulcers. (See Figure 26.29).

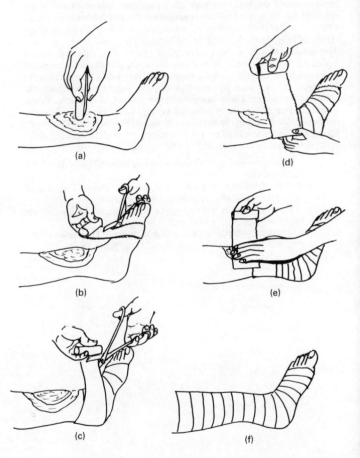

(a)

(b)

(c)

(d)

(e)

(f)

Acknowledgements to Seton Healthcare Group

Figure 26.29 *Application of medicated paste bandage*
(a) The ulcer base should be lightly cleansed and a bland non-irritating medication may be applied. The surrounding skin may be protected from exudate as desired e.g. Siopel
(b) Bandaging should be commenced with the foot at right-angles if possible but chronic cases may present with varying degrees of ankylosis. Take 1½ turns of bandage around the foot at the base of the toes. Cut and repeat about 2 cm further along the foot
(c) Bandage from base of toes, round the heel and back across the dorsum of the foot. Cut and repeat to give adequate coverage of the heel
(d) A final turn is taken around the foot and on to the ankle. Behind the malleolus a fold is formed and a turn in the opposite direction is commenced. Folding and reversing avoids encircling turns and aids removal.
(e) Make 1½ turns, fold back and repeat until the bandage reaches the tibial tubercle and is slightly higher at the back. Avoid tucks and folds over bony prominences.
(f) Compression bandaging is the main method of treatment but cannot be applied directly to friable, inflamed skin. A paste bandage acts as a soothing buffer.

NOTES

Library for an A & E Department

ACCIDENT AND EMERGENCY

Evans, T. R. (1989). *ABC of resuscitation*. BMJ, London.

Kirby, N. G. and Mather, S. J. (1985). *Baillière's handbook of first aid*. Baillière Tindall, London.

Rutherford, W. H. *et al.* (1988). *Accident and emergency medicine* (2nd edn). Pitman Medical, London.

TRAUMA AND ORTHOPAEDICS

Apley, A. G. and Solomon, L. (1984). *Systems of orthopaedics and fractures*. Butterworth, London.

Charnley, J. (1961). *Closed treatment of common fractures*. Churchill Livingstone, Edinburgh.

Kirby, N. G. and Blackburn, G. (1981). *Field surgery pocket book*. HMSO, Norwich.

MacNicol, M. F. and Lamb, D. W. (1984). *Basic care of the injured hand*. Churchill Livingstone, Edinburgh.

McRae, R. (1989). *Practical fracture treatment*. Churchill Livingstone, Edinburgh.

Slater, M. I. (1987). *Hand injuries*. Churchill Livingstone, Edinburgh.

Skinner, D., Driscoll, P., and Brayley, N. (1991). *ABC of trauma*. BMJ, London.

Westaby, S. (1989). *Trauma: pathogenesis and treatment*. Heinemann Medical, London.

GENERAL SURGERY

Cotton, L. and Lafferty, K. (1986). *A new short textbook of surgery*. Hodder and Stoughton, Sevenoaks, Kent.

Kyle, J. (ed.) (1984). *Surgical handicraft*. Wright, London(?).

Bailey, H., Love, R. J. M., Rains, A. J. H., and Mann, C. V. (1988). *Short practice of surgery*. H. K. Lewis, London.

Westaby, S. (ed.) (1985). *Wound care*. Heinemann Medical, London.

MEDICINE

Berkow, R. (ed.) (1982). *Merck manual of diagnosis and therapy*. Merck and Co., Hoddesdon.

Fleming, M. (1979). *Interpreting electrocardiograms*. Update Publications, Guildford.

Rees, J. (1989). *ABC of asthma*. BMJ, London.

Rees, J. and Trounce, J. R. (1988). *A new short textbook of medicine*. Edward Arnold, Sevenoaks, Kent.

Sprigings, D. and Chambers, J. (1990). *Acute medicine: a practical guide*. Blackwell Scientific, Oxford.

Vaccination certificate requirements and health advice for international travel (1990). WHO, Geneva.

Weatherall, D. J., Ledingham, J. G. G., and Warrell, D. A. (1987). *The Oxford textbook of medicine*. Oxford University Press.

DERMATOLOGY

Buxton, P. K. (1988). *ABC of dermatology*. BMJ, London.

Levene, G. M. (1984). *Colour atlas of dermatology*. Wolfe Medical Publications, London.

OBSTETRICS AND GYNAECOLOGY

Anderson, M. M. (1981). *Handbook of obstetrics and gynaecology for the house officer*. Faber and Faber, London.

Rymer, J., Davis, G., Rodin, A., and Chapman, M. G. (1990). *Preparation and revision of DRCOG*. Churchill Livingstone, Edinburgh.

OPHTHALMOLOGY

Bankes, J. L. K. (1982). *Clinical ophthalmology: a text and colour atlas*. Churchill Livingstone, Edinburgh.

Elkington, A. R. and Khaw, P. T. (1989). *ABC of eyes*. BMJ, London.

PAEDIATRICS

Black, J. (1985). *The new paediatrics: child health in ethnic minorities*. BMJ, London.

Hull, D. and Johnstone, D. L. (1987). *Essential paediatrics*. Churchill Livingstone, Edinburgh.

Valman, H. B. (1988). *ABC of one to seven*. BMJ, London.

ENT

Ludman, H. (1981). *ABC of ENT*. BMJ, London.

RADIOLOGY

Clark, K. C. (1986). *Positioning in radiography*. Heinemann Medical, Oxford.

Grech, P. (1980). *Casualty radiology: a practical guide for radiodiagnosis*. Chapman and Hall, London.

MISCELLANEOUS

Anderson, J. E. (1983). *Grant's atlas of anatomy*. Williams and Wilkins, London.

Davies, D. (1985). *ABC of plastic and reconstructive surgery*. BMJ, London.

Duncan, C. (1987). *MIMS colour index*. MIMS Publications, London.

Grundy, D. *et al.* (1986). *ABC of spinal cord injury*. BMJ, London.

McLatchie, G. (1986). *Essentials of sports medicine*. Churchill Livingstone, Edinburgh.

Swinscow, T. D. V. (1983) *Statistics at square one*. BMJ, London.

Walker, E. and Williams, G. (1990). *ABC of health travel*. BMJ, London.

Index

CARDIOPULMONARY RESUSCITATION

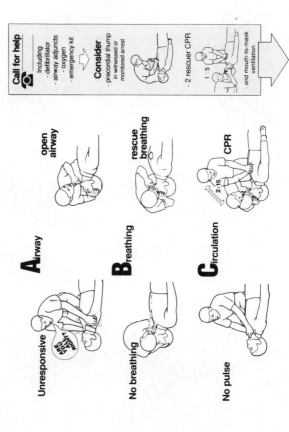

Airway

Unresponsive

open airway

Breathing

No breathing

rescue breathing

Circulation

No pulse

CPR

2:15

Call for help

Including
- defibrillator
- airway adjuncts
- oxygen
- emergency kit

Consider
- precordial thump in witnessed or monitored arrest

- 2 rescuer CPR

1:5

- and mouth-to-mask ventilation

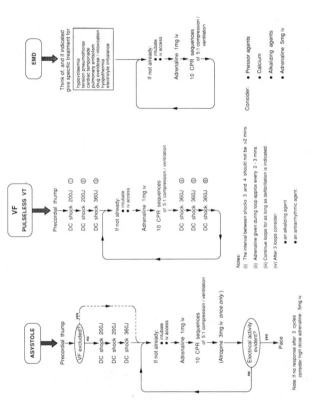

ASYSTOLE

Precordial thump

VF excluded? — yes ·······┐
│ no
DC shock 200J
DC shock 200J
DC shock 360J

If not already:
● intubate
● iv access

Adrenaline 1mg iv

10 CPR sequences
of 5:1 compression / ventilation

(Atropine 3mg iv *once only*)

Electrical activity evident? — yes → Pace
│ no

Note: if no response after 3 cycles
consider high dose adrenaline 5mg iv.

VF PULSELESS VT

Precordial thump

DC shock 200J ①
DC shock 200J ②
DC shock 360J ③

If not already:
● intubate
● iv access

Adrenaline 1mg iv

10 CPR sequences
of 5:1 compression / ventilation

DC shock 360J ④
DC shock 360J ⑤
DC shock 360J ⑥

Notes:
(i) The interval between shocks 3 and 4 should not be >2 mins.
(ii) Adrenaline given during loop approx every 2 - 3 mins.
(iii) Continue loops for as long as defibrillation is indicated.
(iv) After 3 loops consider:
● an alkalizing agent
● an antiarrhythmic agent.

EMD

Think of, and if indicated
give specific treatment for

hypovolaemia
tension pneumothorax
cardiac tamponade
pulmonary embolism
drug overdose / intoxication
hypothermia
electrolyte imbalance

If not already:
● intubate
● iv access

Adrenaline 1mg iv

10 CPR sequences
of 5:1 compression /
ventilation

Consider:
● Pressor agents
● Calcium
● Alkalizing agents
● Adrenaline 5mg iv

Guidelines for advanced life support